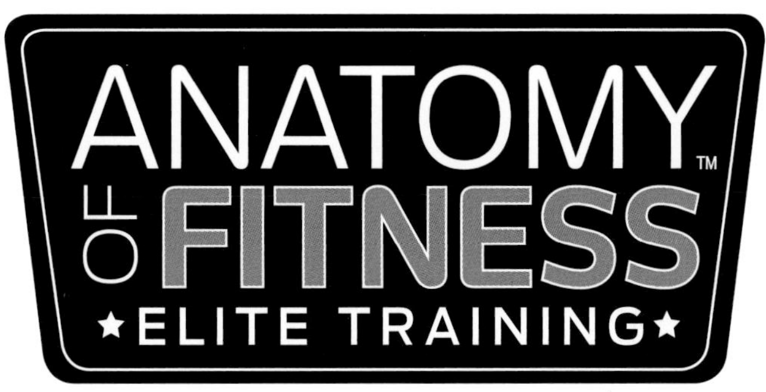


# Navy SEALs Workout

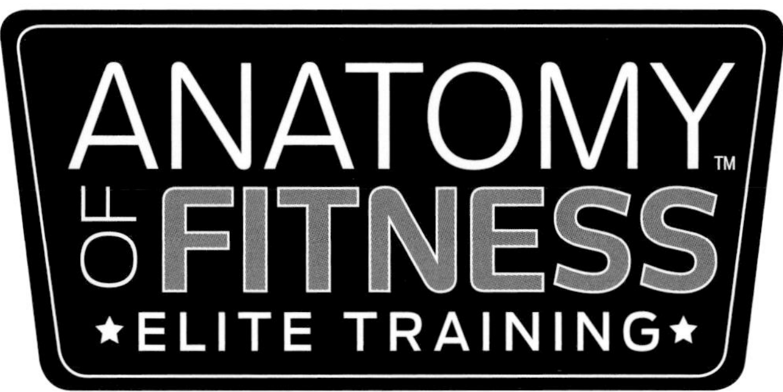


# Navy SEALs Workout

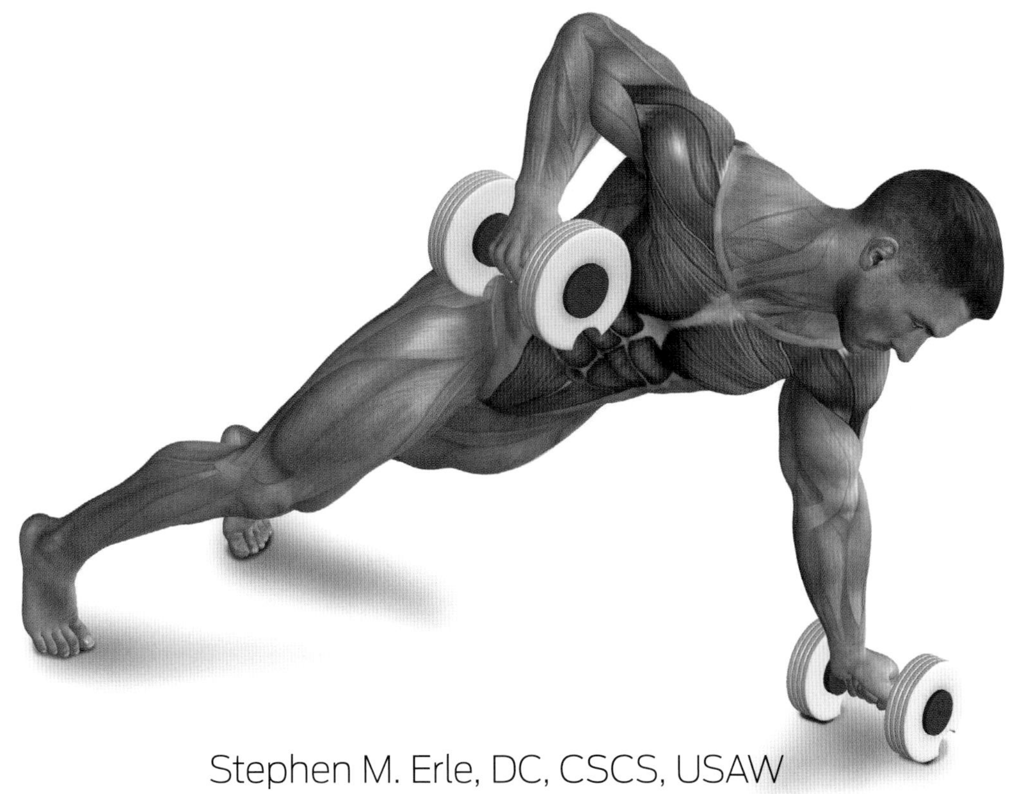

Stephen M. Erle, DC, CSCS, USAW

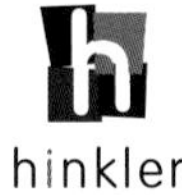

Published by Hinkler Books Pty Ltd 2014, 2015
45–55 Fairchild Street
Heatherton Victoria 3202 Australia
www.hinkler.com.au

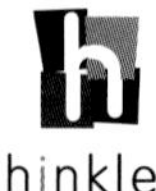




Created by Moseley Road Inc.
President: Sean Moore
Project art and editorial direction: Lisa Purcell Editorial & Design
Cover and internal design: Sam Grimmer
Photographer: Jonathan Conklin Photography, Inc.
Retoucher: Mayoca Design
Author: Stephen M. Erle, DC, CSCS, USAW
Contributing writer: Nancy J. Hajeski
Model: Stew Smith, CSCS
Illustrator: Hector Aiza/3DLabz
Prepress: Graphic Print Group



ISBN: 978 1 4889 0214 7

Printed and bound in China

# Contents

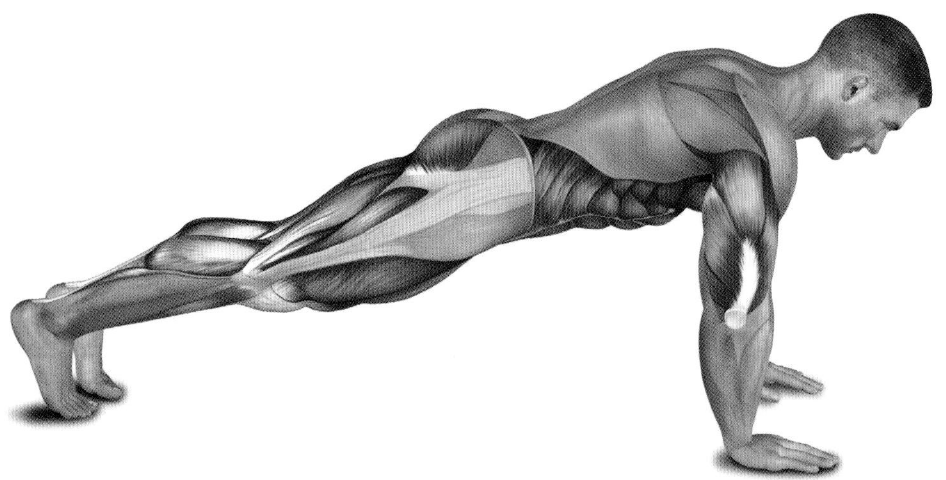

# Train Like a Spec Ops Athlete

Around the world, special operations forces execute high-risk missions. Formed by the armies, navies, and air forces of many nations, these teams are highly skilled and rigorously trained, each member possessing the formidable skills necessary to survive and prevail in the most dangerous situations imaginable.

Specialized units can be found throughout the history of warfare. In ancient times there were the Macedonian Argyraspides, the Theban Sacred Band, and the Persian Immortal Guard, just to name a few. In the early Middles Ages, the Samurai was the elite warrior of Japan, while later, England's King Henry V mobilized his longbow archers against the French.

Special forces as we know them today emerged during World War II, with its multiple fronts involving remote geographic terrain. The United Kingdom's highly regarded Special Air Service (SAS) traces its history back to this era, as does the modern incarnation of the U.S. Army Rangers and the four categories of Australia's special forces that now operate under the Special Operations Command. Similar units exist in nearly every nation, from the Utti Jaeger Regiment of Finland to the Para Commandos of India.

Special operations forces of all nations have one thing in common: their exclusivity. To qualify for entry into these rarified units, a candidate must be in peak physical condition, mentally strong, and highly motivated.

## Why choose a Navy SEALs workout?

You probably picked up this book for several reasons. Perhaps you admire the concept of the SEALs and are curious about how they actually train. Perhaps you believe you have the "right stuff" and can meet their high standards of performance and fitness. Maybe you want to learn how to properly shed unwanted body fat while maintaining muscle mass, or you think it's time that you got both physically and mentally fit. This book provides you with exercises to improve fitness as well as guidelines for increasing your mental strength and tips for reducing stress.

## Get strong mentally and physically

This book gives you the tools necessary to train like a special forces team member. The featured exercises are the very ones performed daily at U.S. Navy SEAL Basic Underwater Demolition School (BUD/S) and by active-duty SEAL platoons working out around the world. The SEALs rely on many basic military exercises such as the Push-Up, Sit-Up, and Pull-Up, performing these and other movements in a way that results in maximum effectiveness.

### Who are the SEALs?

The acronym SEAL stands for Sea, Air, and Land—the three areas from which the men of this elite special military force operate and where their expertise lies.

Formed in 1962 by President John F. Kennedy, the U.S. Navy SEALs are a select maritime force of roughly 2,000 men trained to conduct unconventional warfare. They now embody, in a single force, the heritage, missions, capabilities, and combat lessons learned by five daring groups that no longer exist, but which were crucial to the Allied victory in World War II and to successes in the Korean conflict. These now-defunct organizations were the Office of Strategic Services Operational Swimmer Group, Navy Underwater Demolition Team (UDTs), U.S. Navy Raiders, Naval Combat Demolition Unit (NCDUs), U.S. Army Scouts, and Motor Torpedo Boat Squadron.

The SEALs are the best of the best within the Joint Special Operations Command units (JSOC) for direct-action missions and are therefore the unit of choice among navy personnel. Other JSOC teams, such as the U.S. Army Green Berets, are more adept at foreign internal defense than SEAL teams. Yet, with half the world's infrastructure and population located within one mile of an ocean or river, the ability to maneuver close to the shore is more important now than ever before in history. SEALs conduct small-unit maritime military operations that originate from and return to a river, ocean, swamp, delta, or coastline. Of crucial importance in defense and counter-terrorism, SEALs can negotiate shallow-water areas where large ships and submarines are limited by depth.

SEALs recruits line up at the start of intensive training. By the end, only a quarter of them will have made the grade.

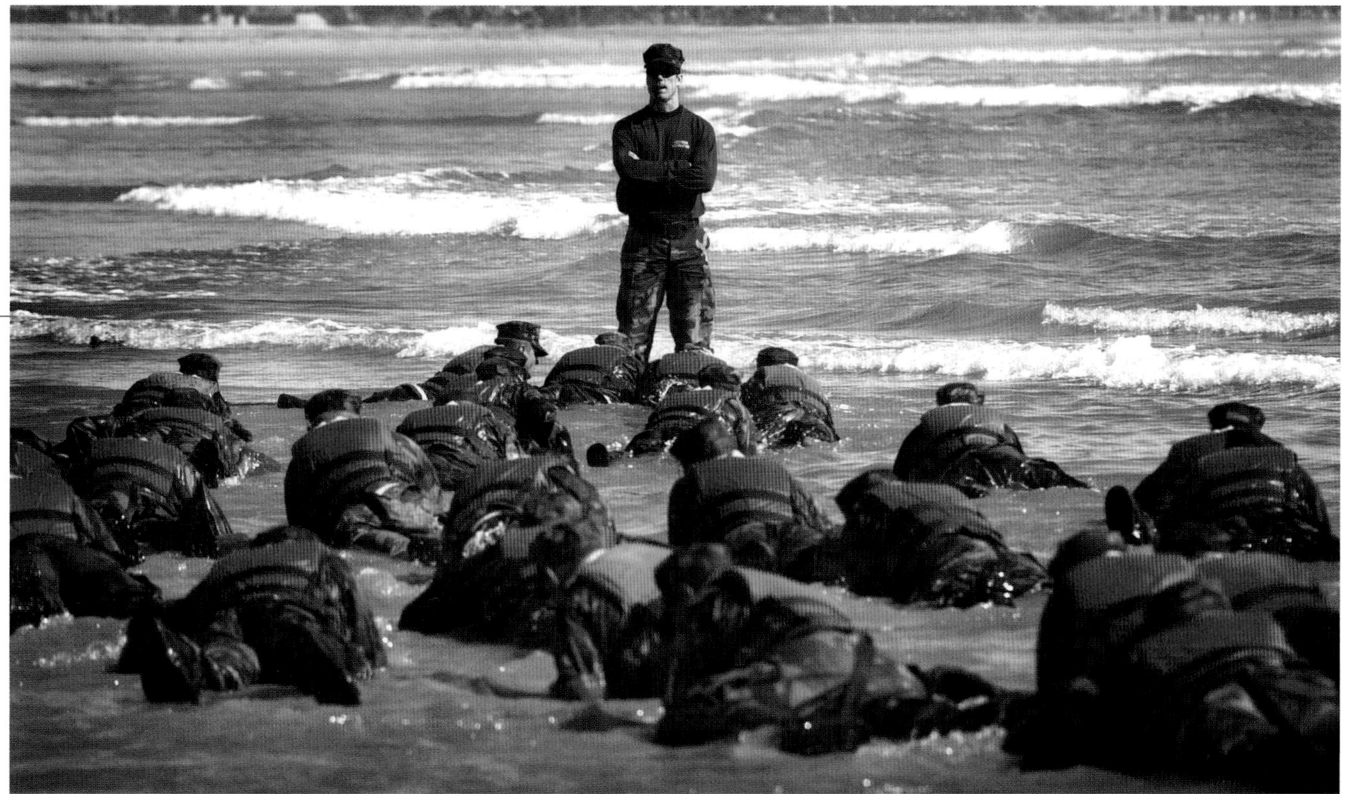

A Navy SEAL instructor drills students from a Basic Underwater Demolition/SEAL (BUD/S) class.

SEALs, or any special forces operatives, must be 100 percent combat effective at all times, both mentally and physically. They must be ready to serve their country at a moment's notice. This takes daily adherence to a very rigid physical training schedule performed both in a group and individually.

Once you are performing the featured exercises (see pages 40–151) as they are written, you will be well on your way to training like an active-duty special forces operative. You will gain greater confidence in your abilities and develop mental toughness well beyond what you previously thought you could achieve. Your physique will be stronger than ever before as you increase your muscle mass and cardiovascular endurance. You will feel at your best as your self-esteem and physical abilities improve.

## How to use this book

Read through and then practice each of the dynamic warm-ups and static cool-downs (see pages 30–37).

Work on your form so that you fully engage the muscles of your chest, legs, back, shoulders, arms, abs, and core, as well as build cardiovascular endurance.

Next, begin to review the featured exercises. Each exercise features a short description, along with step-by-step photos and instructions. Accompanying each exercise is a detailed anatomical illustration that highlights the key muscles used in each set. You'll also find important tips on safe and effective technique and movement patterns to build stable and strong joints.

Alongside each exercise is a quick-read panel that features at-a-glance anatomical illustrations highlighting the targeted areas, an estimate of the level of difficulty, the average amount of time you'll need to complete the recommended reps, and key benefits. The last category is a caution list: if you have one of the issues listed, it is best to avoid that exercise. Of course, check with your doctor before attempting any of the exercises.

Start by trying each exercise once, and then repeat it. When you feel that you have become strong enough, turn to the Workouts section (pages 162–181). Begin with the Phase I Workout (page 164–167), which is designed to give you the initial movements necessary to build an elite level of fitness in a safe manner, while instilling the kind of discipline that special forces are known for. Aim to perform this Phase I workout three times a week, and complete each workout session within 60 minutes.

When you have become comfortable with this routine, you will be ready to tackle the Phase II workouts (page 168–177). As your fitness level increases, you will find that you are ready for the ultimate test—the Phase III Workout. This is the kind of workout performed at the highest levels of special forces training.

Along with exercise instruction, you'll find a section on swimming and running (pages 152–161)—both major components of special forces training.

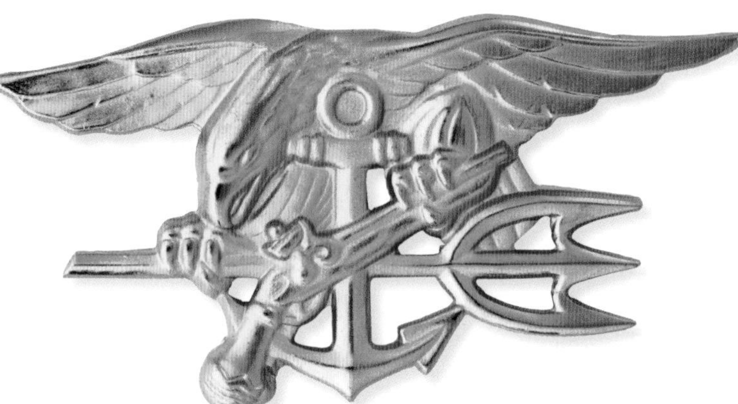

Navy SEAL Trident insignia

## Work out anywhere

Remember, you can perform a Navy SEALs workout just about anywhere—in the gym, at the park, or at home. The great thing about this program is that you don't need much room or need to spend much money to get an amazing workout. Many of the exercises call for you to just use your own body weight as resistance; others require only a set of dumbbells or other hand weights. For the Pull-Ups, if you don't have access to a gym or a park with a bar, reasonably priced Pull-Up bars are available that you can install in a home doorway.

## Warm up, cool down

Be sure to always prepare for your workout with the dynamic warm-up movements included and finish the workouts with the static, cool-down stretches to gain maximum muscle tissue mobility in a full range of motion. If you perform these basic exercises, carefully following the directions, your body will use its energy properly so that body fat will burn and muscle will build.

## Physical Screening Test (PST)

Each branch of the military around the world has physical requirements for all personnel who wear a uniform. In the United States, PT (short for "physical training") is the term used to describe exercise of any type. An official fitness test of military personnel is called a PFT in the Army, Marine Corps, and Air Force, and a PST in the U.S. Navy. Each branch of the service differs in what specific exercises it includes in its respective test.

SEAL teams have a minimum requirement for their PST. Meeting the minimum standard will get you into BUD/S, but it won't guarantee success. Basic Underwater Demolition School has a 75 percent attrition rate. There isn't a test for mental toughness—there is no way to objectively measure a man's heart and guts. Therefore no one knows who will and who will not finish BUD/S and earn a Trident. Research has found, however, that the men who meet the optimum standard are more likely to succeed.

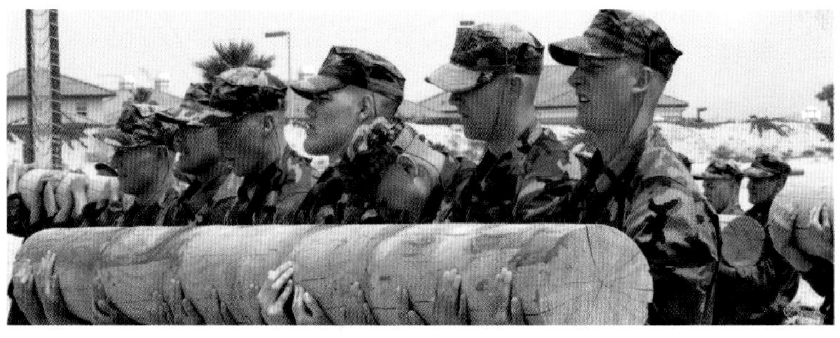

**U.S. Navy SEAL PST standards**

| PHYSICAL SCREENING TEST | MINIMUM | OPTIMUM |
|---|---|---|
| Swim 500-yard (457 m) breaststroke or sidestroke | 12:30 minutes | 09:00 minutes |
| Push-Ups in 2 minutes | 50 reps | 90 reps |
| Sit-Ups in 2 minutes | 50 reps | 85 reps |
| Pull-Ups (no time limit) | 10 reps | 18 reps |
| Run 1.5 miles (2.4 km) in boots | 10:30 minutes | 09:30 minutes |

## The Only Easy Day Was Yesterday

Making the grade and being accepted into the special forces of any military, from the UK's SAS to the Russian Federation's Spetsnaz GRU, means passing a series of grueling tests—both mental and physical. Among special forces, U.S. Navy SEAL training is considered one of the world's toughest military training programs. A SEAL must become the ultimate warrior, remaining combat effective through any level of stress. A candidate must complete six months of BUD/S, followed by six months of SEAL Qualification Training (SQT) before he can enter into an active platoon and wear the Trident.

It is during this training that active SEAL instructors test the limits of a candidate, attempting to push him until he quits. If a man cannot handle the rigors of physical training on a beach in California, he will not be able to handle the rigors of stress in combat overseas. Elevated stress is therefore continually applied, and men are pushed beyond their normal mental capacities in an attempt to simulate combat stress.

The third week of training, known as Hell Week, truly tests a candidate's mettle. He must endure five and half days of cold, wet, brutally difficult training, with fewer than four hours of sleep. SEALs and BUD/S students train the same way they fight, always stressing the motto "The Only Easy Day Was Yesterday."

## Remain hydrated

Plan to spend up to 60 minutes per workout. This requires staying hydrated and motivated. Do not wait until you are thirsty to hydrate—by the time you are thirsty, you are already dehydrated.

Drink only plain water for workouts lasting under 90 minutes. The amount of water needed is dependent upon the level of fitness you possess and the environment you are training in, but here is a general guide:

- 15 to 20 ounces of water one to two hours before your workout
- 8 to 10 ounces of water 15 minutes before you begin
- 8 ounces every 15 minutes during your workout

## Stay motivated

The key to sticking with any fitness program is staying motivated. What motivates you? Movies, music, a workout partner, or training group are great ways to improve the experience of exercise.

Find your purpose and stay on task. In the Warrior Mindset section (pages 12–25), you will find many techniques used in leadership and teamwork seminars and within the military that will allow you to get in touch with your personal sense of purpose and to explore your abilities. These will all help you to stay motivated—and be successful at any endeavor you undertake in life.

You are reading this book because you are looking for a great workout, and you understand that the special ops warriors must reach the very highest fitness levels just to survive the corrosive environment in which they operate. But you can also learn the techniques used by the military not just to get in amazing shape but to also become (and stay) healthy and motivated and master of yourself and your mind. This book will be a mind expander, full of helpful information not readily available in other sources.

Good luck, work hard, and remember what the SEALs say: The Only Easy Day Was Yesterday.

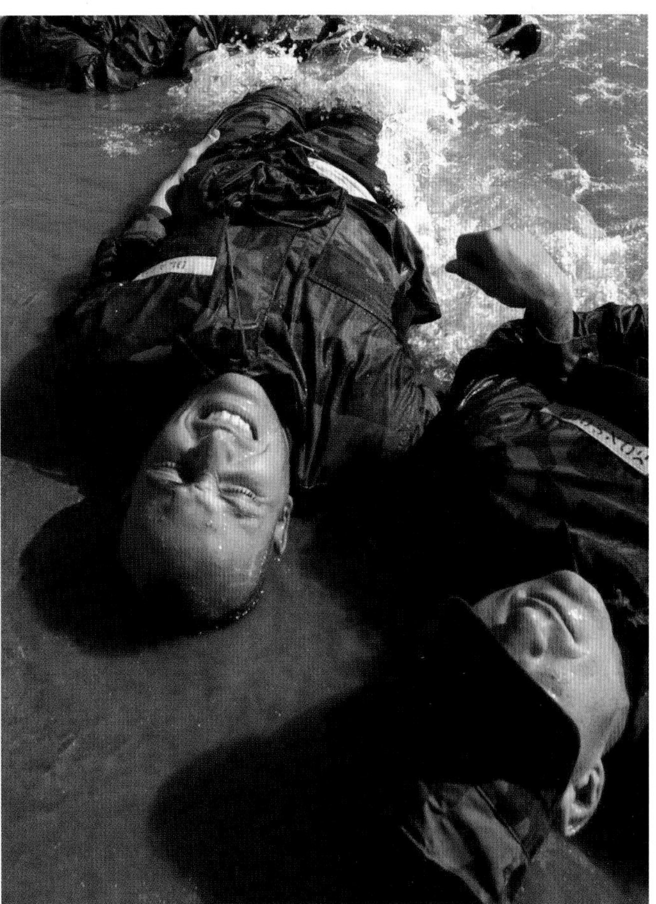

SEAL trainees endure freezing water during Hell Week.

# The Warrior Mindset

If you want the best outcome from your workout program, you must first learn about and master yourself. You must develop the mental toughness of a true warrior.

Anyone seeking the ultimate fitness level must learn not just about the body, but also about the mind. To become a warrior you must first explore the various philosophies of health, the physiology of exercise, sports nutrition, and natural health care.

## Know your mind

Sun Tzu in *The Art of War* states, "If you know the enemy and know yourself, your victory will not stand in doubt." One could say that if you know how your own mind works, figuring out your enemy's mind becomes less difficult. And if you know your own mind, then combating any tendency toward laziness or procrastination you might be feeling becomes easier.

For the purposes of this book, think of fitness and nutrition as enemies you must conquer. You will do daily battle to complete your workout. You will set micro goals in order to achieve victory. With smaller, more attainable goals, you will remain focused and stay motivated. Take a stand or state a definite purpose . . . and then strive daily in every action and thought to reach it, as though it were a fire burning inside you prompting you to completion.

### The scholar as warrior

To many who practice martial arts, the centered individual is one who balances his life of military or combat training with academic or philosophic pursuits. It is only in this way that the enlightened person can become truly rounded, truly centered. This "truth" has been known and accepted by warriors since the dawn of civilization. For instance, the childhood training of the Greek hero Achilles focused not only on skills in the battlefield, but also on scholarship (he was tutored in the arts, medicine, and music by the revered centaur Chiron). Even David, one of the Bible's most successful warriors, was a deeply spiritual psalmist. Pericles, supreme among Greek leaders, was a great patron of music and the arts. T. E. Lawrence (Lawrence of Arabia) was an Oxford-educated archeologist and linguist before he determined to unite the Bedouin tribes and defeat the Turks during World War I.

It may be true that it is the man of action who knows how to fight, but it is the man of intelligence and wisdom who can determine which fights to join in and which to avoid.

A positive mindset is an attitude; when internalized properly it drives you forward and leads to success. It allows you to learn and practice and achieve every micro goal, until they have accumulated into a macro success.

The best part is that you can take this "attitude of accomplishment" into all the arenas of your life—the classroom, boardroom, gym, on the streets, the sports field, your home—just about anywhere.

## The mind–body connection

"The mind and body are connected" gets said so often—at the gym, in the doctor's office, at the weight-loss clinic—that you stop paying attention. But these two are more than connected; they are virtually the same entity.

Way back at the beginning of time, an event occurred that physicists call the Big Bang. It involved the rapid expansion of dense matter in space, the formation of light elements, and the creation of galaxies. Over millions of years, stars formed and died. When these failing stars, called supernovas, exploded, they manufactured atoms of oxygen, carbon, helium, iron and the rest of the periodic table, which traveled light years across the universe to form every atom and energy system on earth. Each of these atoms, which can also be called stardust, is its own energy system. This system of energy links every atom of the universe together as a kind of interdependent engine. All energy in the universe is thereby interrelated.

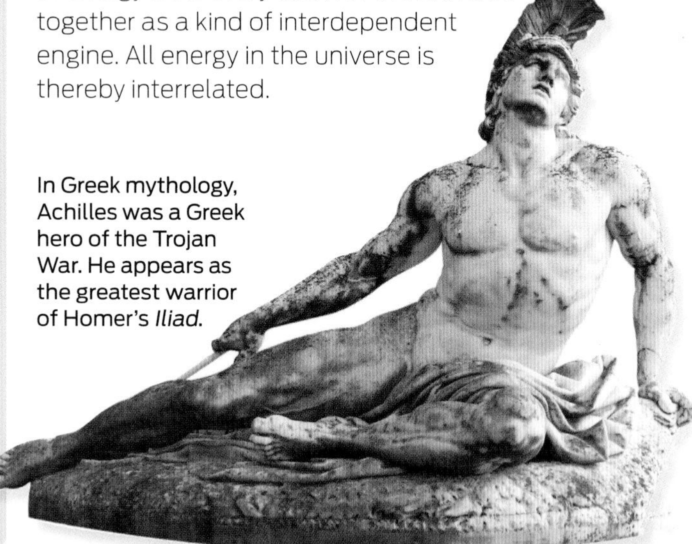

In Greek mythology, Achilles was a Greek hero of the Trojan War. He appears as the greatest warrior of Homer's *Iliad*.

Why is this short physics lesson important in learning about self? Because, as part of that cosmos, humans need to discover that, like the stars and the atoms, everything within them is also interrelated energy: the mind and the body; psyche and structure.

## The weakest link

Even though the mind and body are indelibly entwined, the mind can often act as the weak link when it comes to getting the body fit. It is the mind that breaks down and halts the body, the mind that says "Stop! I can't go on . . . I need a rest . . . I'll work that much harder tomorrow." It is the mind that berates you and says, "You're too old . . . too fat . . . to weak . . . too big . . . too small" or "You'll never be strong enough . . . smart enough . . . rich enough . . . healthy enough . . . or attractive enough." It limits you by manufacturing a dozen excuses to give up on yourself.

The mind seeks the path of least resistance. Most people have a limit to the amount pain or discomfort they will endure. It is, however, a self-imposed limit. A warrior needs to be trained to overcome and master the barriers the brain creates. Tell yourself that you will try to do a tough task, such as a grueling workout, rather than simply saying you can't.

This is the path to self-actualization. This is the path of the motivated; the warrior each of us must find and train. Your mind can be trained to say, "No, I won't quit! I won't accept excuses! I will push through the pain, the sleepiness, the excuses, the barriers. I will endure any hardship, overcome every obstacle, and stay focused on learning and mastering my mind. I will build a cast-iron will. I will seek solutions and embrace problem-solving. I will learn as much as possible about my mind-body connection. I will master myself. I will find my purpose and what motivates me. I will find and push past self-imposed limitations and achieve the fitness level, the health, and the life I desire."

## Exercising the mind

So how do you begin to strengthen the mind in order to better strengthen the body? First of all, by understanding how the mind works and how it controls emotions, thoughts, words, and actions. Every action—positive or negative—begins with a thought. We, therefore, must begin to examine the thought processes that govern our actions and how they are shaped.

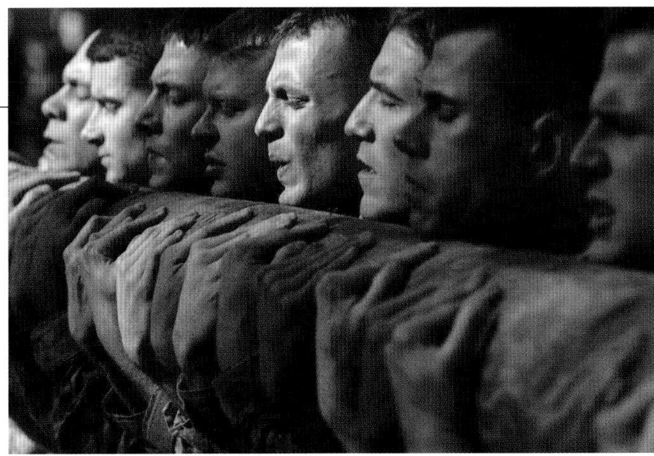

**U.S. Army soldiers in Special Forces Assessment and Selection class participate in grueling log training. Part of their training will include how to overcome physical challenges by attaining a warrior mindset that enables them to push through pain.**

How many people sign up for a gym or physical training program and then lose steam within the first month? This happens so often that it has become a cultural joke. So what is it that prevents so many of us from keeping up with a fitness program? In many cases, we have not paid enough attention to our state of mind. We have not prepped for the "ordeal" by psyching ourselves mentally. A brain that is honed and sharp is eager to improve the form that houses it. A brain that is underutilized and not stimulated grows careless of its body.

It is possible that exercising the mind is more important than exercising the body, because, ultimately, it is a high-functioning brain that will become your greatest ally in getting warrior-fit.

So how exactly do you go about exercising the gray matter? Gaining knowledge and understanding of new topics is one way to give your mind a workout. Doing crossword puzzles, brain teasers, or math problems are a few others. When your brain is engaged, its chemistry actually changes. Its activity speeds up, the synapses begin firing more frequently, and it can even become "toned" through frequent challenges.

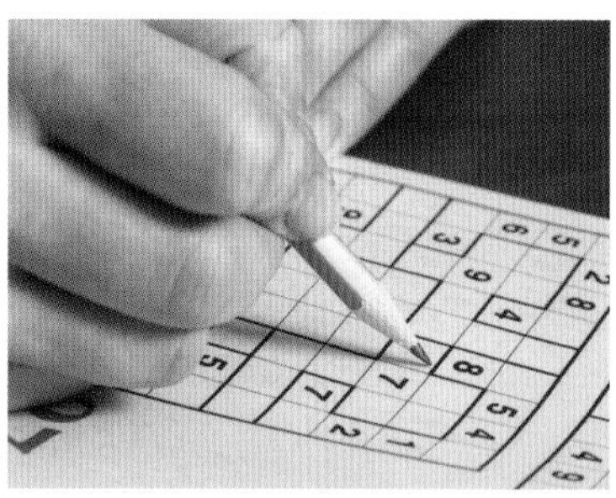

Once you have begun to engage your brain in a variety of healthy exercises—reading, studying, puzzle-solving, pursuing a degree—you can then begin to take on small physical tasks. If your brain begins to object, simply bargain for "another 10 reps," "another 5 minutes." If boredom is the enemy, if your brain insists that exercise is too dull, distract it with a puzzle—count how many of your classmates from third grade you remember, or work out the plot from the latest TV mystery series.

Before long, your stimulated brain will be too busy to object to workout sessions, and you will begin to feel a mastery over your thoughts that you never experienced before. All the excuses and procrastination will evaporate as you alter your patterns of thought and find yourself taking charge of the decision-making process.

## The spiritual link

Another aspect of gearing up for a strict fitness regimen is getting yourself spiritually prepared. Just as the kung fu master meditates before a bout, the warrior must seek answers and insights in order to make the most of the transformative aspects of exercise. Also, once you have engaged your spiritual side, connected with the "true" you, your chances of fitness success are greatly multiplied. Think about it—if the brain can encourage the body to work out, the spirit can certainly reinforce both brain and body.

And, by the way, this concept of spirituality is not a bunch of touchy-feely fluff—the army itself has begun character- and leadership-development programs under the banner of "spiritual fitness," which is part of a larger resiliency program aimed at decreasing incidents of post-traumatic stress and military suicide. These vital programs are based on proven psychological practices. So taking care of your spiritual side is no less important than getting your body fit or flexing your brain.

There are a number of benefits to incorporating spirituality—prayer, Transcendental Meditation, biofeedback, yoga, chanting, or similar pursuits—into your fitness routine:

- *Relief from the stress of the technological world:* By "going deep" into yourself, you can reconnect with your basic or primal nature, critical for shedding daily pressures.
- *A renewed sense of purpose:* You will understand that reshaping your physical self is a way to honor your spiritual self, a means of expressing self-love.
- *The ability to see things in proportion:* You will be able to overcome one problem many people face during physical endeavors—that when the mind sees a normal obstacle, the body sees "a mountain."
- *A strong sense of self:* You will stop comparing yourself to others and realize that your fitness goals are personal and not part of any peer pressure. "You" will be the only person you are competing against.
- *The desire to improve:* You will understand that, while it is important to be accepting of who you were, you are now seeking to become the person you feel you were created to be. Self hate, in the moment, is the great destroyer of goals.

Ultimately, by respecting this triumvirate—body, mind, and spirit—you will be able to create a cyclical exercise/reward dynamic. You will become fitter and feel better. As your confidence increases, so too will your desire for more exercise. You will then become even fitter, feel even better, try out new methods or exercises, heighten your self-image, and so on.

## Preparation

One key element to a successful workout is preparation. Jumping into anything without some forethought is never wise, especially when it is a physically strenuous activity. Just like the professionals from the special operations community prepare their minds and bodies for years to try out for a special ops team, you too must patiently prepare for these exercises.

Study them and learn their form before you begin to actually practice them. Once you think you're ready, try to perform the workouts with as little rest as possible and while using your best-possible form. Remember, the form required of each exercise is more important than reps or speed of the session. As you master the exercises, your speed will increase naturally.

Preparation also means getting the most out of your fitness routine by studying yourself and how you respond to exercise. It means understanding as much about sports nutrition as possible. Seek out books and articles about exercise physiology, combat mindset, and natural healthcare. Be hungry for information from multiple sources.

The more you know about how your body adapts to fitness routines, how to care for yourself, to nourish yourself and the techniques to stay motivated, the more effective your exercise program will be. If you want to train to the level of a special operations warrior, you must become a student.

## Three responses to stress

Mindset, or mental attitude, is also a major part of preparation. Watch any athlete prior to an event and you will see ritualistic behavior: a quarterback running drills with his teammates, a boxer working a speedbag with the eye of the tiger, a martial artist transfigured by meditation. But even the most carefully prepared plans don't always work out.

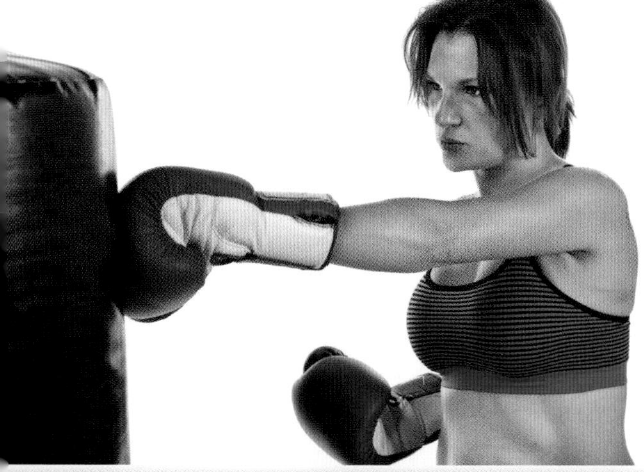

Imagine that you are scheduled to give an important presentation at work. You have prepared well and rehearsed your pitch. You leave the house sure that it will be a success. But on the way to your office, another driver cuts you off, nearly causing a collision. You slam on the brakes, crying out in panic as your laptop hurtles against the dashboard. Suddenly, adrenaline floods your body, and you start to shake. All your confidence from moments before has fled. You now think about your presentation with dread—you're just too shaken up.

So much for all your preparation—stress has just destroyed your feeling of control. No matter how well you prepare, stress can undermine your plans. It affects you on the job, on the road, in the home—even during recreation, while you watch sports or other competitions.

Humans typically have three responses to aggression or stress: fight, flight, or posturing.

- You can choose to *fight* by holding your ground and coping with a situation head-on. It may be a health issue, a verbal attack, job stress, a money problem, or a workout you need to confront. As a warrior, you often have the fighting spirit. You seek a fight or at least never back down from one.
- Sometimes it is smarter and better to opt for *flight*, however, in order to retreat, regroup and fight another day. Wise leaders and warriors know when to fight or flee. In *The Art of War*, Sun Tzu tells the warrior, "He will win who knows when to fight and when not to fight." This lesson can be translated into the boardroom, classroom, or sporting arena, as well as in your daily life and workout.
- A third and less-recognized response to stress or aggression is *posturing*. Most living creatures have an innate resistance to harming members of the same species. A ram will maul predators from the side, attempting to kill them, yet, it will hit another ram head to head in a form of ritualized posturing. Humans, although we do kill each other, have a very low incidence of doing so. We instead assume posturing attitudes every day in multiple ways to avoid interpersonal stress or human aggression.

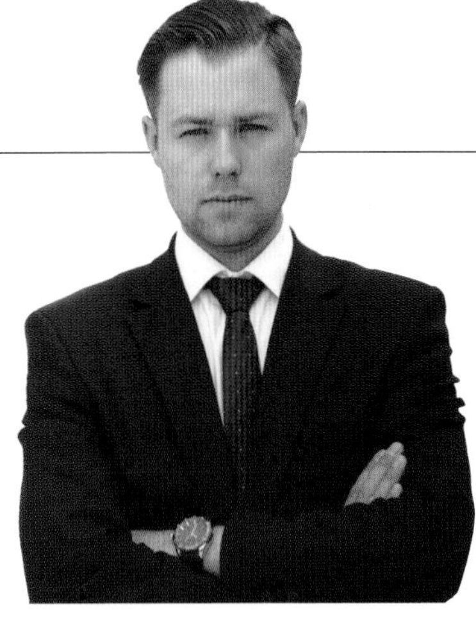

## Posturing

Posturing is a mindset. It is easy to see posturing in humans every day. The way people dress, stand, or interact is often a form of posturing. A businessman might wear a red power tie, a youth may stand up straight with his chest out to impress a girl, and a woman intent on getting noticed by her peers may carry the latest designer bag. Twelve people may show up against seven to negotiate a business deal. Some people walk, stand, or move in submissive postures that they hope will ward off aggressors.

True warriors, however, understand posturing and only use it to motivate themselves or their team and never in place of action. A leader or warrior or seasoned athlete does not tell tales of his or her exploits. He does not boast of his battles or victories. This is for the phony warrior. Boasting of ability or name-dropping is a form of posturing done by those who can only aspire to great things. A true warrior remains a humble and quiet professional.

## Ready for battle

There are a number of activities that warriors perform to prepare for competition or battle—creation of a timetable, assessment of terrain, evaluation of opponent, formulation of tactical logistics, and the gathering of supplies. You must take the same approach toward your daily workout and nutritional requirements.

- *Creation of a timetable:* Establish a schedule for which workout you will be performing each day. As your stamina increases, add more strenuous routines to your workout. Make sure to set aside enough time to complete your chosen exercises, including a warm-up and cool-down period.
- *Assessment of terrain:* Make sure you have a place to work out that is comfortable and relaxing, perhaps with a source for music or a place to watch videos.
- *Evaluation of opponent:* While exercising, your inner voice—telling you it's too hard, it's time to stop—is usually the opponent. Listen to it, but don't necessarily heed it, at least not until you have completed your timetable.
- *Formulation of tactical logistics:* Pay attention to form as you progress through your routine. Don't overextend yourself during any one session, especially during your early routines. Pace yourself and keep track of your pulse. Recheck your responses each week to make sure you are improving in terms of stamina and reps.
- *Gathering of supplies:* Change into your workout gear, and collect your equipment—exercise mat, dumbbells, towels—beforehand. Make sure you have plenty of water on hand. Keep a healthy snack nearby for instant energy in case you feel depleted.

Here are some other tips for making your exercise sessions productive and stimulating:

- Put on your game face and take an attitude of attacking the workouts as if you were attacking an enemy.
- Listen to music and watch movies that motivate you.
- Hang up photos or posters that inspire you in your exercise space.
- Set micro goals while keeping your main goal in mind.

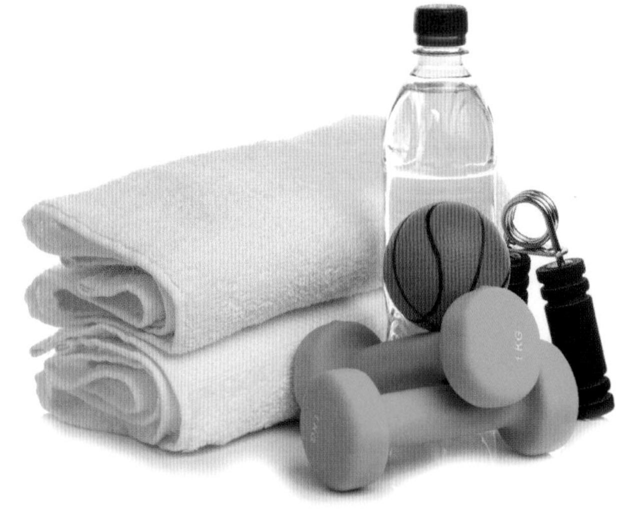

## Determining your fitness goals

What is your primary reason for working out? Do you wish to run a marathon, become a SEAL, compete in an Ironman Triathlon, lose 20 pounds, fight diabetes, or simply return to an earlier state of youthful good health?

When choosing your fitness goals, it helps to keep in touch with reality. Many people shoot for the moon—expecting to lose 50 or more pounds or gain many inches in muscle mass—and become disheartened when their goals aren't swiftly met. Physical transformation is always possible, but for it to be accomplished safely, it has to occur on a healthy timetable. Plus, if you expect too much too soon, you will inevitably be disappointed and your confidence level will plummet.

Here are several things to ask yourself when creating your goals:

- *Are you making a six-month or a three-week goal?* The shorter-term goal is more realistic, and you have a better chance of meeting it. Once you meet your first goal, you can increase your expectations for phase two.
- *What will it take to achieve your fitness goal?* If you plan to do four sessions a week but are also studying for your bar exam or taking your turn as babysitter, you might want to scale back. Start with two or three sessions, and try to add on more time per session—but never more than 10 percent of your previous week's minutes. By gradually increasing your workout time, you will also reduce the risk of injury.
- *Do you actually see yourself achieving your goal?* Be really honest with yourself. Can you stick to the program and visualize your transformation at the end of it? Can you bypass all the goodies you love and try to maintain a healthier diet? Do you have what it takes to increase the level of your workouts until you are starting to feel like a fitness warrior? If you can answer "yes" to these questions, then your goal is probably legitimate.

Don't aim for big rewards in a short time, don't make farfetched promises to yourself, and don't try to recapture past glory through exercise. Also, don't hesitate to tweak a goal a bit if it's not working for you. Sometimes illness intrudes or life gets in the way.

## Meeting your goals

Now that you have chosen specific goals, there are a number of ways to keep yourself on track.

- Keep a journal of your training sessions and post your exercises, times, and reps. Following your progress on paper gives you a concrete reminder of how far you have come and increases your commitment.
- Set up a dedicated workout space at home. Purchase used weights or dumbbells online. Make sure you have an MP3 or DVD player to keep you entertained and upbeat.

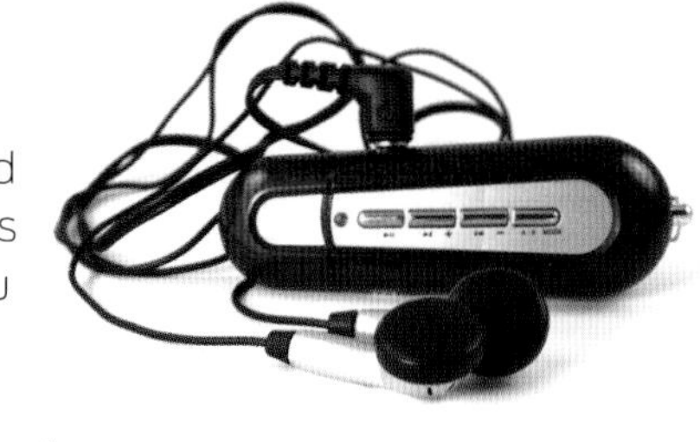

- Add a balance-building element, such as yoga exercises, to your workout. Good balance is vital to most exercises.
- Get a fitness evaluation by a professional trainer. This will allow you to assess your level of preparedness for a specific exercise regimen. Or you can time yourself while walking or running a predetermined 1-mile course as fast as you can. Check your pulse at the end, then again one minute later. Redo the test two months later after your exercise program has begun and compare your time and heart rate. Both should have decreased.
- Go public with your fitness goals. Let friends and family know that you are taking your health seriously. They can also become a cheering section if you start to flag or feel overwhelmed.
- Challenge yourself. As part of your new exercise regimen, why not plan to participate in a 5K-charity walk or run? That way your weekly schedule of workouts becomes a "training" session—allowing you to become a road warrior for a good cause.

Another factor to consider when trying to meet your goals is your specific fitness style. Are you one of those folks who leap out of bed at dawn and hit the rowing machine? Or are you a night owl who goes for long runs at dusk to work out the stresses of the day? Or maybe you enjoy spending your lunch hour at the gym rather than at the hot dog cart?

It's not only the time of day that affects your exercise outlook. Your personality can also dictate what types of exercises you prefer—slow, endurance-based ones; mid-rate, repetitive ones; weight-based ones that enhance your strength; combinations that include isometric and isotonic movement; stretching and flexing routines; or good, old-fashioned aerobic workouts that increase your heart rate and flush you with endorphins. If you notice that one type of exercise typically leaves you cold, you might just have a natural aversion. Determine what body part it or specific motion it pertains to and look for another exercise that works the same area.

## Outcome goals

These are the goals that address the big picture, the long-term results of your fitness routine. Some competitive people have higher expectations than others when it comes to these goals. Some are happy if they achieve 60 or 70 percent, while many are not satisfied unless they reach 100 percent. Some people tend to "push" the goals; that is, if they achieve one completely, they will set the bar even higher in the next set of goals. This is not always productive and can even be self defeating.

### The big three motivators

Numerous studies indicate that these three things most heavily motivate people to begin a fitness routine:

1. Vanity, or the desire to look good, or at least look better.

2. Health, or the desire to improve longevity, lower cholesterol and blood pressure, and decrease chances of developing diabetes or cancer.

3. Performance, or the desire to improve the ability to walk, run, swim, or lift weights, and to increase levels of energy and vitality.

The main thing when dealing with outcome goals is to keep your focus on the process, not on the result. This takes you back to your micro goals—or short-term "process" goals. These goals not only work for exercise plans but for nutrition and diet as well. If you are a snacker or fast food fan, cut down gradually or replace your bad-food habit with something healthier over a period of time.

The good news is that these incremental process goals eventually feed into your outcome goals—a person who starts out with 30 minutes of exercise a week and adds on five minutes each week (a bit over the 10 percent limit recommended earlier), will be exercising nearly five hours a week within a year.

Perhaps the most important thing when dealing with goals is remembering to reward yourself when you reach one. A small treat after accomplishing a process goal—a movie, a bottle of wine, new workout gloves—reinforces your success and sends you toward your next goal with renewed enthusiasm. After completing an outcome goal, a larger reward might be in order—a short fishing vacation, the latest MP3 player, or a cutting-edge pair of training shoes, for instance.

Never become so focused on the goal that you forget to acknowledge the hard work and determination that got you there.

## The way of the warrior

Perhaps the most important mindset you can adopt is that of the well-balanced warrior. Whether you are preparing for competition, combat, covert ops, or simply the conflicts of the boardroom, the lessons and attitudes of the warrior are always useful. The confidence you will experience once you are centered in mind, body, and spirit can carry you through job interviews, yearly evaluations, project deadlines, vendor mix-ups, office politics, and any number of other stressful situations in the workplace.

Simply put, the warrior is in command of his environment as much as himself. He controls what

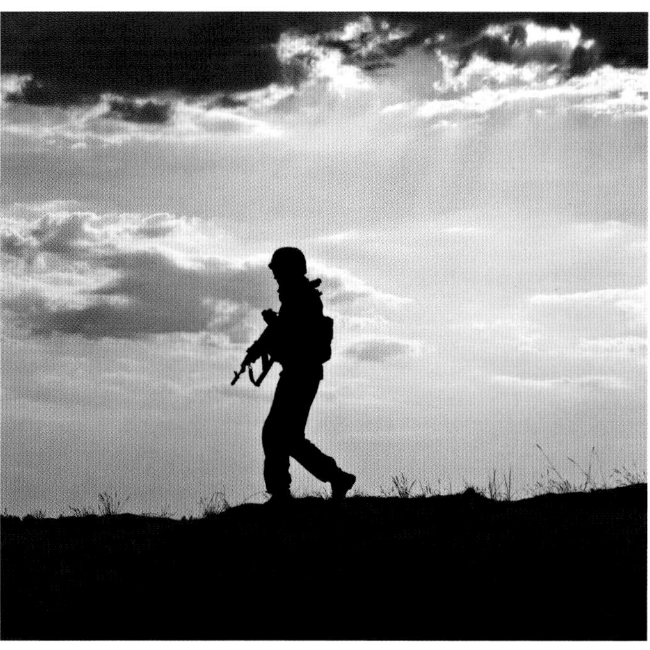

he can and rolls with whatever outside influences keep trying to distract him. This intense focus and the ability to improvise a successful outcome do not develop overnight. But they are yours to acquire if you combine the exercises in this book with a program of stimulating your mind and nurturing your spirit.

## Qi and yin-yang

One of the most important aspects of becoming a warrior is that the title must be earned. Being able to do 100 push-ups or having the fastest, most powerful karate chop are not the only criteria. In addition to mastering combat training or the art of self-defense, the true warrior must also present an air of serenity and control. When she enters a room, it stills for a moment. When he catches and holds someone's eye, they feel a soothing effect. This is because the true warrior's inner strength is outwardly conveyed by a healing presence.

This inner energy is called "qi," and when it touches other people—even though they don't feel anything physical—they immediately begin to experience a sense of peace. Perhaps you yourself have felt this restful calm after meeting a particularly spiritual or self-aware person.

The warrior also relates strongly to the world around him, to all living things as well as inanimate objects. The trees, the sky, the rocks in a stream, the insects in the forests, and the creatures of the ocean all have meaning. He understands how this world is interconnected just as the world of atoms and space are interconnected. And that he is, in turn, connected to all of it.

The warrior communicates on some level with everything around him. That way he gains an understanding of the forces on earth, the limitations, which he must accept or perish. He does not walk knowingly into danger, but respects it and sidesteps it. Although he has the power to change many things, he also has the wisdom to recognize the times he cannot make a difference.

Yet for all the gifts the warrior possesses, he knows there is a price to be paid. That nothing comes without a downside. This system of cosmic giving and taking is referred to as yin and yang. For each moment of happiness, a moment of sadness is required. For each victory, there will be a reciprocal defeat. This is not necessarily a bad thing—it teaches the warrior the power of sacrifice and the concept that he must lose in order to gain. He will do without food, do without comforts, or do without consolation, but he will prevail and become stronger. When the warrior has reached this point, he knows there are few challenges he cannot surmount.

## Master and student

Another quality of the warrior is that he welcomes instruction. In spite of all the knowledge and power he has accumulated, he recognizes that there are still individuals who are wiser and more powerful, those who are farther along the warrior's path from whom he can learn. The warrior also knows that those who help him along this path are guides rather than teachers. And in turn, the master offers his friendship and dedication to the student. They both understand that they are at different stages of the same journey and can benefit from each other.

This is a helpful attitude to adopt when beginning this—or almost any—workout program. As a true warrior, trust that your guide will have your best interests at heart, that he or she will not ask for more than you can give, and that having once been where you now are, they will feel empathy for your struggles to master the program. Your humility will ultimately result in newfound strength of purpose and revitalized confidence.

## Visualization

One of the most successful tools used by fitness or sports pros is visualization—the ability to envision the act of surmounting a problem or achieving a goal. In your case, it might be imagining yourself working out three times a week or completing one level of an exercise plan, and eventually seeing yourself 25 pounds lighter or able to bench press twice your own weight.

It might sound a bit crazy to insist that a person's imagination is linked to their physical capabilities, but it's already been established that when a fitness goal is established, all parts of the body—including the mind and spirit—can and will work in collaboration.

Visualization also works well to control negative behaviors or damaging urges. This removal or redirection of counterproductive thoughts is sometimes called "scrubbing." If you are an exercise-phobe, imagine yourself happily working out, enjoying the rhythm of your movements, savoring the new strength in your arms, legs, and core. If you indulge yourself with sweets or fast food, visualize yourself sitting down to a delicious serving of grilled salmon or a low-calorie angel-food slice laden with fresh strawberries.

Ideally, a combination of visualization and guided activities will speed you toward your fitness goals.

### *The steps toward visualization*

In addition to the specific fitness goals you might have—becoming a better tennis player, losing a specific amount of weight around the middle, building up muscle mass on your legs and arms—there are also basic goals that visualization will help you achieve:

- You will replace unhelpful or negative thinking with affirmative thoughts and emotions.
- You will increase your ability to commit to your current training plan as well as to other projects in your life.
- The visualization process will inspire more calmness and confidence in your life and work.

When beginning to visualize, you need to be in a comfortable, relaxed state. Initially, it helps to have another person's voice guide you through the stages of visualization. Eventually, you will be able to take yourself to that quiet place of positive energy, but, at first, it is much easier to make the journey with someone who understands the steps.

*Just prior to the experience:*

- Determine your specific goals.
- Replace negative thoughts with positive ones.
- Begin thinking of yourself as a warrior, an athlete, an Olympian, or some other fitness role model.
- Prep by eating healthy foods.

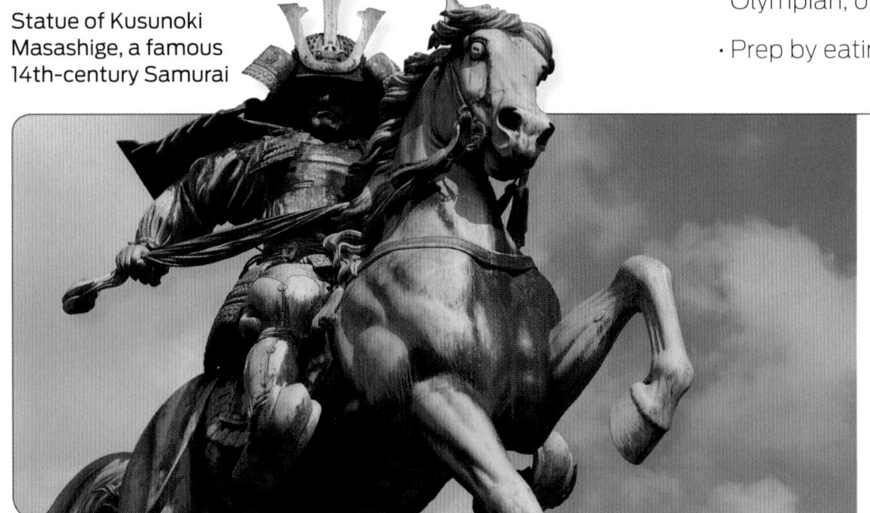

Statue of Kusunoki Masashige, a famous 14th-century Samurai

### Bushido

In Japanese, *bushido* literally means "the way of the warrior." It specifically refers to the Samurai way of life, which embodies a set of principles similar to those Europeans call "chivalry." Bushido reflects a moral code of conduct that emphasizes the mastery of martial arts, loyalty, frugality, and the notion of honor unto death. Bushido further calls for intense training sessions (using thousand-year-old methods), strict obedience, and devotion to duty, a kind of schooling that begins in early childhood.

*Getting started:*

- Find a softly lit, quiet spot to sit, and then arrange yourself in a comfortable upright position on a chair or small couch. Do not recline.
- Determine how long you would like the experience to last.
- Close your eyes.

*Learning to relax:*

- Hear yourself breathing. Feel the rise and fall of your chest. Try to slow your breathing using yoga or other relaxation aids.
- Count down from 200, telling yourself with each new number that you are becoming increasingly relaxed. Or imagine you are in a down elevator, and that with each floor you pass, you feel a greater sense of peace.
- Visualize a wave lifting away your stress as it passes through your body. Feel the muscles of your face relax. Feel your shoulders drop. Feel your arms become limp and heavy. Your hands relax into your lap. Your legs and feet become weighted and still.

*Beginning visualization:*

- Now you are ready to listen to the person who is guiding you through this session or to begin on your own. One suggestion, if you are trying this alone, is to think of 10 adjectives to describe how becoming warrior-fit would make you feel. Or use all your senses to see yourself as the true warrior—supremely healthy, capable, informed, spiritual, in control of your life, and balanced in all things. It is important not only to view the new you, but to also experience how achieving this goal would make you feel.
- Take some time to acknowledge the changes that you are already undergoing. Even just planning a life-changing exercise and fitness program is deserving of praise.
- Bring yourself back to full awareness by counting forward from 1 to 20.

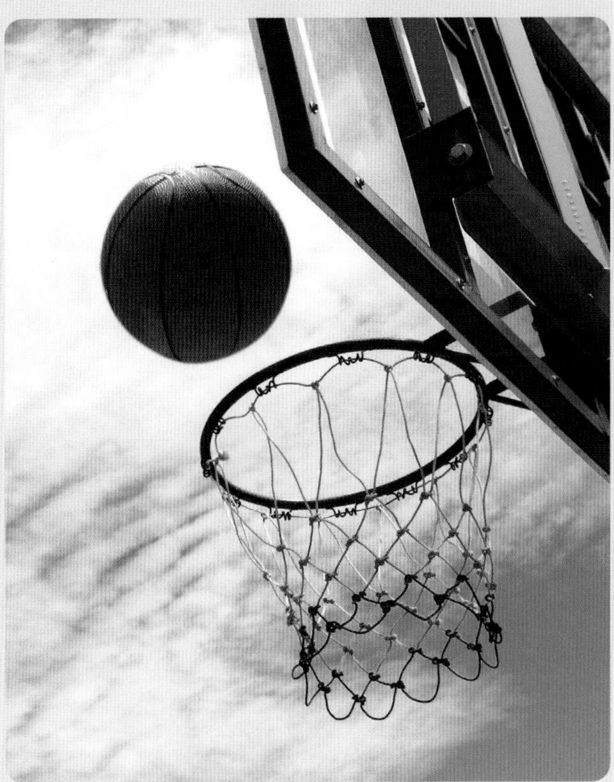

### The basketball study

Tests have repeatedly proven that visualization works. One notable example is a study on visualization and muscle memory conducted by Australian psychologist Alan Richardson.* As a baseline, he first asked a group of subjects to shoot 100 basketball foul shots, or free throws. He then randomly divided the subjects into three groups.

Over four weeks, Group A practiced free throws for 20 minutes a day, 5 days a week. Group B did nothing basketball related—not even think about it. Group C was guided in visualizing shooting free throws for 20 minutes, five days a week.

At the end of the four weeks, Richardson had each subject again shoot 100 free throws. Those in Group A had improved in their ability by 24 percent. Group B made no improvement. Group C, although they had never actually touched a ball, improved by 23 percent, nearly as much as Group A. Psychological research indicates that visualization actually creates an impression on the brain that simulates real practice. In other words, the thought is equal to the deed.

* Richardson, Alan, "Mental Practice: A Review and Discussion: II." *Research Quarterly*, Volume 38 (2), 1967, 263–273.

- Shift your focus from your breathing to your whole body. Feel it touching the chair and the floor.
- Open your eyes and look around. You will probably still feel heavy limbed and slightly fuzzy-headed. You should also feel a sense of great calm.

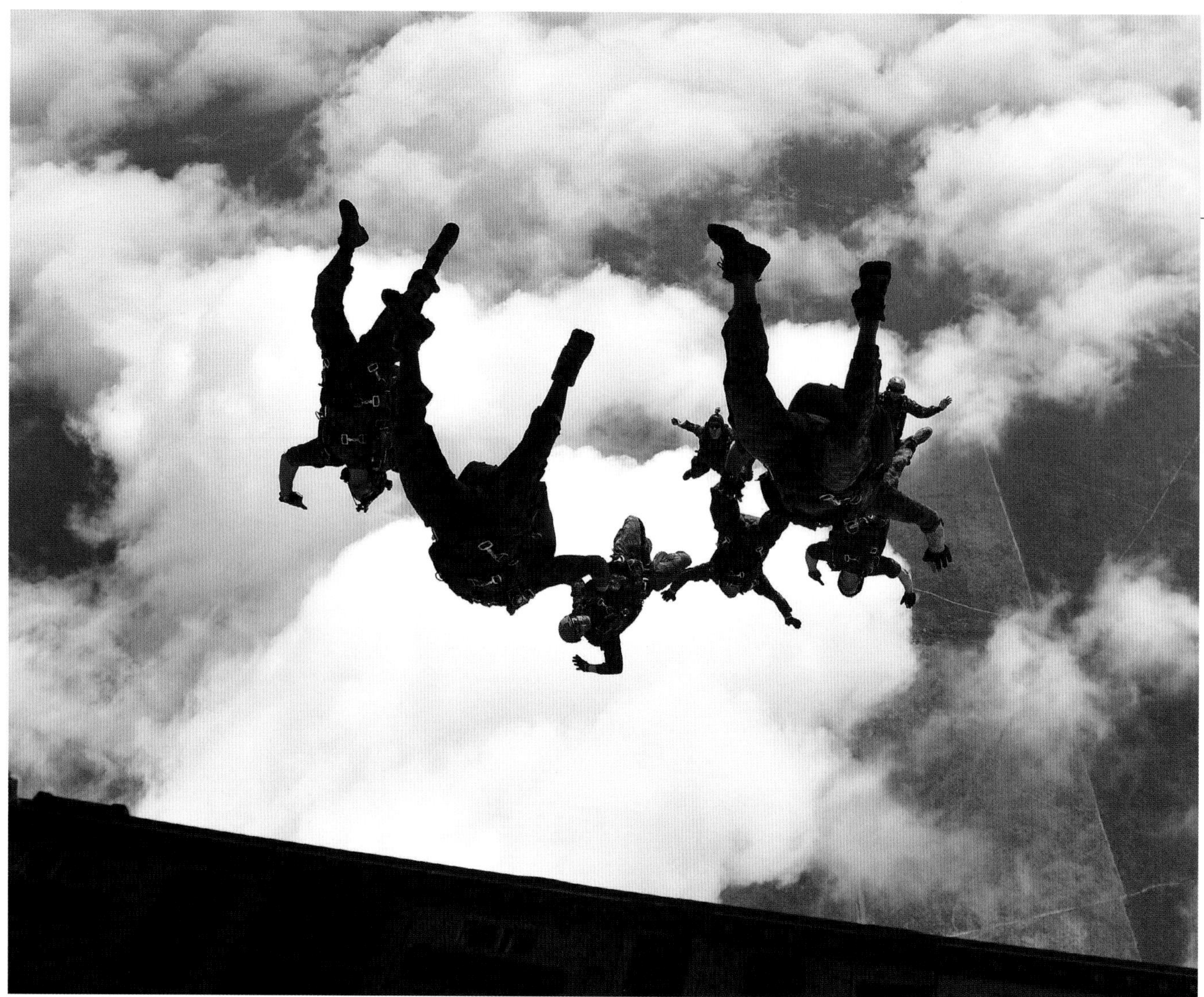

Canadian special operation regiment members conduct a free-fall jump during tactical exercises. Special forces training includes tough mental tests that teach recruits how to overcome their fears and self-imposed limitation. They learn how to adopt a warrior mindset that will see them through even the most challenging assignments.

## Autosuggestion

Visualization is only one way to coax the brain into improving the body. Other techniques include relaxation therapy, meditation, self-hypnosis, and autosuggestion. The latter term was coined by French psychologist and apothecary Emile Coué (1857–1926), who began to comprehend that if he praised a medication's effectiveness, the patient had a noticeably better response to it than if he just dispensed it without comment.

His study of this phenomenon led to the discovery of what is now called the placebo effect. Coué discarded hypnosis as a means to reach the subconscious mind, believing that if a patient repeated a positive mantra—for instance, "Every day, in every way, I'm getting better and better"—the mind would begin to replace "thoughts of illness" with "thoughts of a cure." There is much clinical evidence that he was correct, that the subconscious does eventually absorb encouraging words and react to them.

Inspirational leaders like Tony Robbins and Joel Osteen, as well as seasoned SEAL Commander Mark Divine, all teach Positive Mental Attitude (PMA) via autosuggestion. Autosuggestion uses many of the same steps as visualization, while placing an even greater emphasis on repetition of the healing or beneficial mantra. Instructors suggest repeating it morning, noon, and night, and some even recommend recording the message on a tape and playing it at night while the subject sleeps.

## Using your gifts wisely

Each person on the planet has gifts; most of us possess innate abilities and some, rare skills. One purpose of life is to understand these gifts and link them to the desire to improve yourself and the world around you.

Beyond this, most of us also possess spiritual gifts—our moral code or sense of ethics. This could also be known as our "stand" or "definitive purpose."

Our stand reflects our core values and indicates who we were meant to be. It is a set of principles, virtues, the code we live by. In a sense, it is the way we were programmed from birth, by family and by the forces around us. Nurture *and* nature.

This programming has created the person you are today. If you want to improve that person, you must reprogram. Yet you cannot reprogram without knowing your current state of mind, your core thoughts.

So how do you gain insight into your core being, the engine that drives your actions? It's not that difficult. If your actions are dictated by your thoughts, then guard your thoughts from negative influences. If you fill your mind with violence, negativity, gossip, anger, or doubt, these are the things that your psyche will crave. If you fill your mind with love, forgiveness, faithfulness, gentleness, kindness, self-control, joy, love, and peace, these will become your sources of sustenance.

If you can manifest a spirit of self-discipline—sometimes translated as "a sound mind and body"—you will be freed from much internal strife. In return, you will find your life being filled with all the positive virtues that lead to success.

### The Cooper Color Code

An excellent example of a man who understood his gifts and studied himself thoroughly, was Jeff Cooper; small arms expert and the creator of the "Modern Technique" of handgun shooting. Cooper broke down the alertness levels for the use of deadly force into four colors, indicating escalating degrees of preparation. This color-coded system is a mental process, not a physical one, and can be utilized whether or not you are armed. Being alert may help you to avoid a deadly threat in the first place, which is always the best outcome.

**Condition White**

- You are unaware of and unprepared for whatever is going on around you. You are probably in a safe environment like home or work. If attacked, you may freeze in panic.

**Condition Yellow**

- You are relaxed, but aware of who or what is in the surrounding area. In a restaurant, you may take a seat with a minimum number of people seated behind you so that you are more aware of the surroundings. This is not paranoia or panic you feel, but a state of surveying and assessing the environment.

**Condition Orange**

- A potential threat has entered into your radar area, and something has piqued your interest. You are mentally preparing for a threat, and, if attacked, you would be expecting it. You know where your weapon is and what you may have to do if attacked.

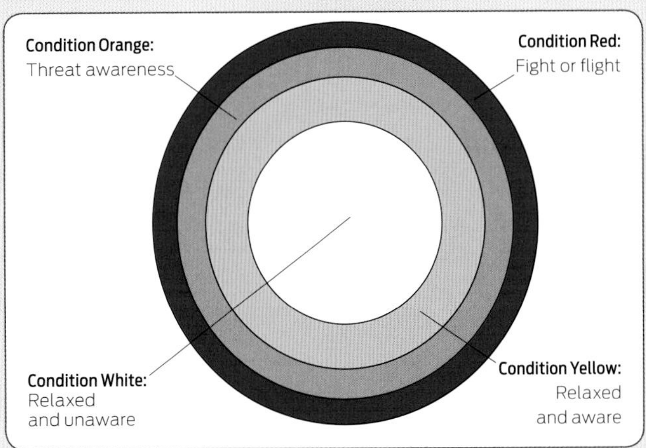


**Condition Red**

- Your mental trigger has been activated. You are very aware of what or who the threat is, and you have made all mental preparation to react to the danger. You may have started advancing to the target but have not yet engaged the target.

The U.S. Marine Corps also has a status it calls Condition Black. This involves a catastrophic breakdown of mental and physical performance in the subject. This can occur when there is a rapid progression from Condition White or Yellow straight to Condition Red, when the subject has not had time to acclimate to the threat.

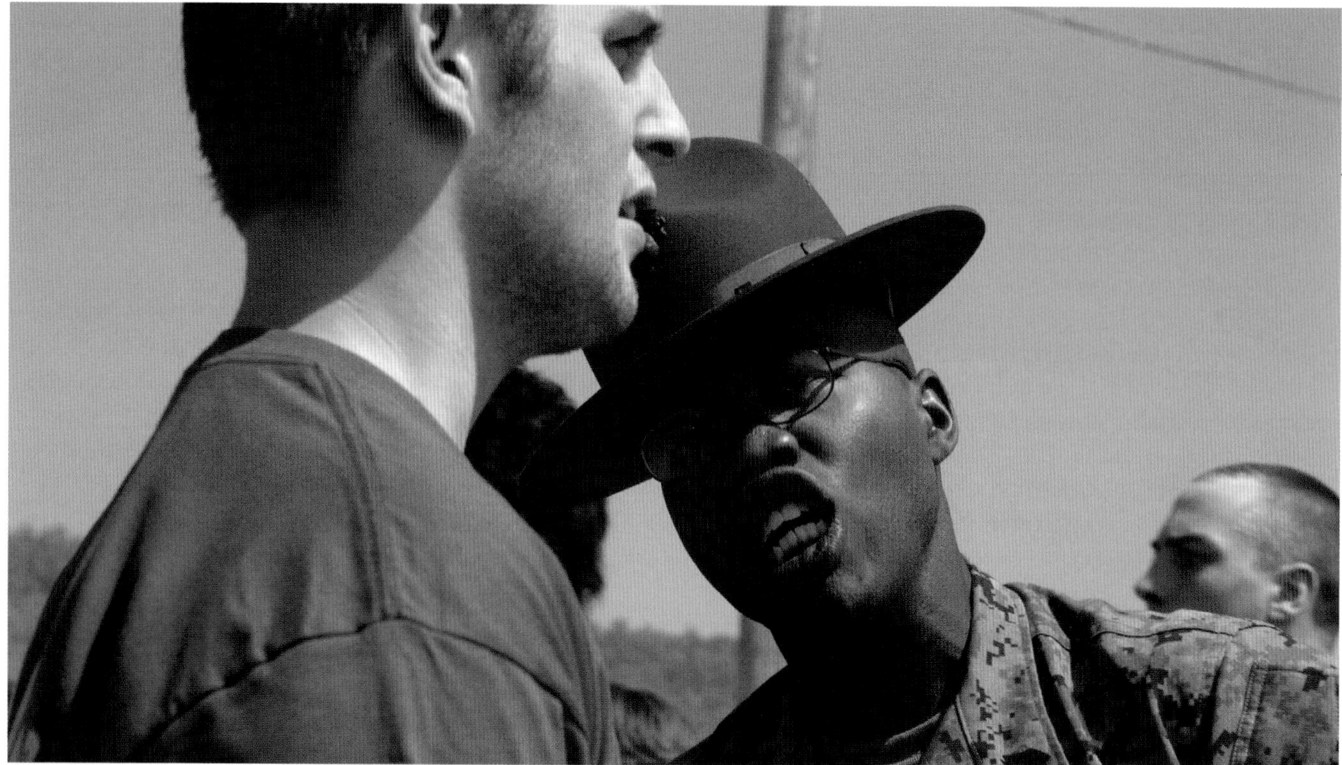

A Marine drill instructor shouts at a new recruit during basic training. The instructor is not being cruel, but instead beginning the process of stress inoculation that will help this soldier meet the stresses of real assignments on the front line.

## Stress inoculation

Everyone has seen war movies that include a drill instructor screaming in a new recruit's face, calling him names like "maggot." You might wonder if all that yelling is necessary. Why must they yell so much?

All that yelling is really part of a mental-training technique known as "stress inoculation." Warriors have always known and practiced the art of subjective mind-building along with physical training. And in the military, mind-building is conducted daily, starting on day one in boot camp. If a recruit can't handle the stress of someone yelling at him or her within the confined quarters of stateside training, it is not likely he or she could deal with the stress of combat overseas. Much like an inoculation or vaccine gives a small dose of a disease to build immunity in preparation for large exposure, stress inoculation provides small but constant doses of stress to prepare the recruit for large stresses.

Yelling in a recruit's face at boot camp is a small dose of stress. Yelling does not produce a physical injury; however, yelling constantly elevates the recruit's mental threshold for stress. A recruit is stressed out past his or her mental limits and then brought back to reality. This routine is performed over and over during many weeks of training. The final result is a mind inoculated against stress, which is then combat effective.

Disciplines such as daily PT, shining shoes, folding clothes, frequent visits to the barber, marching, standing at attention, and saluting are minor disciplines for training the mind. These disciplines are important because they not only prepare the mind and body for combat, they also enable those who enter the military and work on "the pointy end of the spear" (the front line) to learn how act upon any order given by his or her nation.

Physiologically, stress inoculation affects the central nervous system. Stress comes in three forms: physical, like PT; chemical, like food deprivation; and emotional, like being yelled at constantly. All three have the physiological effect of elevating the heart rate. If a person has never been inoculated for stress, he or she is going to respond to that stress with an elevated heart rate.

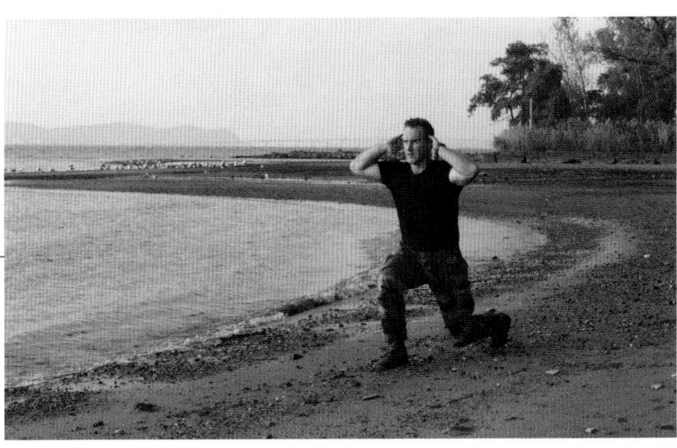

This is not acceptable in a combat situation. For example, studies have shown that with a sustained heart rate of 115 beat per minute (bpm), fine motor skill deteriorates. At 155 bpm gross (large muscles) motor skill deteriorates. With a count of 175 bpm, thinking deteriorates, tunnel vision begins, loss of depth perception, tunnel hearing, and loss of near vision. With sustained heart rates above 175, freezing occurs, as well as irrational fight or flight, loss of bowel or bladder control, vasoconstriction (reduced bleeding), and submissive behavior.

On the other hand, a mixed martial arts fighter who has been stress inoculated for hand-to-hand combat maintains a heart rate of about 115 beats per minute during a fight. If the stress is altered, however, from hand-to-hand fighting to a gun battle, his heart rate jumps into the 200-plus range. He gets tunnel vision, freezes, loses motor coordination, and is completely useless during the firefight. Still, his prior inoculation quickly helps him acclimate in a firefight—much more quickly than someone without prior stress inoculation. One stress inoculation builds upon another during training.

## The tactical athlete

The U.S. military is beginning to take a more holistic approach to training those who live at the point of the spear. The term "tactical athlete" is now used to describe the training of these personnel. Although military healthcare continues to be dominated by the allopathic philosophy, the men and women at point are working out with professional strength coaches and now have access to chiropractors, massage therapists, and nutritionists. Psychologists are appointed for not only post-traumatic stress disorder (PTSD) but also for the purpose of allowing the soldiers to verbalize their emotions. Self-actualization is advocated by building up the mind-body connection.

Within Special Operations Command, standard levels for physical fitness have been enhanced. Use of complex technology and understanding of multiple languages and cultures have become part of the training of the mind for a special forces warrior.

## Start your quest

Whether you seek health, wealth, or fame in your life, the lessons you have learned in the quest to adopt a warrior's mindset will remain with you and aid you in your other pursuits.

You now understand the mind-body-spirit connection and how you can make all three into your greatest allies as you strive for ultimate fitness. You know all the steps necessary to prepare for a successful physical transformation. You understand how to set up realistic goals and how to meet them and chart them. You have encountered the way of the warrior and realize how important it is to become a well-rounded individual. You understand the benefits of pain and sacrifice and how they actually help you to become stronger.

You will now be able to visualize any improvement you want to make in your life, and use autosuggestion to keep your positive mantras going. You now see all the possibilities that exist in making holistic choices, whether they involve medicine, fitness, or nutrition.

Perhaps most important, you now have that "fire in your gut" to commit yourself to the rigorous, yet rewarding, fitness routines contained in this book. You have the hunger to become one of the few, one of the best. You fully understand the Buddhist philosophy that when "the student is ready, the master will appear."

You are the student, and you are ready. This book is the teacher, appearing right when you need it. Work hard, stay committed, focus on your goals, but don't forget to have fun.

As a SEAL Team Six Ops Officer once told me, "Life's journey is not about arriving safely at the grave in a well-preserved body, but rather to skid in sideways, totally worn out, shouting 'Holy **** . . . what a ride!'"

# Nutrition

Just as you must master your mind, you must also master your body. Becoming a student of nutrition is one of the most important things you can do to affect your overall health.

Everything you ingest into your body is considered nutrition: food, liquid, medications, vitamins, supplements, and air. You are not only what you eat, you are also what you digest.

Ideally, your diet should provide your body with enough nutrients to maintain good health and proper energy levels to stay active.

## Nutrition and sports performance

Nutrition plays two main roles in our lives. First, for the purposes of this book, is the role it plays in sports or exercise performance. The second, much broader role is how nutrition affects our health.

In the world of fitness, diet can be adapted to meet the needs of many different types of athletes. For instance, endurance aerobic athletes such as military special operatives, swimmers, tri-athletes, and adventure racers should eat differently from anaerobic athletes such as football players, power lifters, baseball players, or sprinters.

Energy in diet comes from only three sources: carbohydrates, protein, and fat.

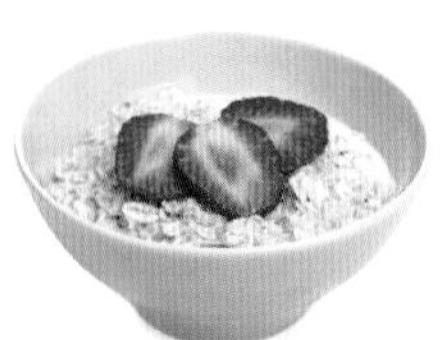

- *Carbohydrates:* Sources include items made from grains, like bread, cake, pastries, bagels, pasta, and oatmeal, plus white or sweet potatoes, vegetables, and fruit.

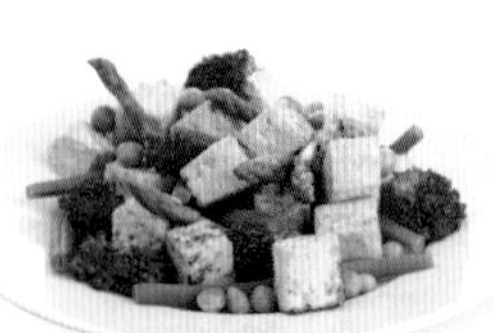

- *Protein:* Sources include meat, chicken, eggs, fish, beef, turkey, lamb, organ meat (offal), and pork, plus vegetable sources like soy, legumes, and broccoli.

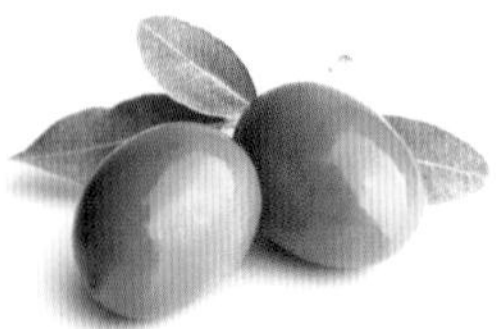

- *Fat:* Sources include peanut butter, olive oil, olives, nuts, seeds, vegetable and nut oils, and fatty fish (like sardines, tuna, salmon, and mackerel).

Vitamins, minerals, and electrolytes serve to help cellular function, but they do not supply energy.

## Anaerobic and aerobic diets

An athlete develops a diet that is right for his or her performance by determining the energy needs of a particular sport. The two main types of sports (or exercises)—each requiring different levels of nutrients—are anaerobic and aerobic.

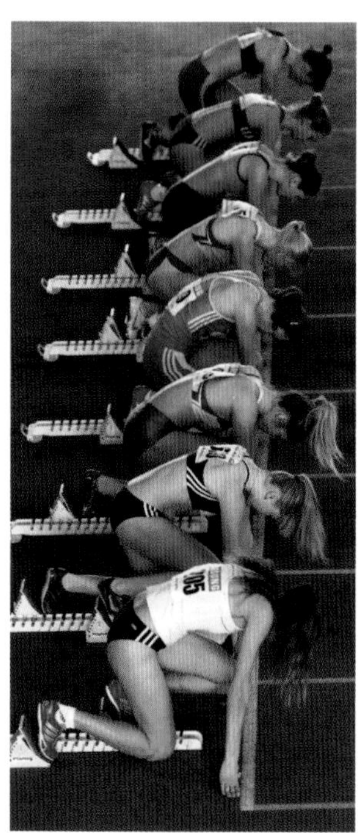

Are you an anaerobic athlete? This means your sport does not require long periods of sustaining an elevated heart rate. Anaerobic athletes are American football linemen, shot putters, baseball outfielders, lacrosse or hockey goalies, power lifters, weight lifters, sprinters, and body builders. These activities may very well require the heart rate to shoot up, but only for brief periods. An anaerobic athlete's diet should reflect the following breakdown:

- *Carbohydrates:* 55 percent.
- *Protein:* 30 percent.
- *Fat:* 15 percent.

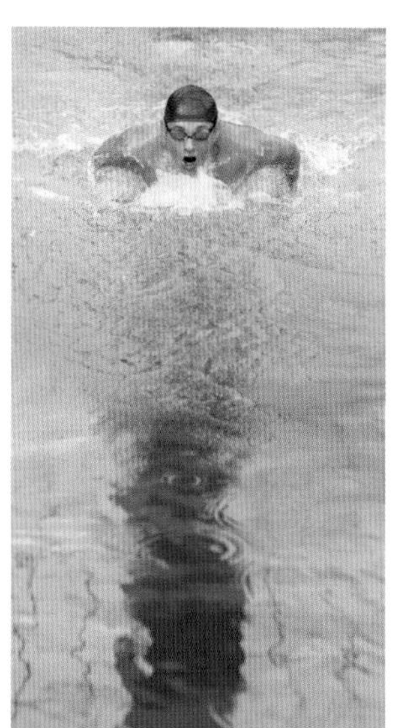

Aerobic athletes compete in events that require a sustained elevated heart rate. They are the distance or marathon runners, tri-athletes, swimmers, competitive cyclists, adventure racers, speed skaters, and rowers. Their nutrient breakdown should look like this:

- *Carbohydrates:* 65 to 80 percent.
- *Protein:* 20 to 35 percent.
- *Fat:* 10 percent.

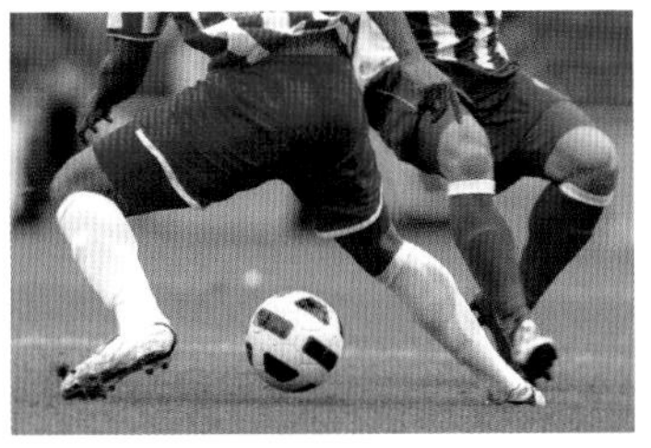

There are also combination athletes, whose sports consist of a mix of aerobic and anaerobic activity. These include mixed martial arts fighting, CrossFit, boxing, wrestling, tactical athletics, military PFT, soccer, lacrosse, basketball, baseball, and hockey, plus American football running backs, defensive backs, and wide receivers. Their ideal food intake should be broken down into:

- *Carbohydrates:* 60 percent.
- *Protein:* 30 percent.
- *Fat:* 20 percent.

As you can see, in all three diets, the main energy source comes from carbohydrates, however, the percentages change for each event. A less aerobic sport like baseball requires less energy and therefore less carbohydrate intake in the diet compared to a highly aerobic pursuit like running.

## Fat loss and lean muscle gain

The most common goal within the fitness community is to lose body fat and gain lean muscle. How does someone with this goal adjust his or her diet to achieve it?

To begin with, you must understand two key principles of weight loss:

- The first principle is that *the body does not want to burn body fat.* Fat is its best energy source, and your body is, above all, geared toward survival. It is going to store up its best energy source in case of emergencies. You, therefore, must trick your body into burning fat. In tricking your body, you will also gain lean muscle.
- The second principle is that *the body does not spot-reduce body fat.* Doing ab crunches or butt extensions will not make those areas leaner. There isn't a sports shoe that will make your butt lift or a new ab exercise that will give you a six-pack.

## Allopathic philosophy vs. holistic medicine

During the 19th century, doctors practiced what has been referred to as "heroic" medicine, relying on extreme measures, such as bloodletting to treat illnesses. Allopathic medicine, a term created by alternative or homeopathic doctors, refers to this type of mainstream medicine, which today is also called Western medicine or biomedicine.

The problem with the allopathic approach is that it segregates different parts of the body for treatment. Each system is understood chemically as separate from other bodily systems. Medical providers seek to manipulate the chemical balance of the body with drugs to suppress symptoms.

This philosophy of modern medicine has bled into the fitness and nutrition world. We seek to manipulate our bodies for appearance or performance with little attention paid to the entire mind-body system and overall health.

Physical performance or the appearance of strength is not the same thing as good health. A bodybuilder can look lean and healthy, but his muscular form may be due to diet manipulation and synthetic steroids. A star athlete can perform fantastic maneuvers on the field but die from heart disease or cancer. True health is not merely the absence of infirmity or disease, it is the body working together physically, chemically, and emotionally.

Those in the health field who speak of energy systems, innate intelligence, disease prevention, or whole-food diets and wellness are thought of as "alternative." Over the past 15 to 20 years, however, people have been starting to realize that the allopathic philosophy is very limited in its ability to cure or prevent most disease or promote sustained health.

In increasing numbers, people are now seeking alternatives to Western medicine. Eastern medicine has used chiropractors, acupuncturists, yoga, massage therapy, meditation, homeopathy, and naturopathic methods for centuries. These are examples of natural healthcare, which operates on a "holistic" philosophy. It is healthier and much more cost effective to promote health and education about fitness, nutrition, and prevention of disease than to suppress symptoms with medications and surgeries.

Within the fitness and nutrition industry a shift in philosophy is also occurring. A concentration on the use of body-weight exercises and on endurance sports is growing. Over the past decade, there has been a change in attitude from exercise being only about vanity. The old image of muscle heads standing in the mirror performing single, joint-controlled biceps curls is changing to a concept of sport-related fitness. Sports performance gyms and group exercise classes are increasing in popularity. The holistic philosophy leading people to seek function and performance has taken root in the fitness community.

Within the nutrition industry, the same is true. Rather than simply seeking weight loss via portion control, people are opting for healthier choices. The grocery chains that promote whole and natural foods have a large portion of the grocery market share. Gaining in popularity are so-called paleolithic diets, which try to replicate a hunter-gatherer diet, promoting nutrition based on fundamentals of genetic digestive evolution. This is evidence of people seeking a more holistic approach to life and fitness and health care.

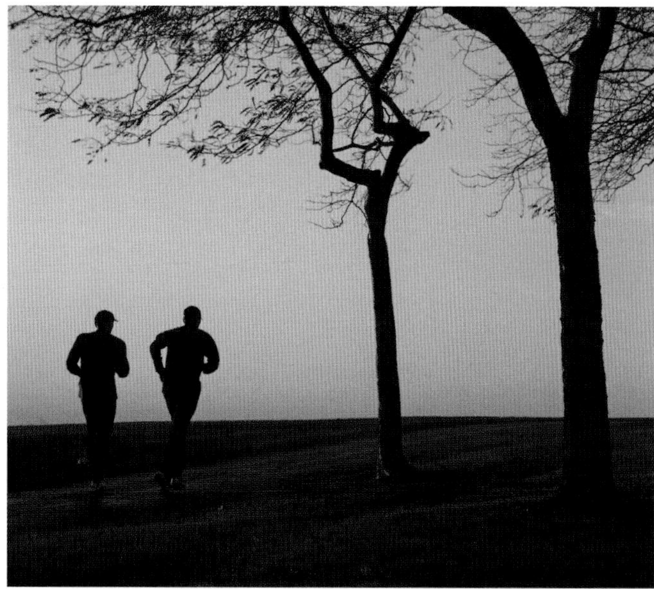

A early-morning run before breakfast takes advantage of your already-low blood-sugar level to help burn fat.

## The blood-sugar solutions

If you really want to lose body fat, there are two easy ways to do so. One way is to manage blood sugar (carbs) by working out with weights. A normal blood sugar reading is 120 milligrams per deciliter (mg/dl). The body does not tap into stored fat sources until it gets to about 80 mg/dl. If you work out with weights, you will gain muscle and lower your blood sugar to that level.

Once your blood sugar reaches 80 mg/dl, you should move on to cardiovascular exercises. Make sure that you can carry on a normal conversation as you perform your cardio—this is the best low-tech measure for making sure that you are at the target heart rate and burning body fat.

Another easy way to trick your body into burning fat is to do cardio in the morning before breakfast. No weight training is necessary. When you first wake up, your blood sugar is already at about 80 mg/dl from fasting all night, so you can be assured that you are burning fat. Again, be sure to stay in your target conversational heart rate.

## Muscle fiber types

While these tricks for burning fat and saving lean muscle—lowering blood sugar by lifting weights first and cardio workout second, doing cardio before breakfast—are effective, eating properly for a specific athletic goal is different from burning fat and gaining lean muscle. Athletic or sports nutrition requires not only knowledge of the first and second principles, blood sugar levels, and target heart rates, but also an understanding of the types of muscle fibers used during an event.

There are three types of athletic muscle fibers: type 1, type 2a, and type 2b.

- Type 1 is aerobic. These fibers are red because they use a lot of red, oxygenated blood.
- Type 2a is anaerobic. They are white due to a lack of blood supply.
- Type 2b is a combination . They are pink. They have less blood and use less oxygen than type 1 fibers and more blood and more oxygen than type 2a fibers.

All athletic events use all three muscle fiber types, but each event has a dominant type.

The aerobic endurance athlete predominantly uses type 1 fibers and requires 65 to 80 percent carbohydrates. The anaerobic athlete uses type 2a fibers and requires a lower 55 percent carbohydrates, and the combination athlete uses type 2b fibers and requires about 60 percent carbohydrates.

The chart below shows what sorts of muscles are used for specific events and the amount of carbohydrates required as a general percentage for each.

| FIBER TYPE | CARB % | MAIN ENERGY SOURCE | BY-PRODUCT | EXERCISE TYPE |
|---|---|---|---|---|
| Type 1 | 65–80% | oxygen + carbs + fats (red) | sweat | endurance—competitive biking, marathon running, triathlons, swimming, adventure racing, crew rowing |
| Type 2a | 55% | sugar (white) | lactic acid (burning muscles) | football (linemen), shot-put, baseball (outfielders), hockey (goalies), Olympic lifting, sprinting, bodybuilding |
| Type 2b | 60% | oxygen + carbs (pink) | sweat + lactic acid | mixed martial arts fighting, CrossFit, boxing, wrestling, tactical athletics, military PFT, soccer, lacrosse, rugby, football, basketball, hockey |

Experiment with these percentages in your own nutrition program to see what works best for you. Once you master the amounts of each energy source you require, you will have a better chance of consistently performing at your best.

## Nutrition and health

The other part of the nutrition equation is how diet and nutrition affect your health. An improper diet can contribute to the development of heart disease, diabetes, and cancer, while a proper diet, or a specialized diet, can aid in the battle against these diseases.

Nutrition also plays a key part in controlling another health risk—obesity. For those with weight issues, the goal should be not merely eating less in order to lose pounds, but rather eating healthier foods, learning to read labels, (for instance, many low-fat foods are high in sugar, i.e., carbs), and retooling dietary habits and choices so that the weight will stay off.

## Keep learning

It should be clear that nutrition is one of the most effective means for ensuring health, preventing disease, and maximizing optimal function of the body. If you become more than a casual student of nutrition and continue to explore how it can help you reach your fitness goals, you will be well on the way to mastering yourself—and your body.

### Superfoods in your fridge

It seems like every month or so the public latches onto the latest low-fat, disease-fighting "superfood"—a fruit, vegetable, herb, or spice that nutritionists or infomercial health gurus tout as a miracle worker. Acai and goji berries, pomegranates, kale, collard greens, ginger, turmeric, and cumin have all had their 15 minutes of fame. While these are all fine dietary choices, some of them are a bit exotic . . . and chances are you already buy and consume quite a few less trendy superfoods, such as those listed below:

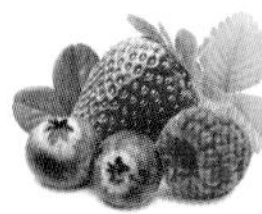

- Strawberries, blueberries, and raspberries contain fiber, antioxidants, and vitamin C.
- Eggs offer protein and a more lasting sense of fullness at breakfast than toast or a bagel.

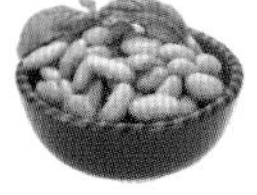

- Beans contain fiber and are a source of iron (especially when combined with a vitamin C-rich food like sweet potatoes).

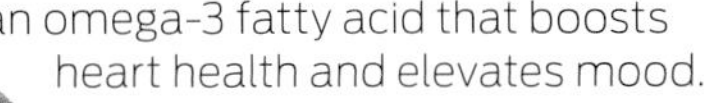

- Nuts are a source of healthy unsaturated fat; walnuts in particular contain alpha-linolenic acid, an omega-3 fatty acid that boosts heart health and elevates mood.

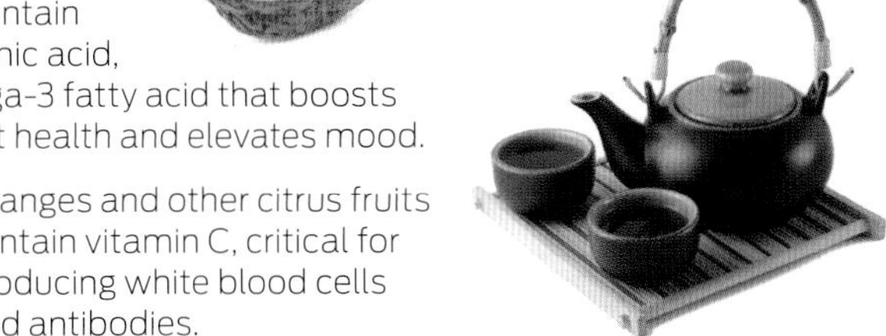

- Oranges and other citrus fruits contain vitamin C, critical for producing white blood cells and antibodies.

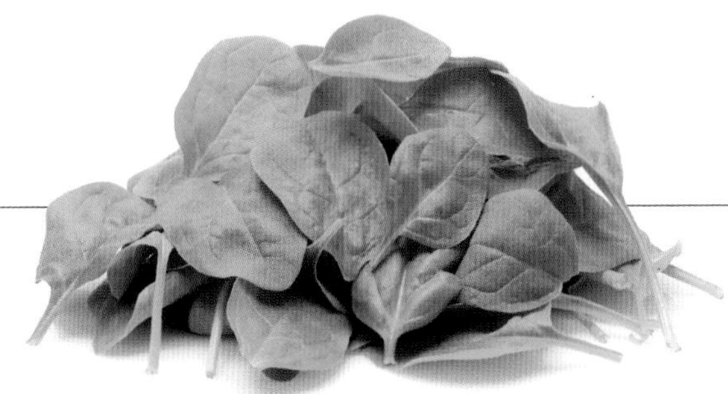

- Spinach is packed with vitamins—A, C, E, and K—as well as fiber, iron, calcium, potassium, magnesium, and folate, which helps produce healthy new cells.

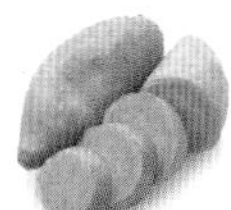

- Sweet potatoes are extremely nutritious, and contain alpha and beta carotene, which are converted into vitamin A, important for your vision, bones, and immune system.

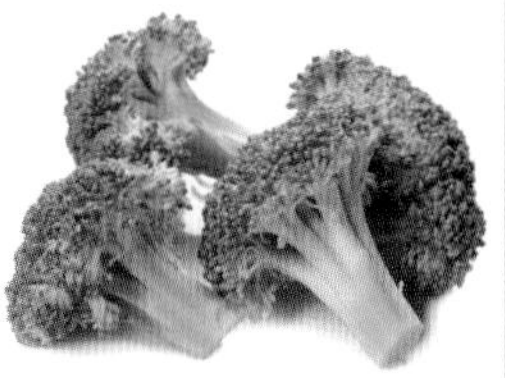

- Broccoli offers vitamins C, A, and K (increases immunity) and folate; it also delivers sulforaphane, which stimulates detoxifying enzymes.
- Tea is rich in antioxidant flavonoids that can reduce risk of Alzheimer's, diabetes, and some cancers.

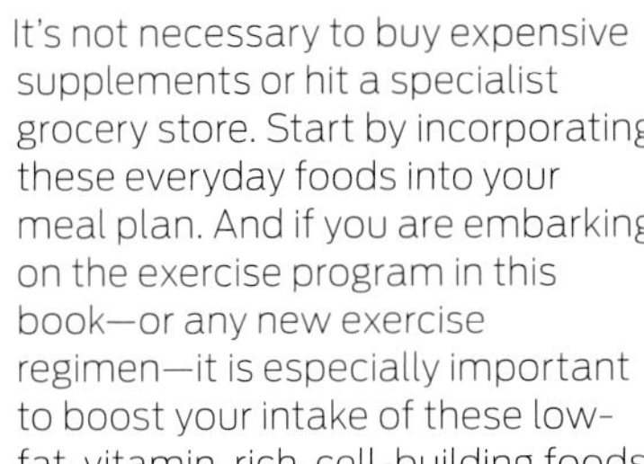

It's not necessary to buy expensive supplements or hit a specialist grocery store. Start by incorporating these everyday foods into your meal plan. And if you are embarking on the exercise program in this book—or any new exercise regimen—it is especially important to boost your intake of these low-fat, vitamin-rich, cell-building foods.

# Warm-Ups and Cool-Downs

When scheduling your workout, leave a few minutes before your exercise session to properly prepare your muscles. Add a few at the end to give yourself time to execute a few cool-down moves that will allow your muscles to recover for your next workout.

Before you begin your main workout, perform a few simple warm-up stretches and exercises. A warm-up prepares muscle groups for exercises of greater intensity.

## Dynamic warm-up

The following stretches and exercises are all dynamic—meaning that they get the joints and muscles moving. A dynamic warm-up stimulates the central nervous system to pump blood to working muscles, which warms them for increased and safe contraction.

### *Neck Stretch*

To prepare the muscles of your neck, use this simple dynamic stretch. To begin, lie on your back. You can fold your arms across your chest or rest them at your waist. Lift your head forward. Try to touch your chin to your chest, and then extend it back. Forward and back is one rep. Perform 10 reps.

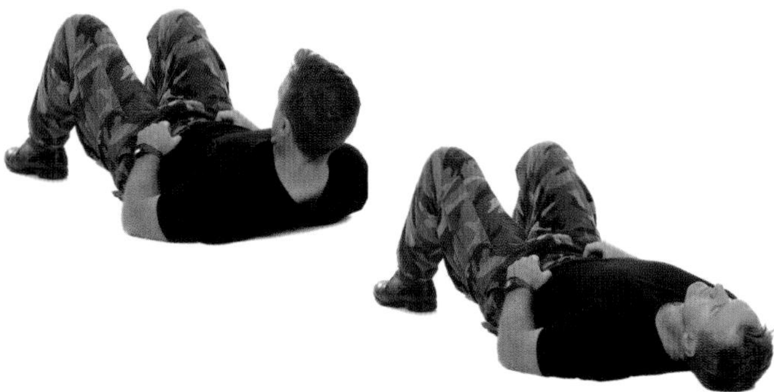

Next, lift your head, and then move your head side to side. Both right and left equal one repetition. Perform 10 reps.

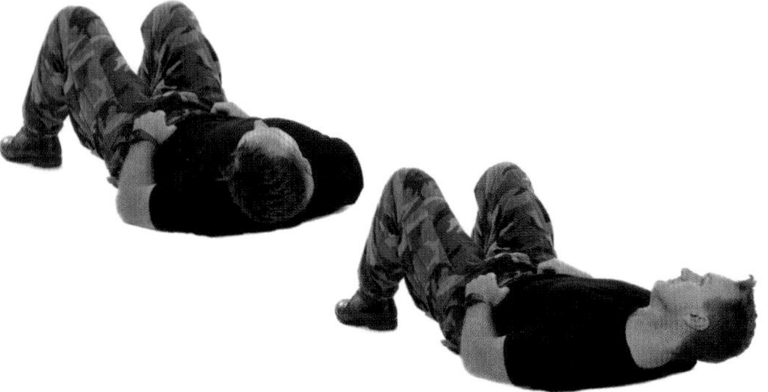

### *Shoulder Circles*

To warm up your deltoids, stand straight and extend your arms to the side at shoulder height. Rotate your arms forward in small concentric circles 10 times and then backward 10 times.

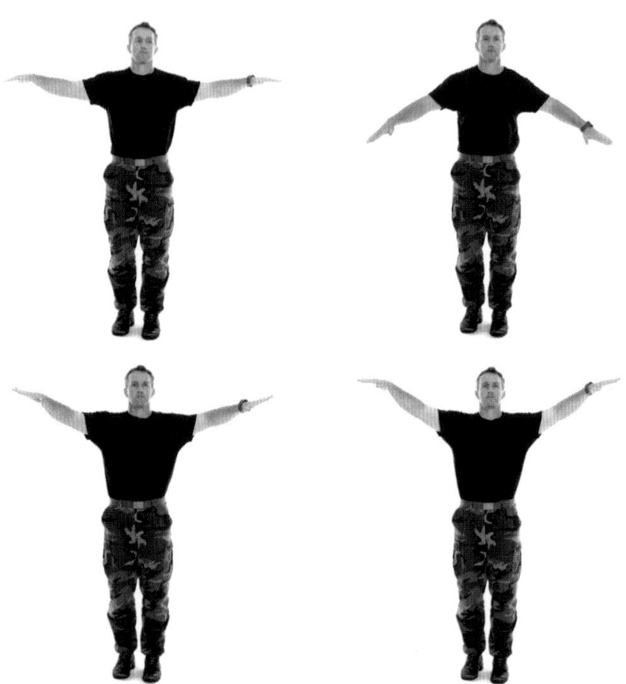

Next, extend your arms forward, and rotate them inward 10 times and then outward 10 times, making small circles.

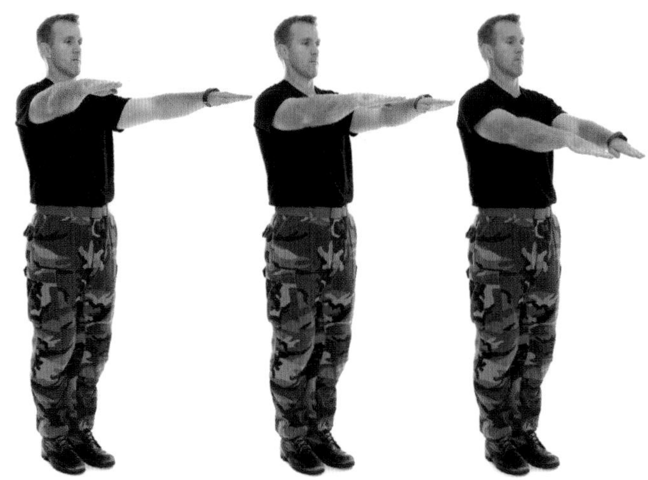

## Dynamic versus static

Dynamic exercise, also known as "ballistic," involves continuous movement of both joints and muscles. During a dynamic exercise, your muscles repeatedly alternate between concentric and eccentric contractions. A concentric contraction shortens your muscles, and an eccentric contraction lengthens them.

Static, or "isometric," exercise exerts muscles at high intensities, without movement of your joints. During a static exercise, the targeted muscles will contract only.

The high-intensity workout featured in this book calls for a dynamic warm-up. Your goal is to bring your heart rate up and to increase the speed of the contraction and relaxation of your muscles, which warms them up. Active movements will do just that—with the added benefit of stoking you mentally to prepare for the challenge ahead.

When you've completed your workout, your goal is just the opposite: you want your body and mind to relax and return to a resting state. A cool-down session composed of static stretching decreases the tension in your muscles, allowing them to relax and recover. It also works to calm you mentally.

### *Chest Fly*

To warm up the pectoral muscles of your chest, stand with your arms at your sides. Swing both arms out as far as possible, and then swing them back inward. Perform the motion quickly enough to stretch the chest muscles but slowly enough not to cause pain in your chest. Swinging in and out is one rep. Perform 10 reps.

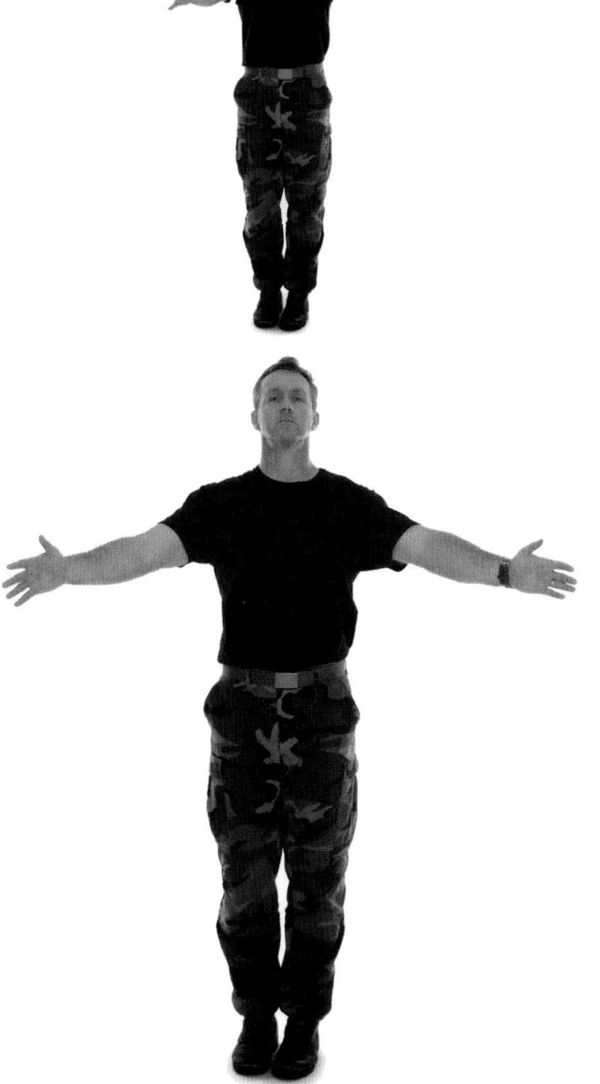

### *Lower-Back Stretch*

To prepare the vulnerable lower-back area, stand with a slight bend in your knees. Bend forward from the hips as far as possible, and then rise quickly, leaning back with a slight extension in your lower back. Perform 10 times.

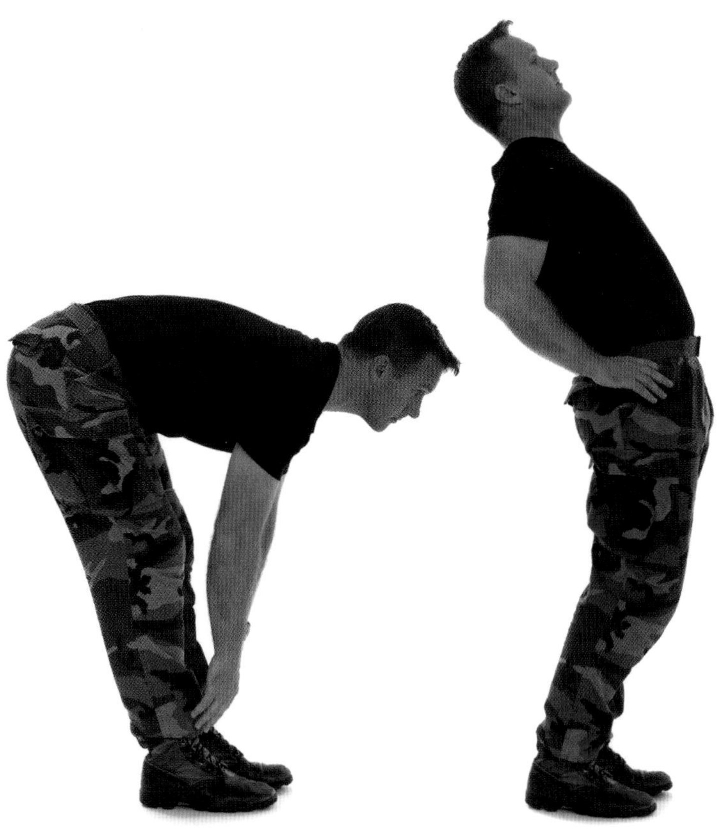

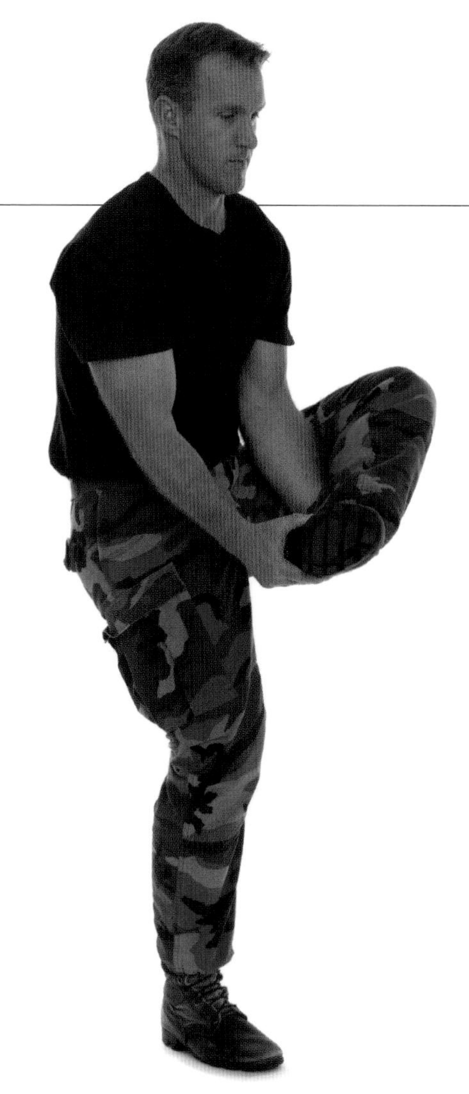

## *Glutes Stretch*

To warm up your glutes, use this dynamic stretch. Walk in place, and with each step grab one foot with your hands and pull it toward your belly button while your knee rotates away from your body. Alternate holding each foot. Perform 10 times on each leg.

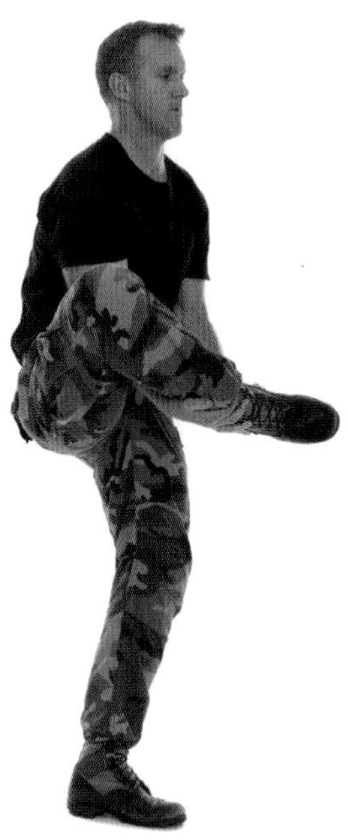

## *Monster Walk*

It is essential to keep your hamstrings, the group of muscles at the back of your thigh, supple. To warm them up, walk in place, kicking each leg out straight in front of you. As you elevate your leg, attempt to touch your foot with the opposite hand. Perform 10 times on each leg.

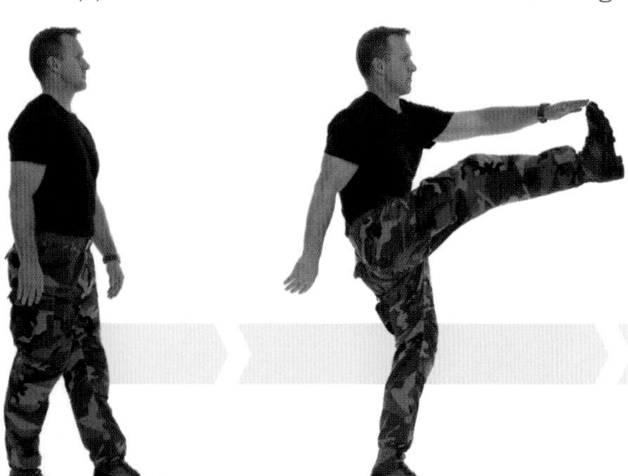

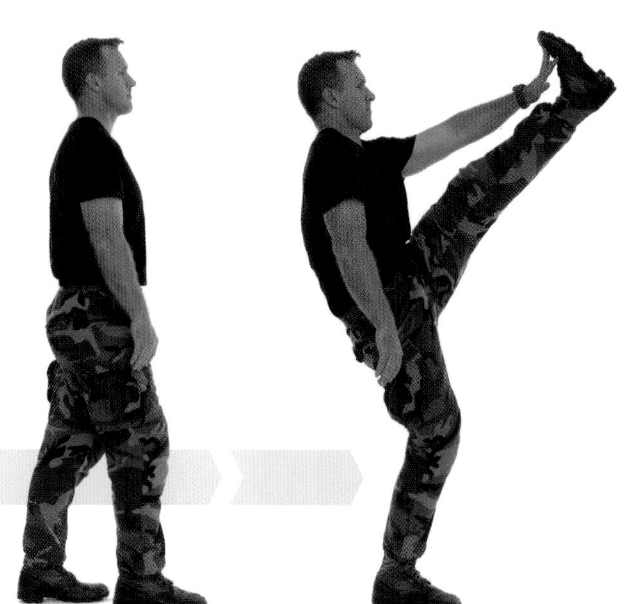

### *Butt Kicker*

This exercise will warm up your quadriceps femoris, the large muscle group at the front of your thigh. To perform this move, run in place while attempting to kick yourself in the butt. Kick each foot 10 times.

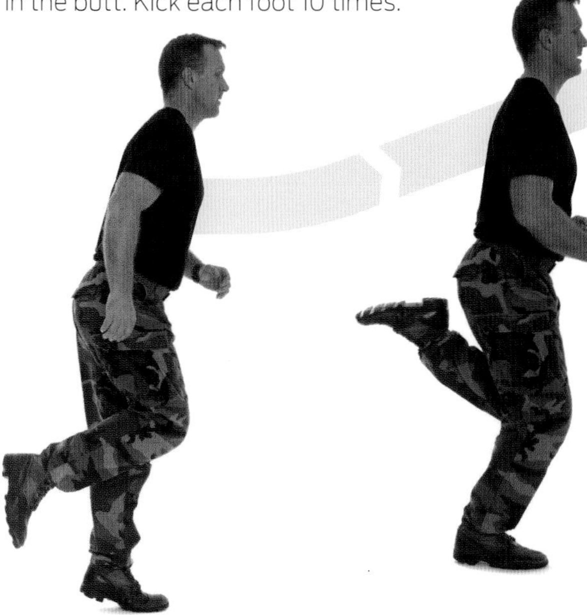

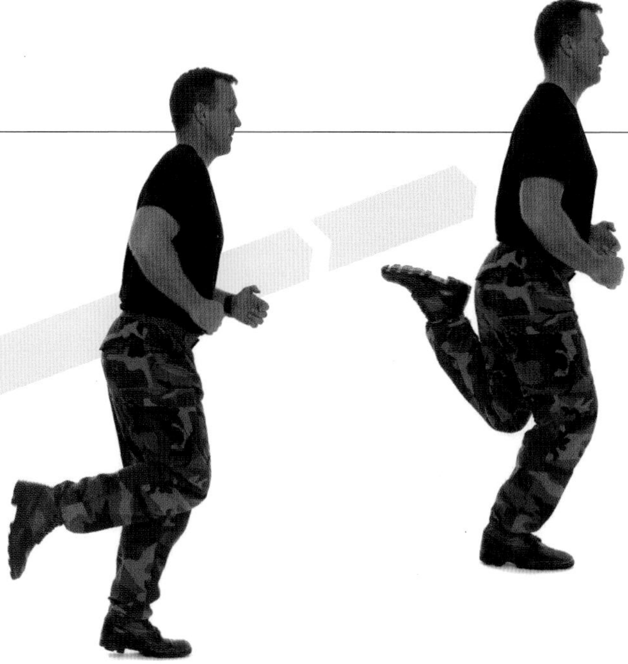

### *Calves Jump*

To warm up the soleus and gastrocnemius muscles of your calf, perform this simple move. Stand straight with your feet close together, but not touching. Jump up slightly, and land without touching your heels to the floor, attempting to bounce off the balls of your feet. Perform 10 jumps.

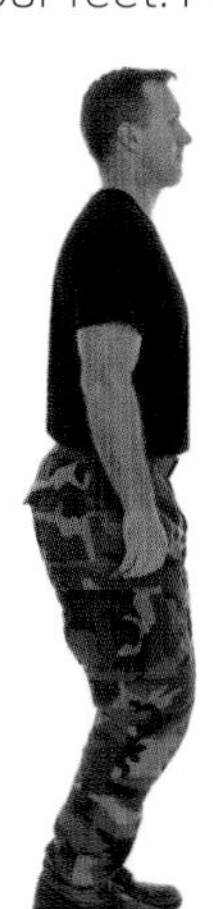

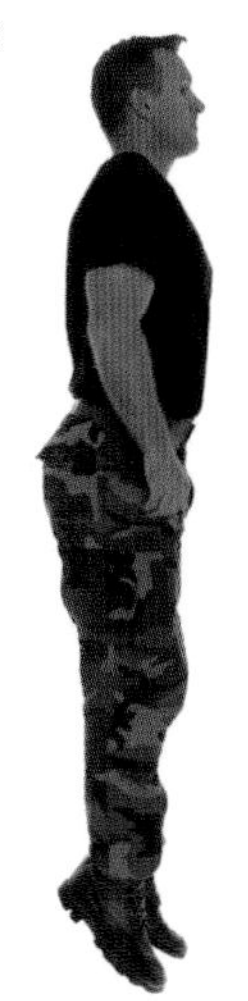

### *Jumping Jacks*

Jumping Jacks are a simple but effective cardiovascular endurance exercise that warms up just about every muscle in your body. It is also a weight-bearing movement, which helps make your bones stronger and denser. To execute, stand with your hands at your side and your feet together. Jump and spread your legs while simultaneously placing your arms over your head. Repeat 10 times.

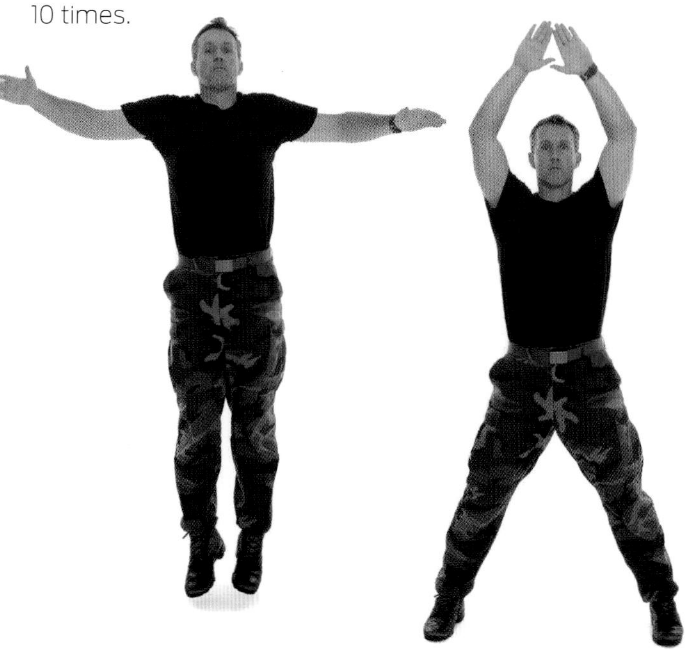

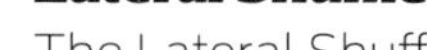

## *Rocking Chair*

To keep your back limber, warm it up with the Rocking Chair exercise, which stretches your paraspinal muscles, the band of muscles next to the spine that support and move the spine. It will also stretch your gluteus maximus, preparing this large muscle for further activity. To begin, lie on your back, and bring both knees to your chest. Wrap your arms around your legs, and roll backward and forward 10 times.

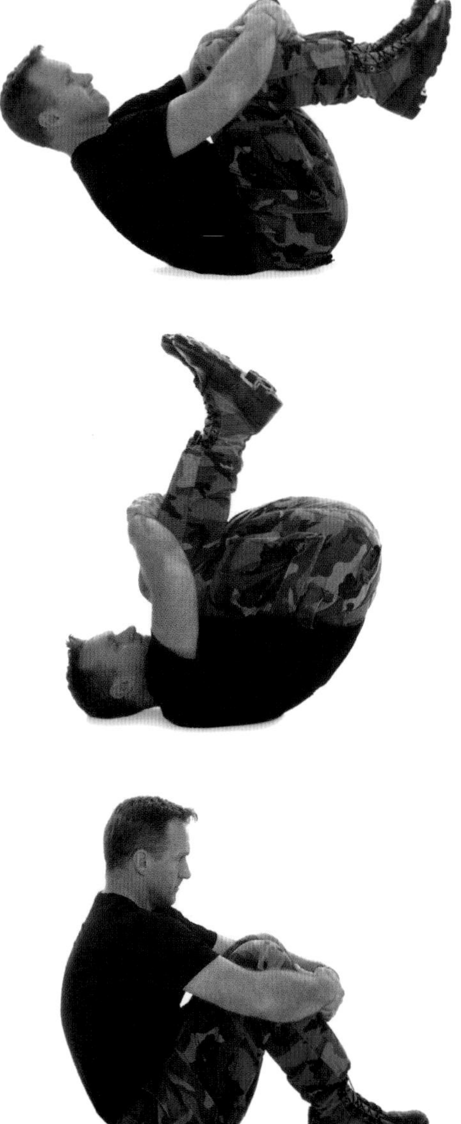

## *Lateral Shuffle*

The Lateral Shuffle will warm up the muscles of your inner thighs—the hip abductors and adductors. The abductors pull a limb or other bodily structure away from the midline of body, as when you separate your legs. The adductors do the opposite, pulling your hip joint inward, as when you cross your legs. To perform this exercise, stand with your legs open and bend your knees to assume a half-squat stance. Stay in the squat position while bringing your left foot to your right and then your right foot to your left. Hold the squat position while shuffling 10 times in each direction.

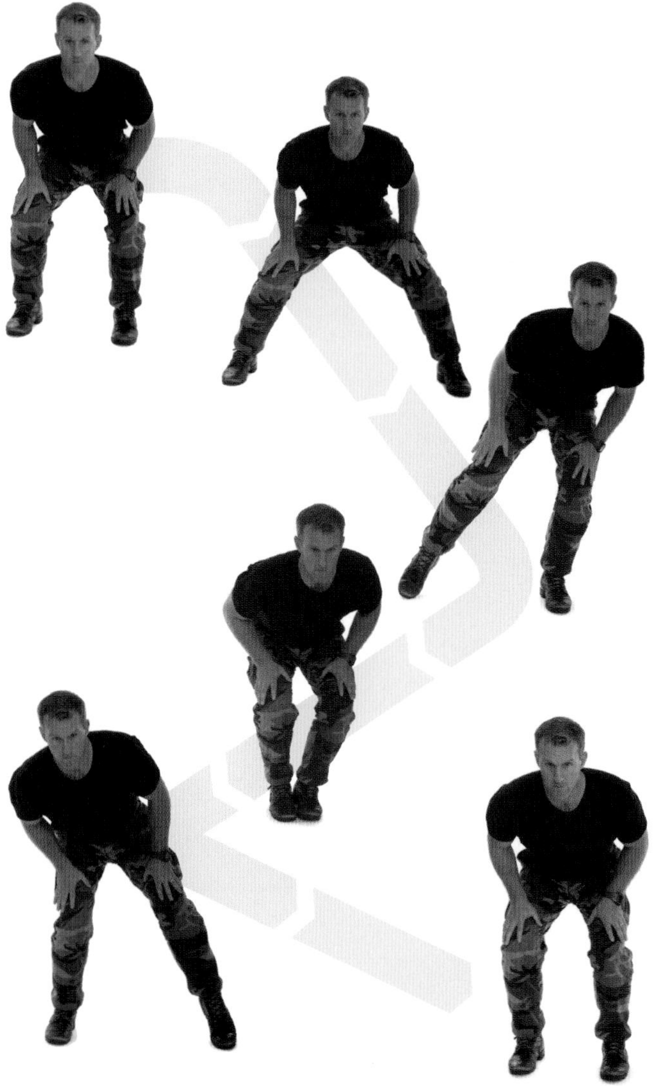

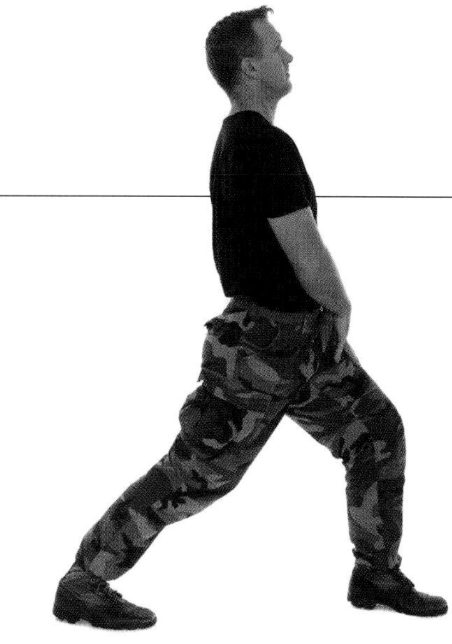

## Static cool-down

Cooling down after working out is an essential part of any fitness program, and performing a series of static stretches is a great way to achieve this. Static exercises, also known as isometrics, allow high-intensity muscle exertion without movement of the joints. The stretches featured here aid in preventing muscle soreness and allow fresh blood to fill fatigued muscles, preparing them for the next day's workout.

### *Seated Hamstring Stretch*

For a hamstring cool-down, sit on the floor with your back straight and your legs extended in front of you in parallel position. Bend your left leg outward, and rest the bottom of your left foot on your right inner thigh just above the kneecap. Placing your hands on either side of your right knee, bend from your waist and lean forward over your right leg. Hold for 15 to 30 seconds. Switch legs, and repeat the stretch on the other side.

### *Calf Stretch*

To cool down the muscles of your calves, stand with your legs straight, your right foot behind the left. Bring your left leg forward, slightly bending your knee. Keeping both heels on the floor, lean into your left leg until you feel the stretch in your right calf muscle. Hold for 15 to 30 seconds. Switch sides, and then repeat sequence three times on each leg.

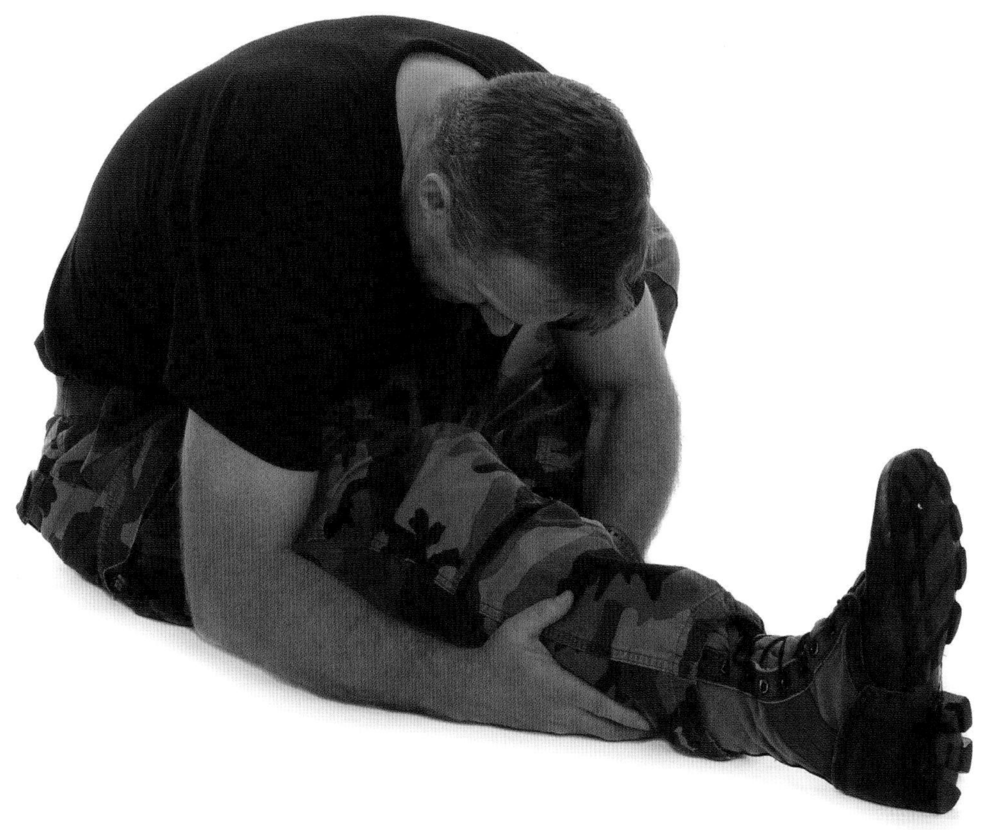

## *Quadriceps Stretch*

This stretch targets the muscles at the front of your thigh. Stand with your feet together. Bend your right leg behind you, and grasp your foot with your right hand. Pull your heel toward your butt until you feel a stretch in the front of your thigh. Keep both knees together and aligned. Hold for 15 to 30 seconds. Repeat sequence three times on each leg.

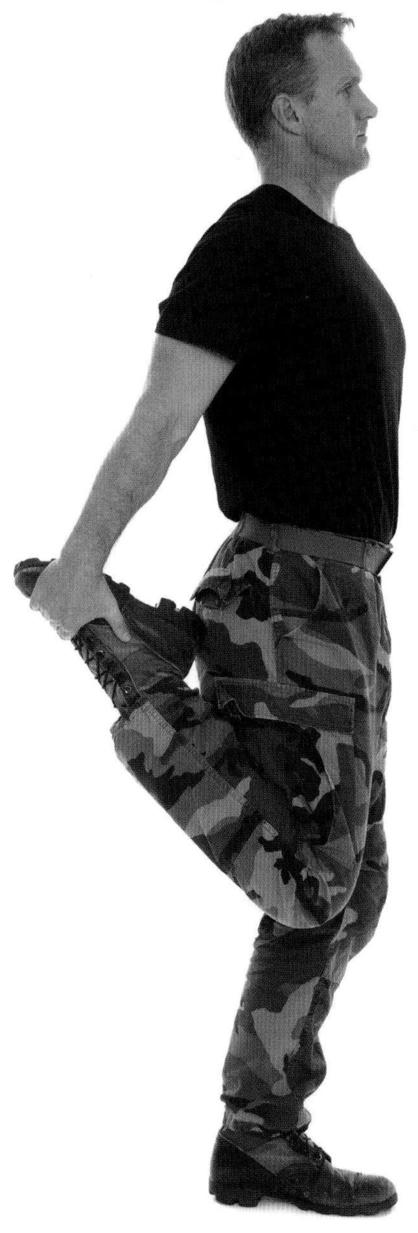

## *Lower-Body Stretch*

This multipurpose stretch targets your lower back, glutes, hips, and iliotibial band. To perform it, sit on the floor, sitting up as straight as possible with your back flattened and your legs extended in front of you in parallel position. Extend your left leg straight in front of you, and bend your right knee. Cross your bent knee over your left leg, and keep your foot flat on the floor. Wrap your left arm around your right knee so that you are able to apply pressure to your leg to rotate your torso and head to the right. Keeping your hips aligned, rotate your upper spine as you pull your chest in toward your knee. Hold for 15 to 30 seconds. Slowly release, and repeat on the other side.

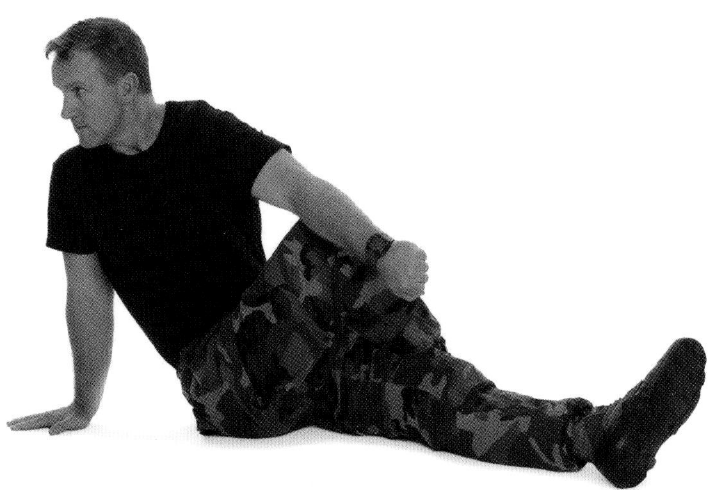

### You can do it!

With no reveille or bugle call to jolt you out of bed at sunrise and no drill sergeant to put you through your paces, you may sometimes lack the motivation to get yourself exercising. Starting out with the less-demanding warm-ups revs you up, preparing your muscles for the challenges ahead while preparing your mind to persevere. Special forces workouts are designed to push you to your limits. Completing them will make you stronger, both physically and mentally. Besting your previous day's times and reps will give you a sense of satisfaction.

Cooling down has similar benefits—it allows your muscles to recover and gives you a chance to reflect on your progress. You won't be heading out into the field, but you will be facing the day armed with the knowledge that you can achieve whatever you set your mind—and body—to.

### *Pectoral Stretch*

To cool down your chest muscles, stand straight with your feet together. Extend your arms out and pull them back until you feel a deep stretch in your pectoral muscles. Hold for 15 to 30 seconds.

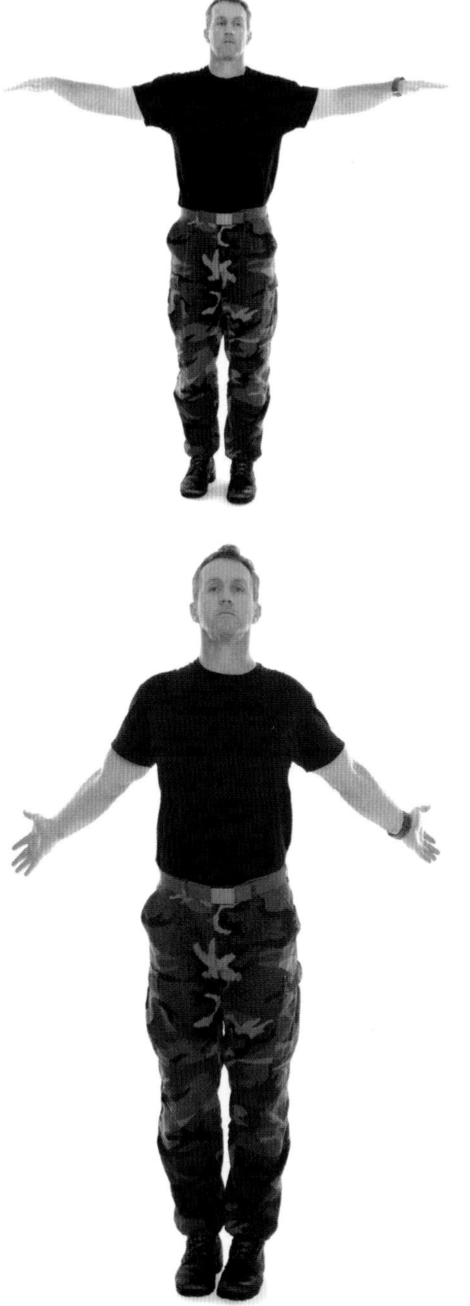

### *Latissimus Dorsi Stretch*

Your latissimus dorsi (commonly known as the "lats") is the broad muscle that covers your lower back. To cool this muscle down after your workout, perform this soothing stretch. With both hands, grasp a steadying object, such as a broom handle, doorknob, or chair back, and bend forward as deeply as you can, and then bend your knees until you feel a comfortable stretch. Hold for 15 to 30 seconds.

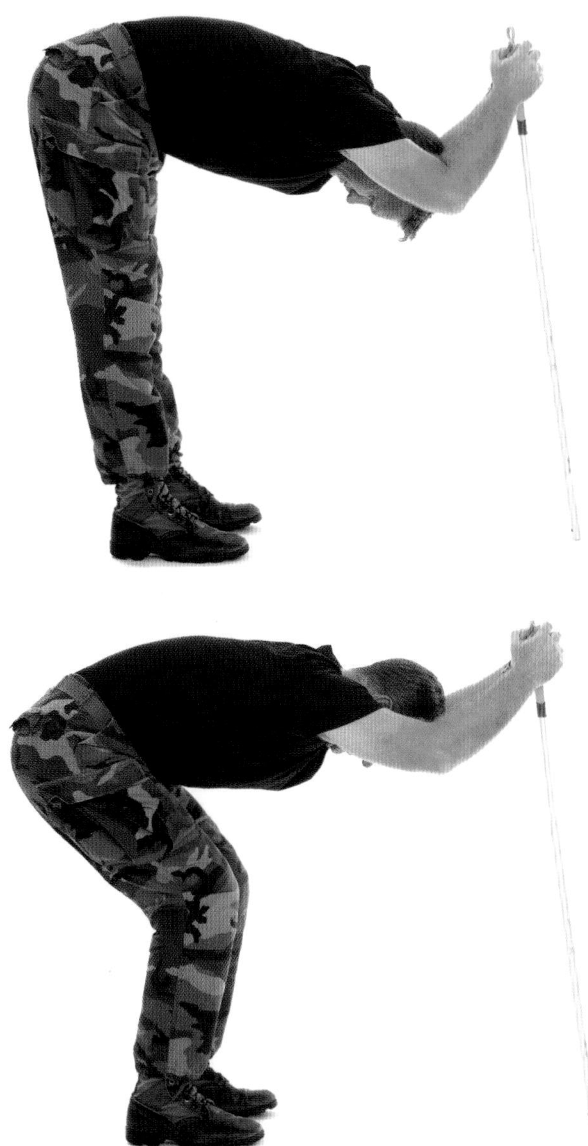

# Full–Body Anatomy

## Front View

**Annotation Key**
* indicates deep muscles

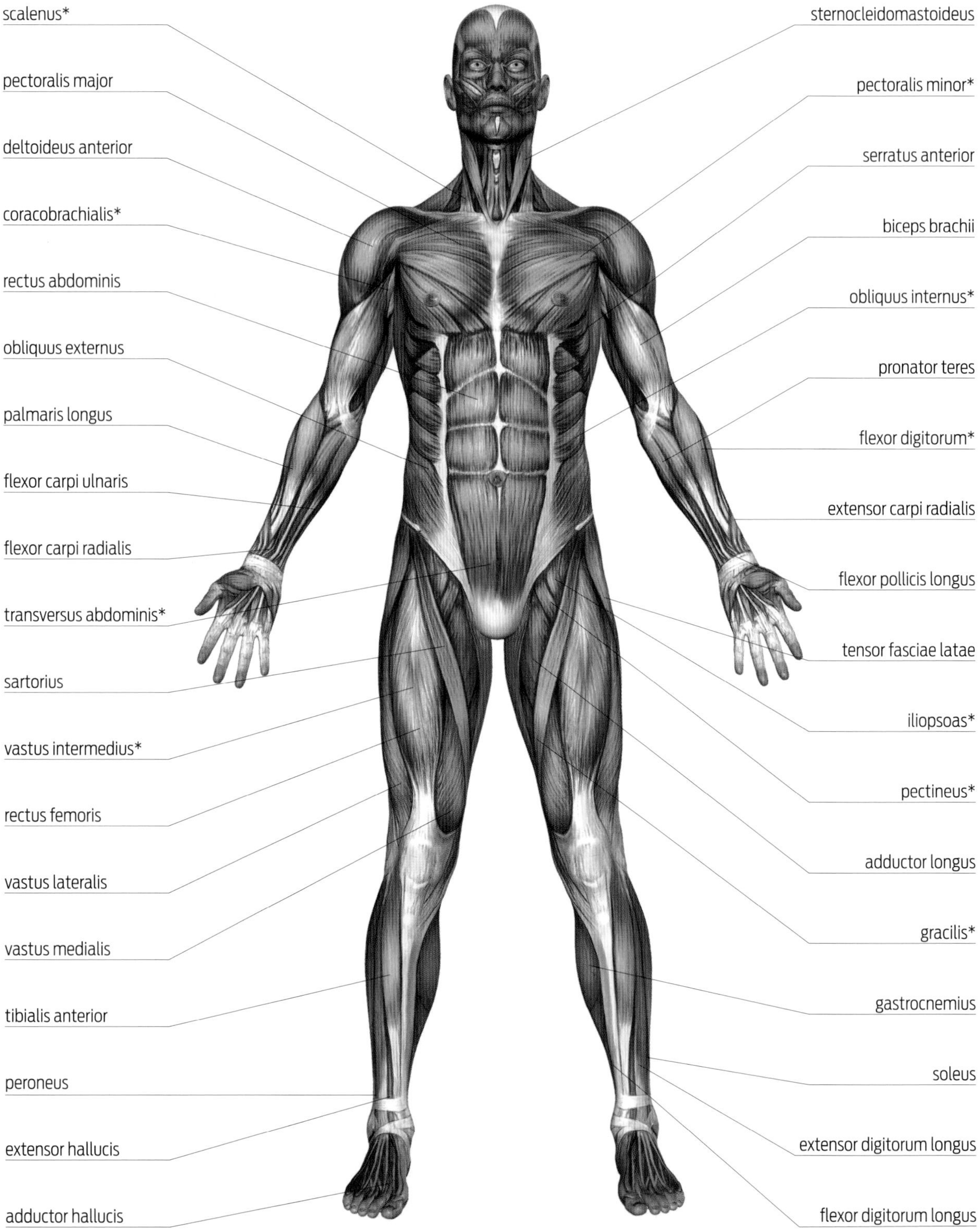

scalenus*
pectoralis major
deltoideus anterior
coracobrachialis*
rectus abdominis
obliquus externus
palmaris longus
flexor carpi ulnaris
flexor carpi radialis
transversus abdominis*
sartorius
vastus intermedius*
rectus femoris
vastus lateralis
vastus medialis
tibialis anterior
peroneus
extensor hallucis
adductor hallucis

sternocleidomastoideus
pectoralis minor*
serratus anterior
biceps brachii
obliquus internus*
pronator teres
flexor digitorum*
extensor carpi radialis
flexor pollicis longus
tensor fasciae latae
iliopsoas*
pectineus*
adductor longus
gracilis*
gastrocnemius
soleus
extensor digitorum longus
flexor digitorum longus

Annotation Key
* indicates deep muscles

## Back View

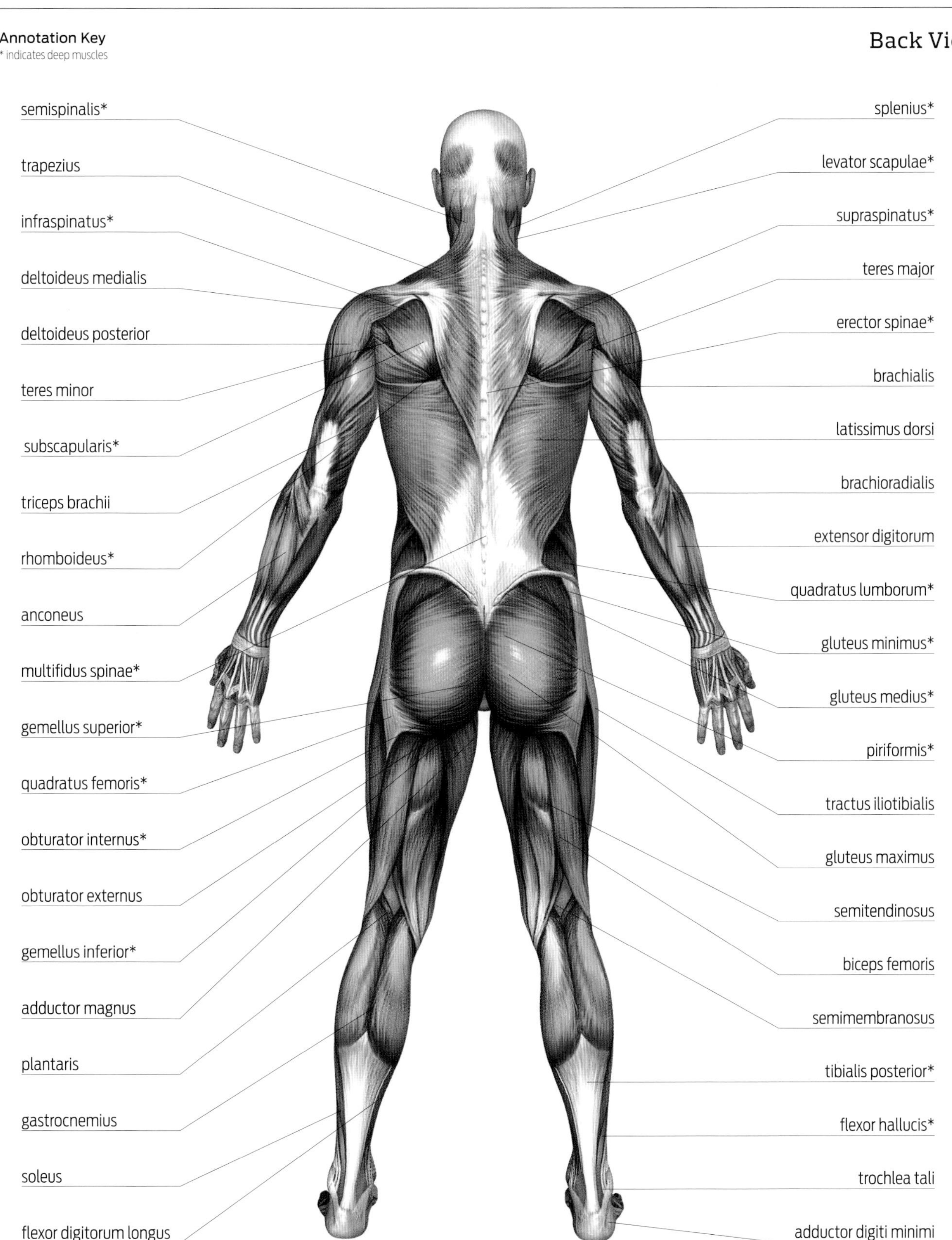

## Contents

# Exercises

Are you ready to work out like a special forces operative? The following 55 exercises will help get you into the peak shape required of all special forces personnel.

These exercises will strengthen and tone your muscles, reduce body fat, and build lean muscle tissue. They will also promote cardiovascular endurance, core stability, balance, coordination, and agility.

Start your workout program by trying out a few of the beginner exercises, and then gradually work your way to the more advanced ones. Once you feel comfortable executing them with good form, turn to the Workouts section (pages 162–181) to learn how to put them all together.

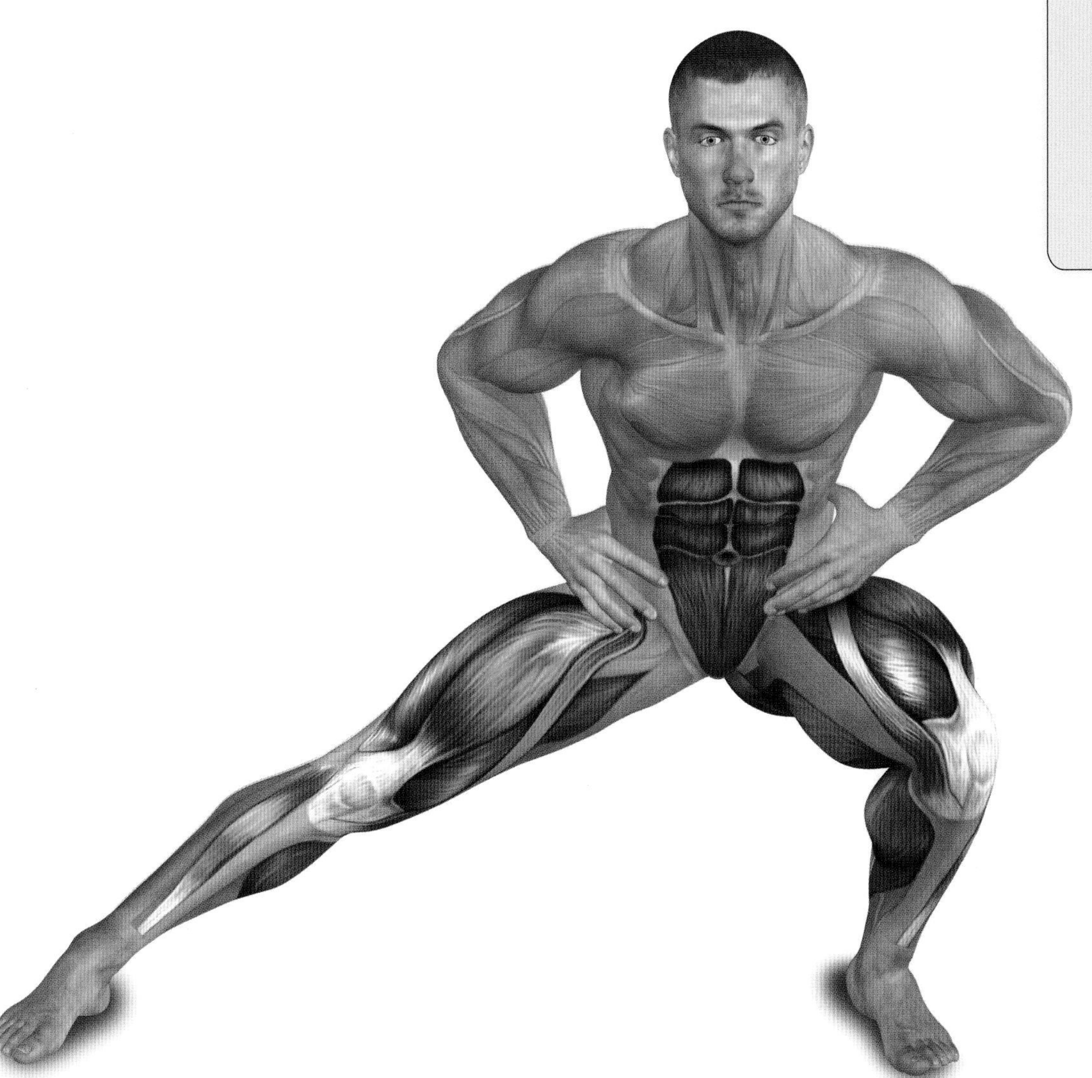

# Push-Up

The Push-Up is a fundamental component of just about all military basic training and is one of the exercises commonly used in military physical fitness tests. Push-Ups target the pectoral muscles, triceps, and anterior deltoids, with secondary benefits to your entire midsection. The starting position, with your legs extended and arms straight, is known as the "Drop" Position, and it is one you will assume many times during your workout.

1 With your hands shoulder-width apart, place your palms on the floor, keeping your feet together and back straight. Push your body up until your arms are straight. This is your start position.

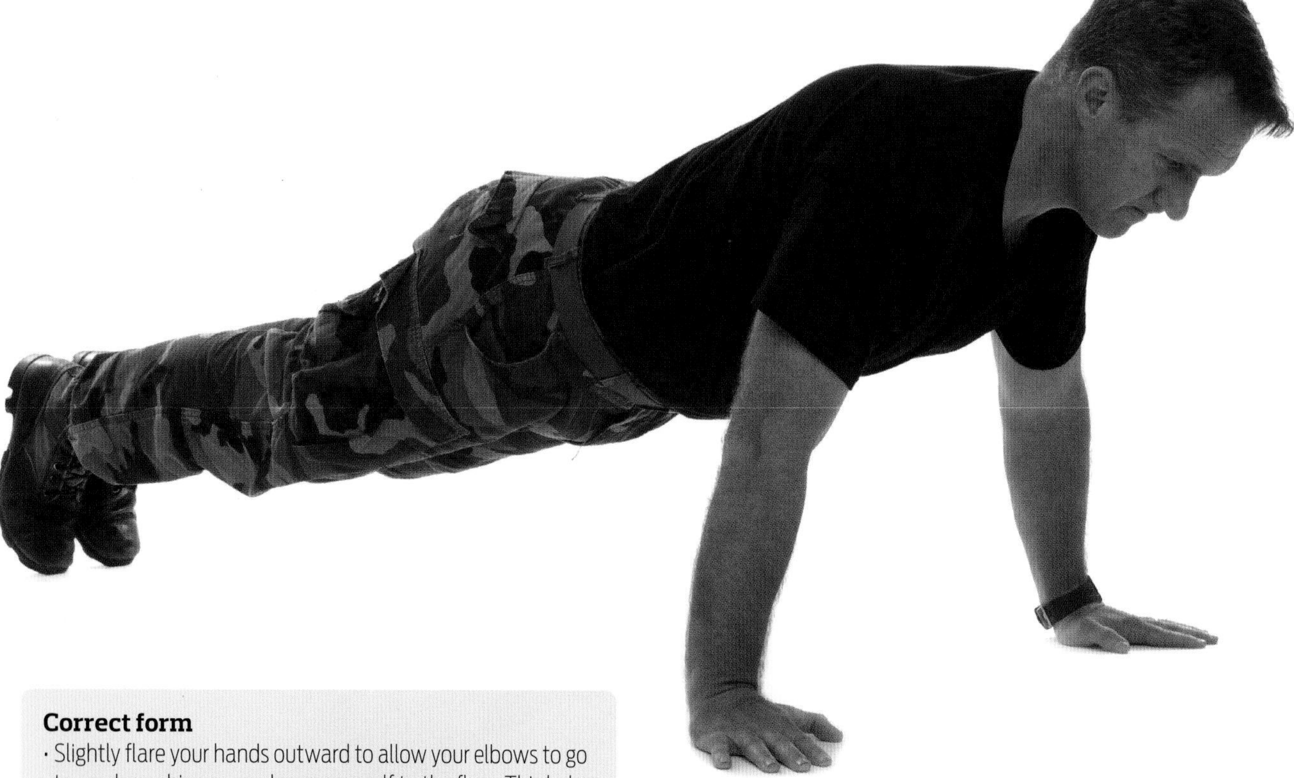

**Correct form**

- Slightly flare your hands outward to allow your elbows to go toward your hips as you lower yourself to the floor. This helps prevent shoulder tendonitis.
- If you cannot keep your back straight during the entire movement or you experience back pain, start this exercise on both knees and do a modified push-up.

**Avoid**

- Pushing your hips into the air.
- Pointing your elbows to the side during the down movement. This places undue stress on the anterior deltoids.

2 Bend your arms, and lower your torso until your chest touches the floor. Straighten your arms to rise back up to the starting position to complete the repetition. Perform 10 reps.

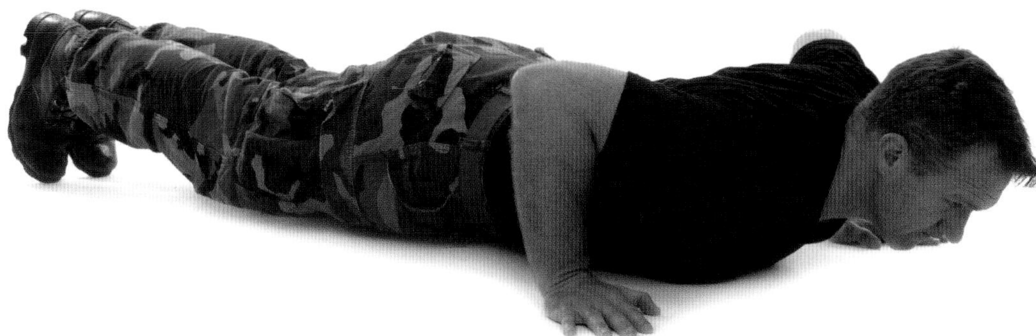

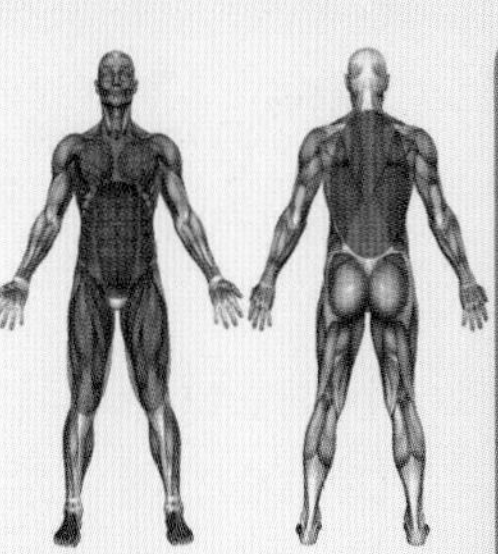

**Level**
- Beginner

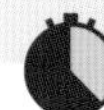

**Duration**
- 45–60 seconds

**Benefits**
- Strengthens upper body

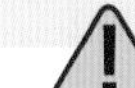

**Caution**
- Shoulder issues
- Wrist issues
- Lower-back pain

**Annotation Key**
* indicates deep muscles

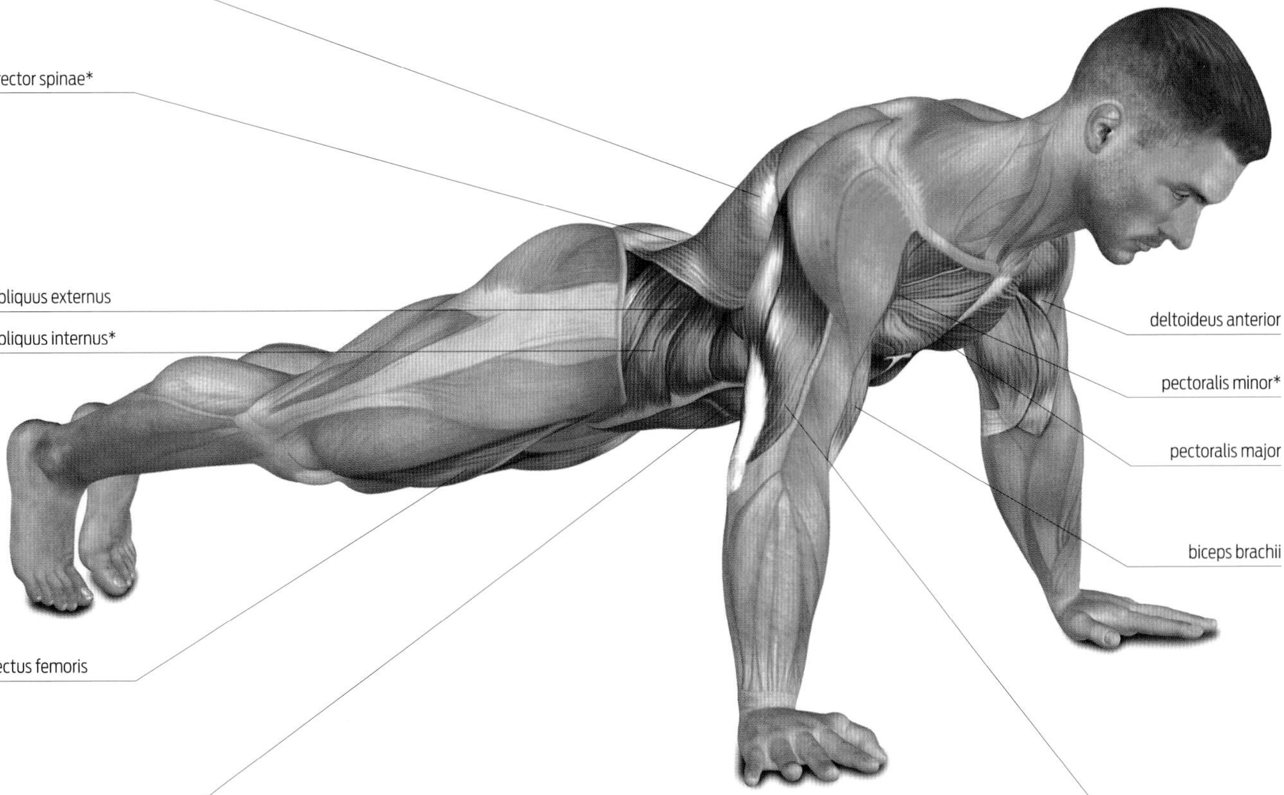

latissimus dorsi
erector spinae*
obliquus externus
obliquus internus*
rectus femoris
rectus abdominis
deltoideus anterior
pectoralis minor*
pectoralis major
biceps brachii
triceps brachii

# Triceps Push-Up

The Push-Up is a versatile exercise, and just changing your hand position can emphasize different muscle groups. In the basic Push-Up, the pectoralis major and minor muscles are the primary movers, but in a Triceps Push-Up, the closer hand placement means that there is more shoulder flexion and elbow extension, which places greater emphasis on the shoulders and triceps.

1 With your hands close together, place your palms on the floor, keeping your feet together and back straight. Push your body up until your arms are straight. This is your start position.

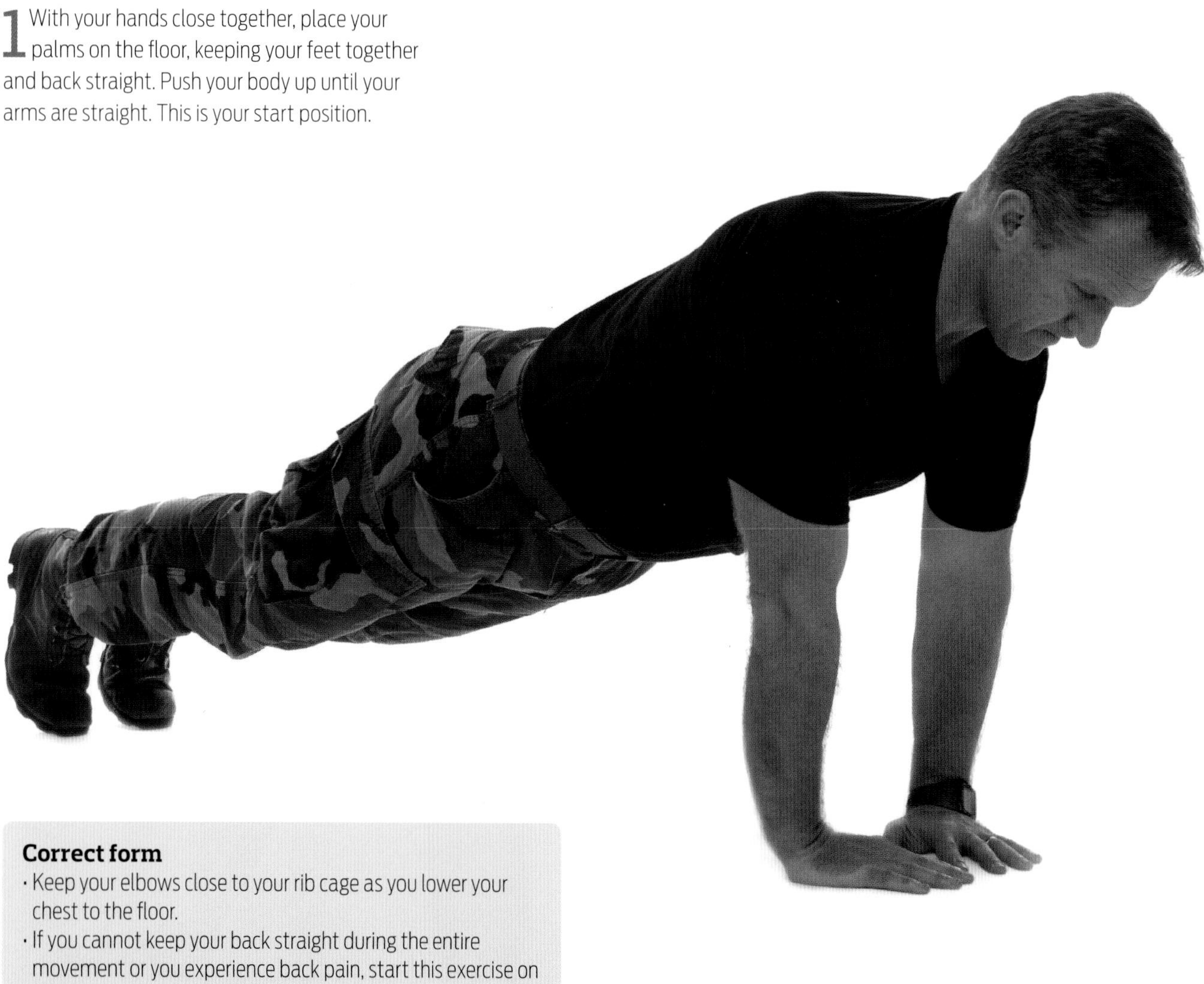

**Correct form**

- Keep your elbows close to your rib cage as you lower your chest to the floor.
- If you cannot keep your back straight during the entire movement or you experience back pain, start this exercise on both knees and do a modified push-up.

**Avoid**

- Pushing your hips into the air.
- Pointing your elbows to the side during the down movement. This places undue stress on the anterior deltoids.

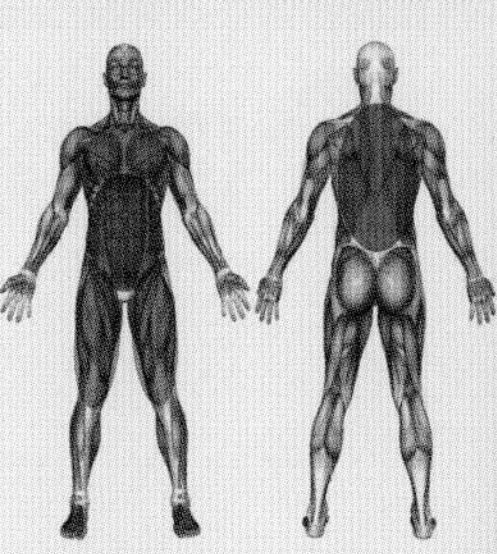

**Level**
· Intermediate

**Duration**
· 45–60 seconds

**Benefits**
· Strengthens upper body
· Tones triceps

**Caution**
· Shoulder issues
· Wrist issues
· Lower-back pain

2 Bend your arms, and lower your torso until your chest touches the floor. Straighten your arms to rise back up to the starting position to complete the repetition. Perform 10 reps.

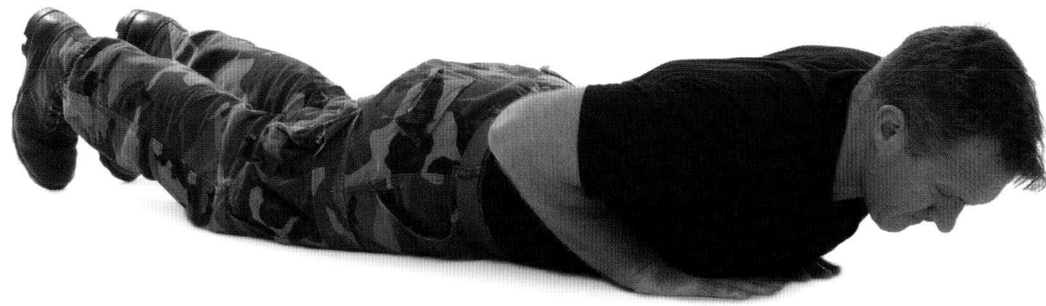

**Annotation Key**
* indicates deep muscles

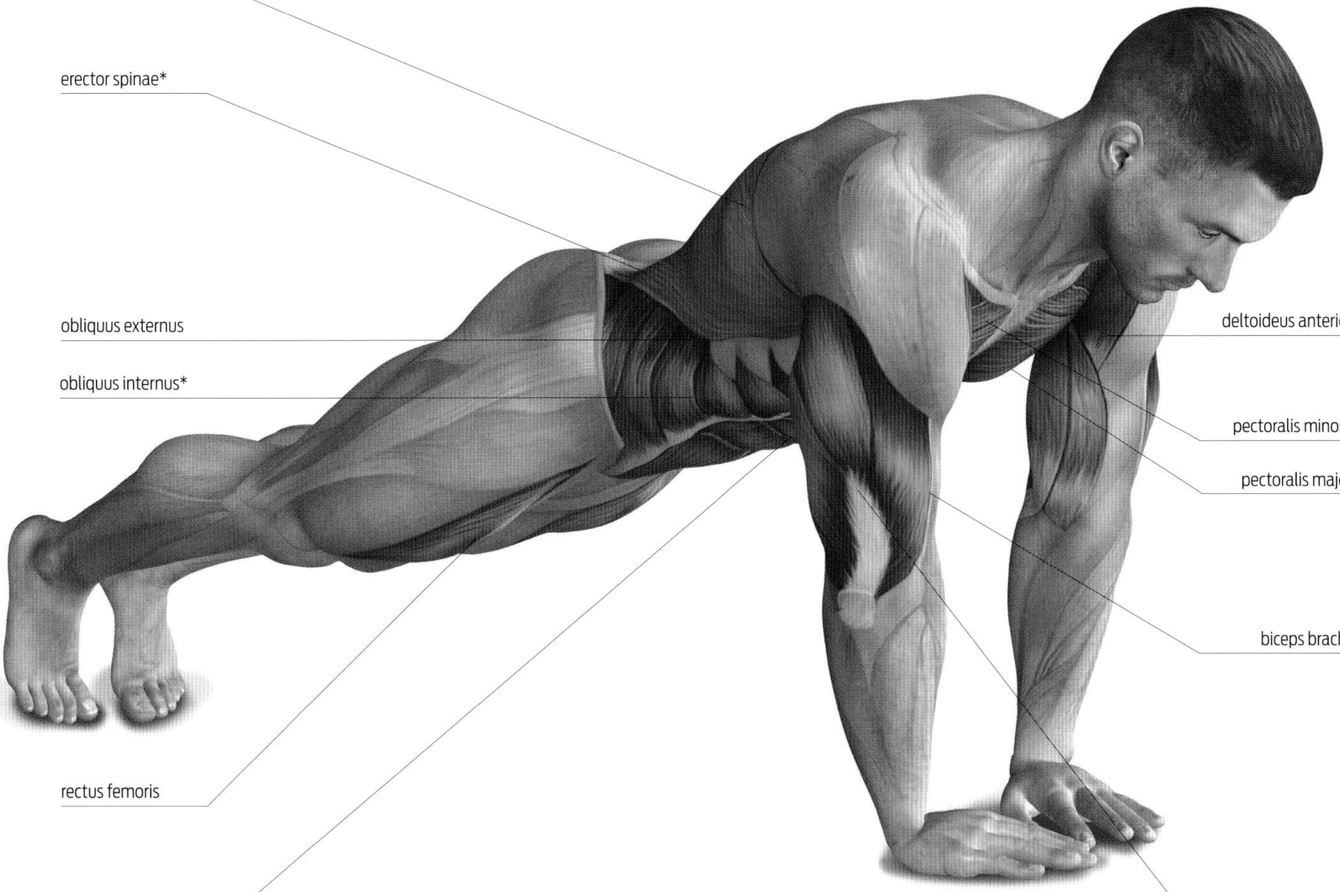

latissimus dorsi
erector spinae*
obliquus externus
obliquus internus*
rectus femoris
rectus abdominis
deltoideus anterior
pectoralis minor*
pectoralis major
biceps brachii
triceps brachii

# Decline Push-Up

The Decline Push-Up is another variation of the fundamental military Push-Up. The decline position, in which you place your feet higher than your hands, applies greater pressure to the upper chest and the front of the shoulders and isometrically contracts the core muscles during the movement. You can vary the height of the decline, starting with your feet on a step and working your way to a higher surface, such as a bench or chair.

1 Start on your hands and knees, with your hands about shoulder width or a little wider. Extend your body, and carefully prop your feet up, one at a time, on an elevated surface.

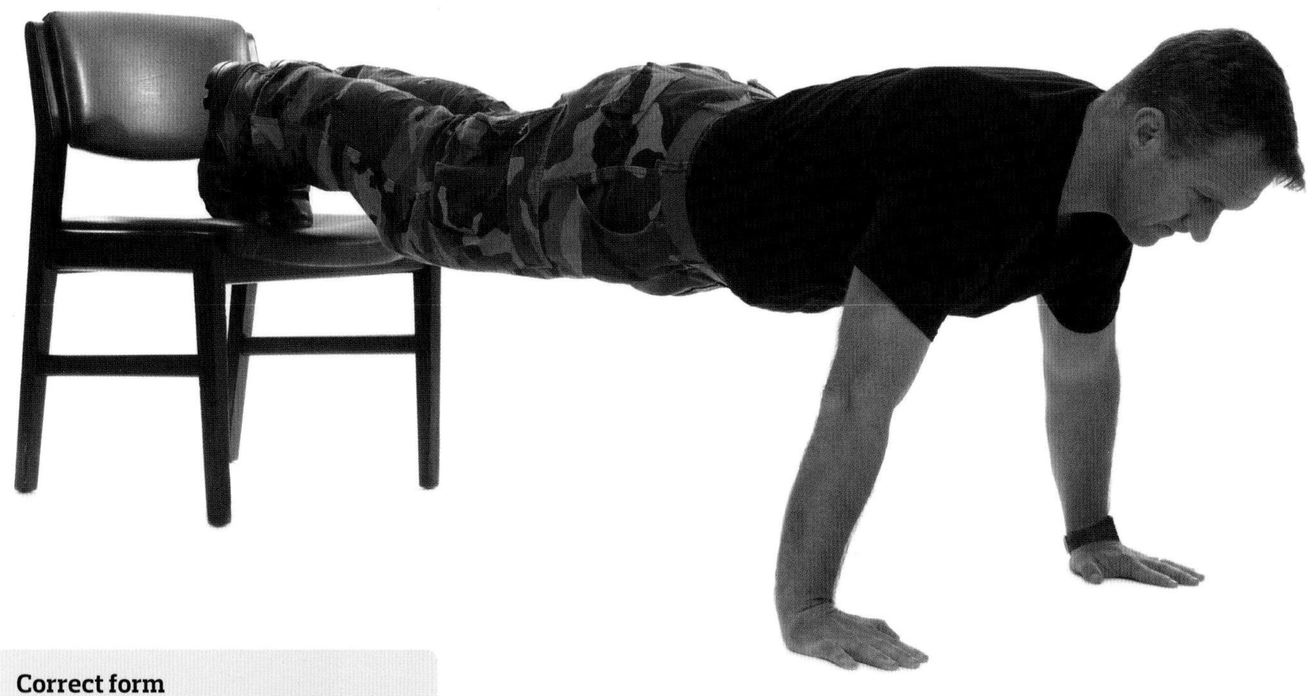

**Correct form**

- Keep your legs and back straight.
- Tighten your glutes.
- Until you build adequare strength, perform only as many reps as you can do without compromising your form.

**Avoid**

- Arching your back.
- Locking your elbows in the Drop Position.

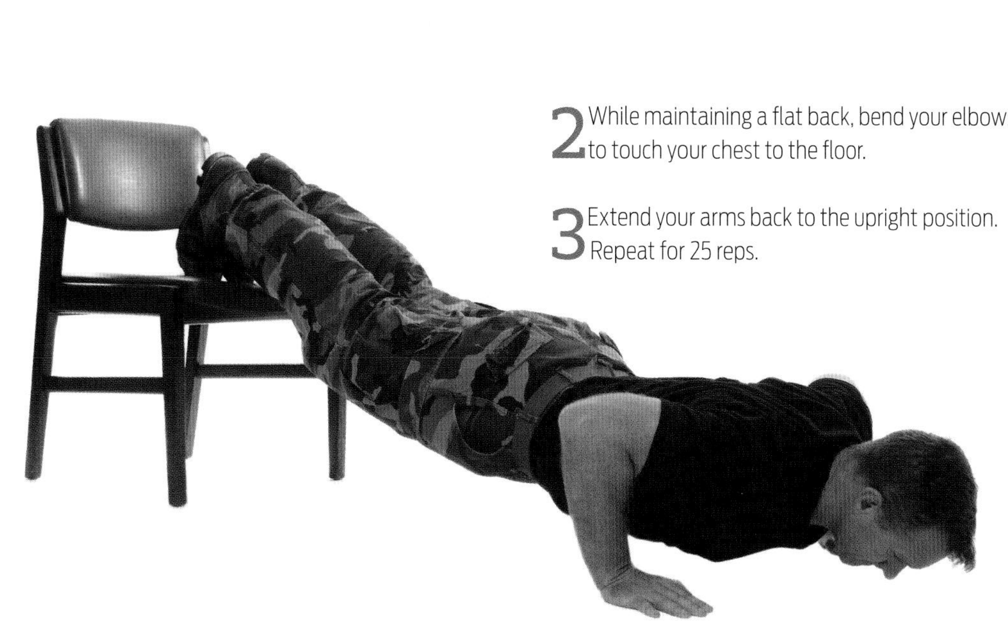

**2** While maintaining a flat back, bend your elbows to touch your chest to the floor.

**3** Extend your arms back to the upright position. Repeat for 25 reps.

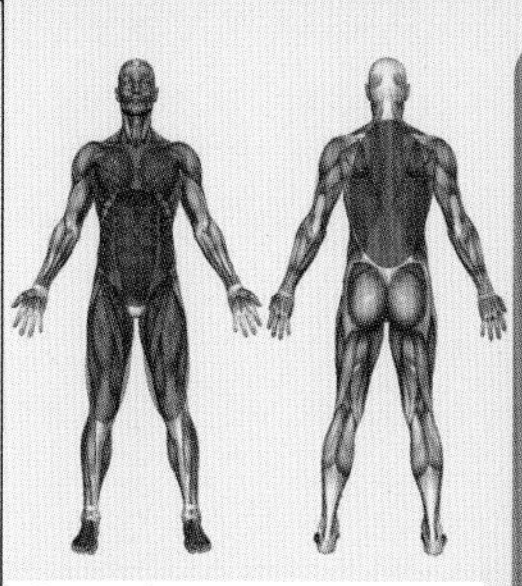

**Level**
- Intermediate

**Duration**

- 45–60 seconds

**Benefits**
- Strengthens upper body
- Strenghtens core stabilizers

**Caution**
- Shoulder issues
- Wrist issues
- Lower-back pain

**Annotation Key**
* indicates deep muscles

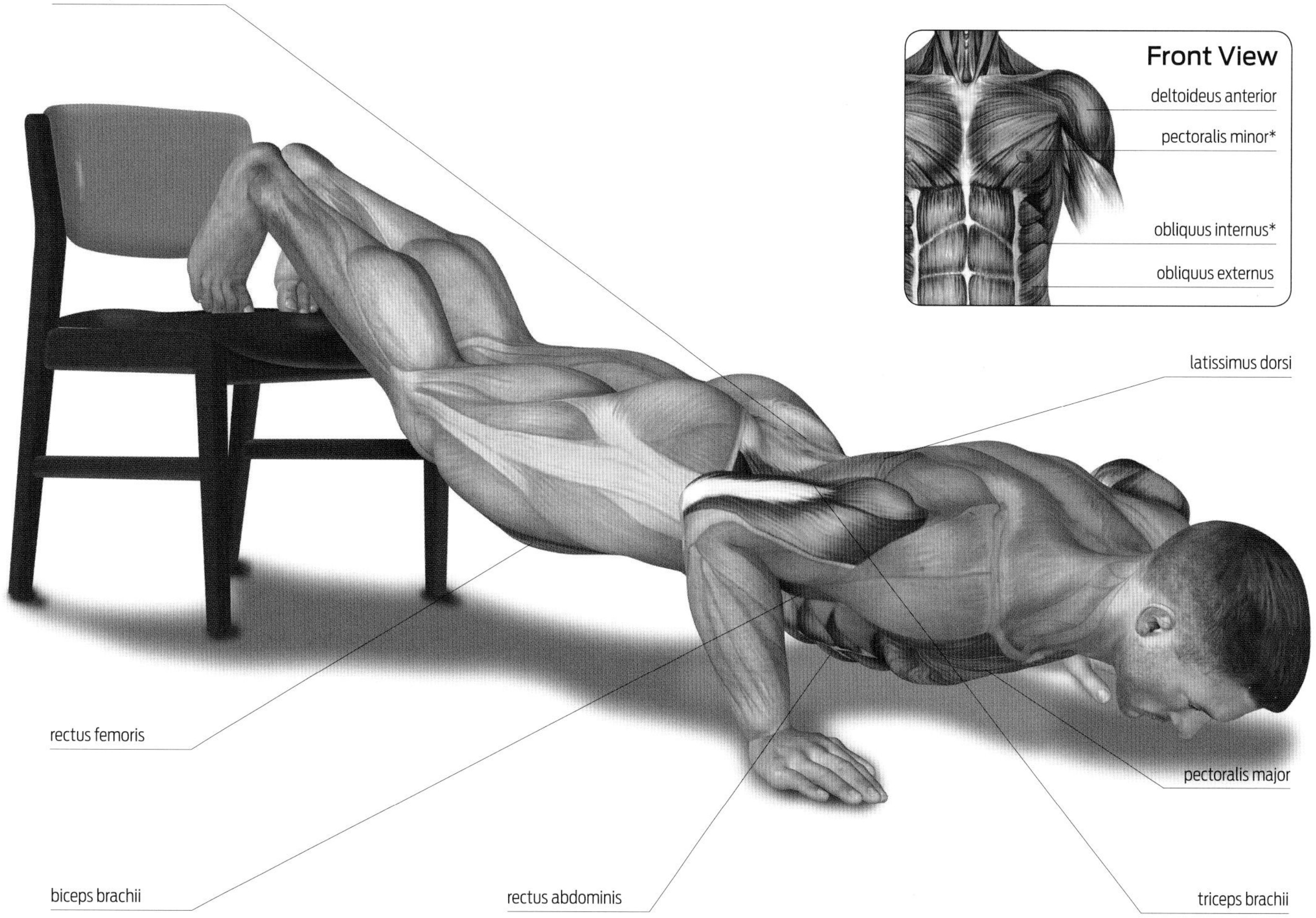

erector spinae*

**Front View**

deltoideus anterior

pectoralis minor*

obliquus internus*

obliquus externus

latissimus dorsi

rectus femoris

pectoralis major

biceps brachii

rectus abdominis

triceps brachii

# Wide Push-Up

The Wide Push-Up takes your shoulders and chest through a different range of movement than the basic Push-Up, isolating the lateral part of the pectoralis major. This can add size and shape to the outer ridge of your chest.

1 With your hands spread wider than shoulder width, place your palms on the floor, keeping your feet together and back straight. Push your body up until your arms are straight. This is your start position.

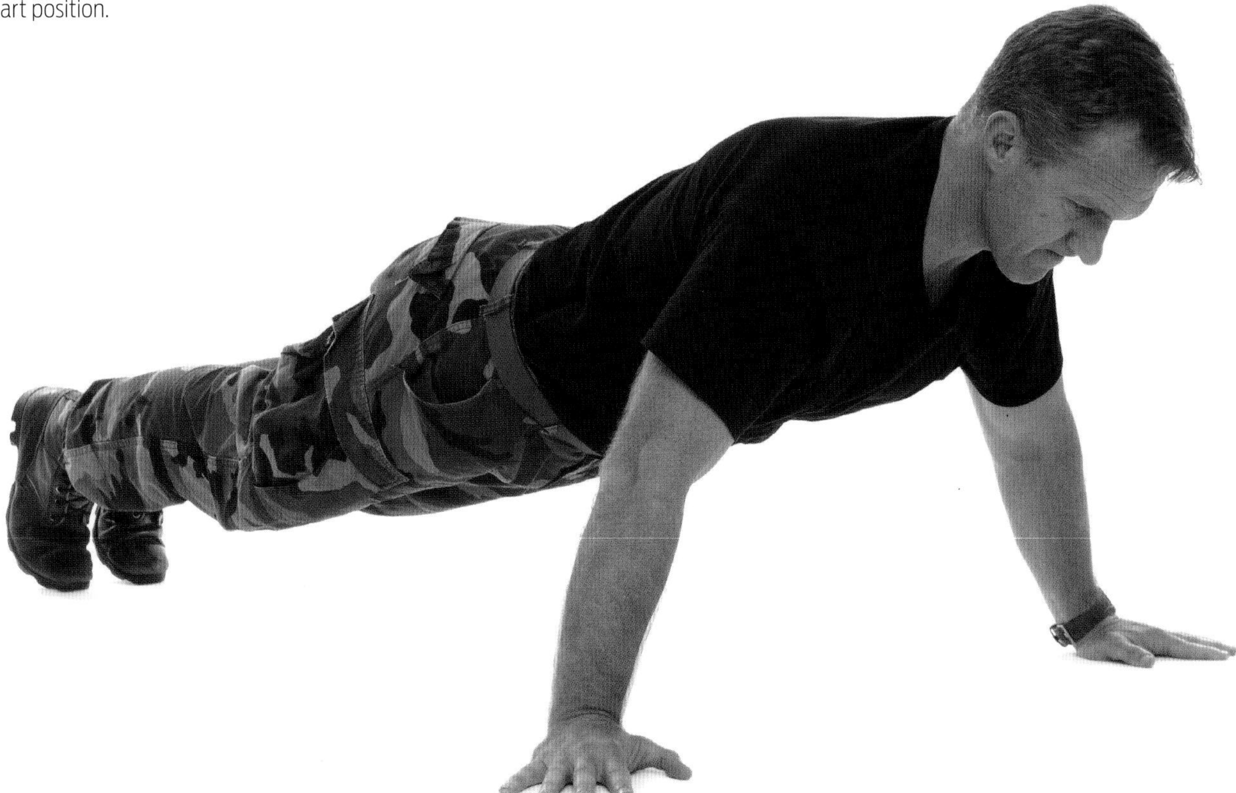

**Correct form**

- Slightly flare your hands outward to allow your elbows to go toward your hips as you lower yourself to the floor. This helps prevent shoulder tendonitis.
- If you cannot keep your back straight during the entire movement or you experience back pain, start this exercise on both knees and do a modified push-up.

**Avoid**

- Pushing your hips into the air.
- Pointing your elbows to the side during the down movement. This places undue stress on the anterior deltoids.

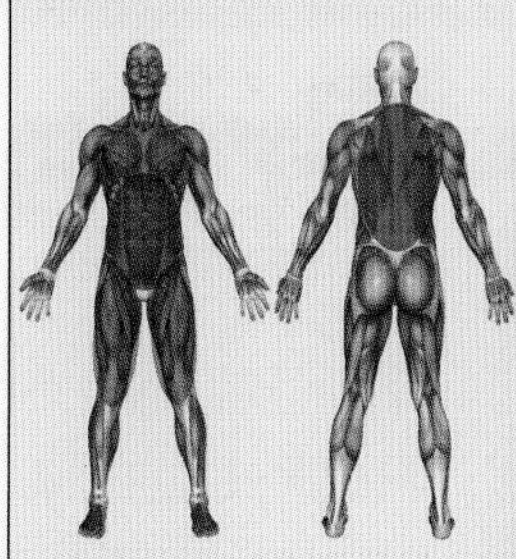

2 Bend your arms, and lower your torso until your chest touches the floor. Straighten your arms to rise back up to the starting position to complete the repetition. Perform 10 reps.

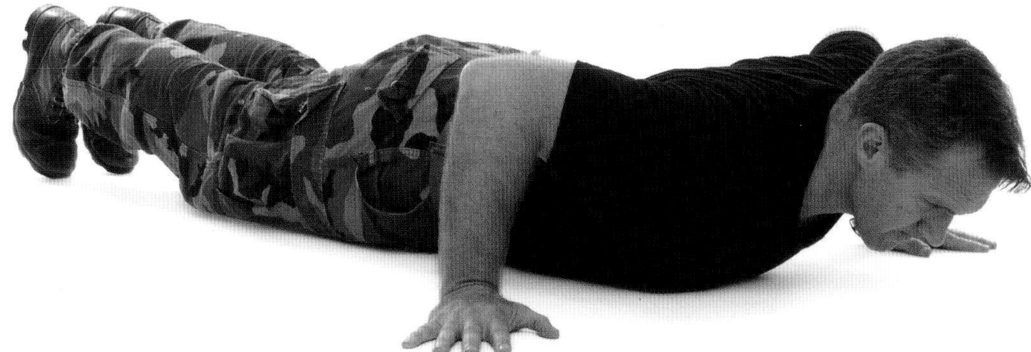

**Level**
- Intermediate

**Duration**
- 30–45 seconds

**Benefits**
- Strengthens upper body
- Strengthens shoulders

**Caution**

- Shoulder issues
- Wrist issues
- Lower-back pain

**Annotation Key**
* indicates deep muscles

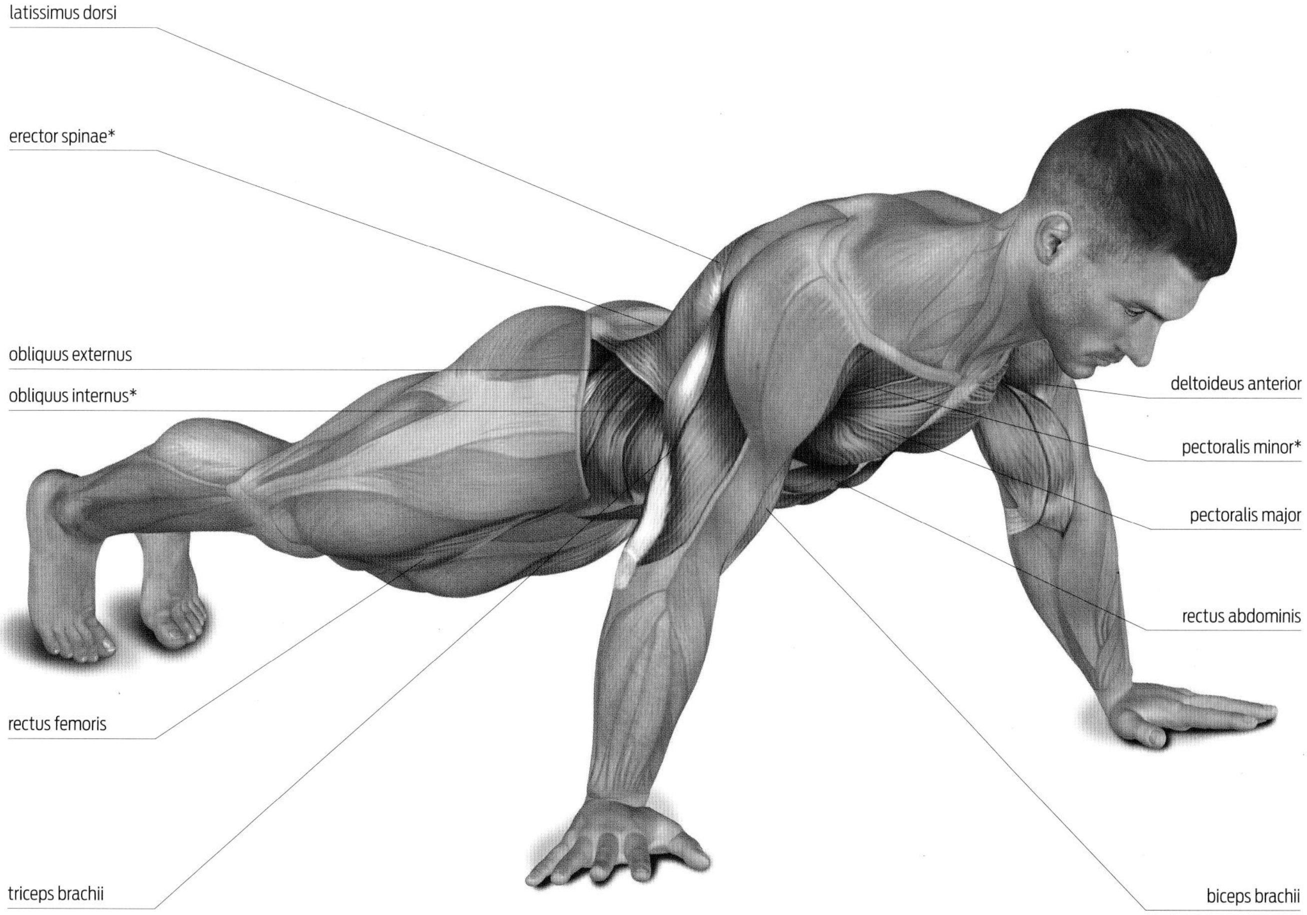

latissimus dorsi

erector spinae*

obliquus externus

obliquus internus*

rectus femoris

triceps brachii

deltoideus anterior

pectoralis minor*

pectoralis major

rectus abdominis

biceps brachii

# Sprawl Push-Up

The Sprawl Push-Up is a more cardio-intensive version of the basic Push-Up. Try to perform this exercise as quickly as possible to increase the demand on your cardiovascular system.

1 Start in the standing position.

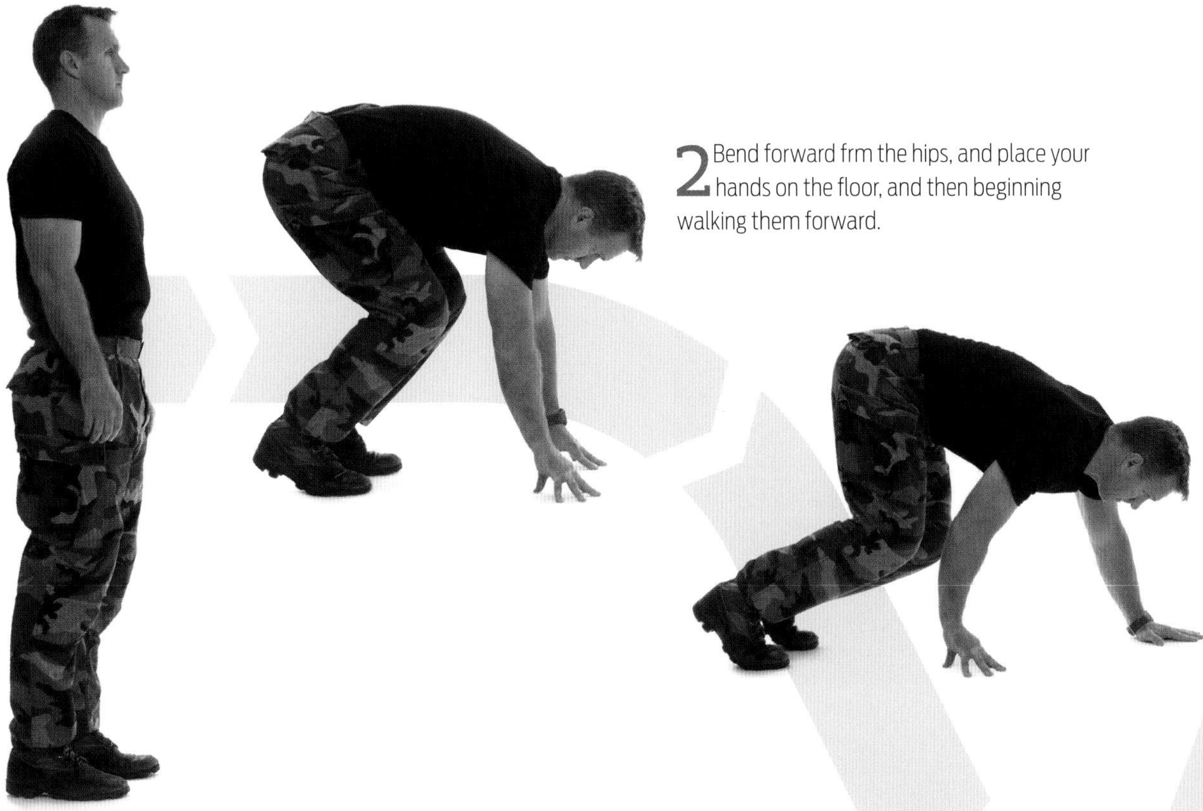

2 Bend forward frm the hips, and place your hands on the floor, and then beginning walking them forward.

3 Continue walking your hands forward until you are in a flat Push-Up position.

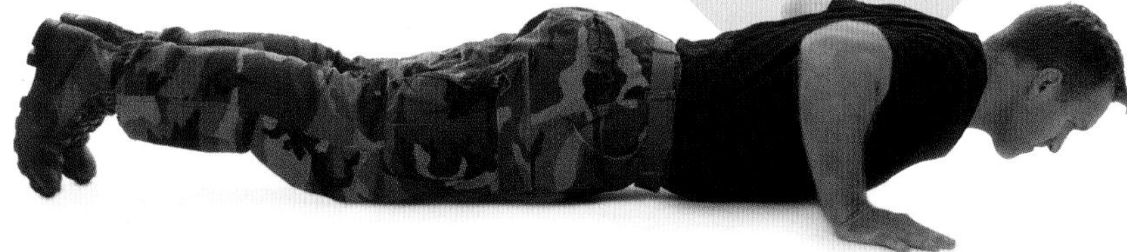

**Correct form**

- Keep your legs and back straight. in the Push-Up portion of this exercise.
- Challenge yourself to walk your hands out into the Drop Position in four or fewer steps.

**Avoid**

- Pointing your elbows to the side during the down movement. This places undue stress on the anterior deltoids.

4 Raise your body to the Drop Position.

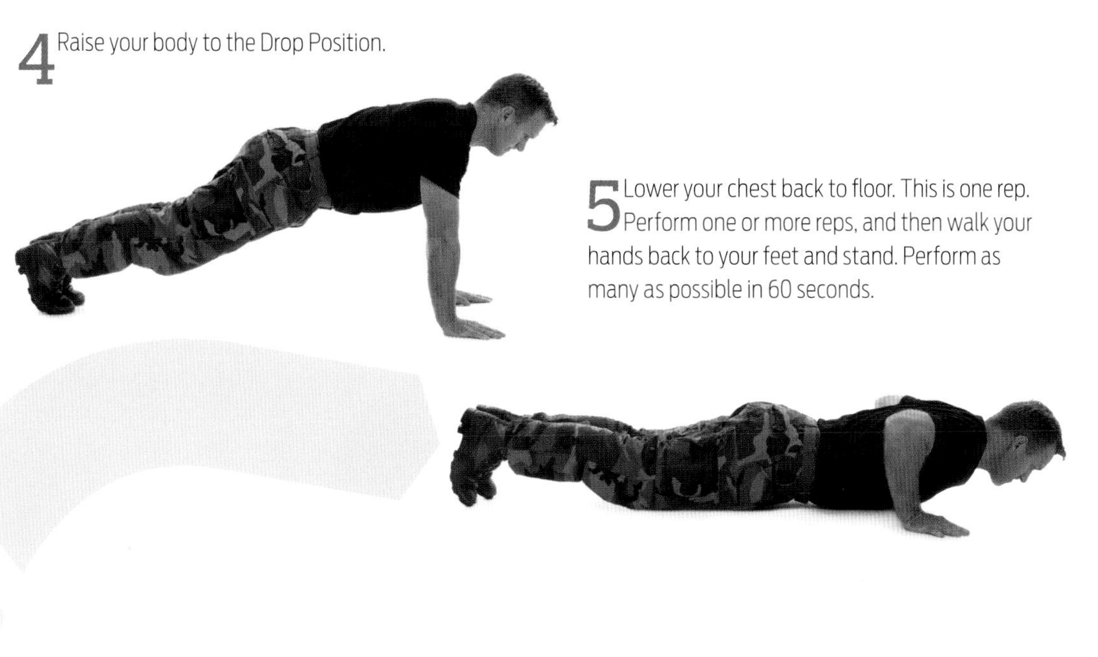

5 Lower your chest back to floor. This is one rep. Perform one or more reps, and then walk your hands back to your feet and stand. Perform as many as possible in 60 seconds.

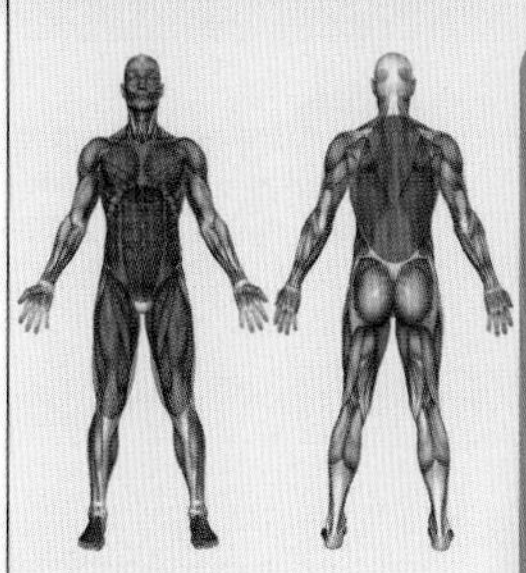

**Level**
- Advanced

**Duration**
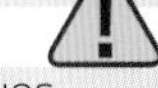
- 60 seconds

**Benefits**
- Strengthens upper and lower body
- Builds cardio and muscle endurance

**Caution**
- Shoulder issues
- Wrist issues
- Lower-back pain

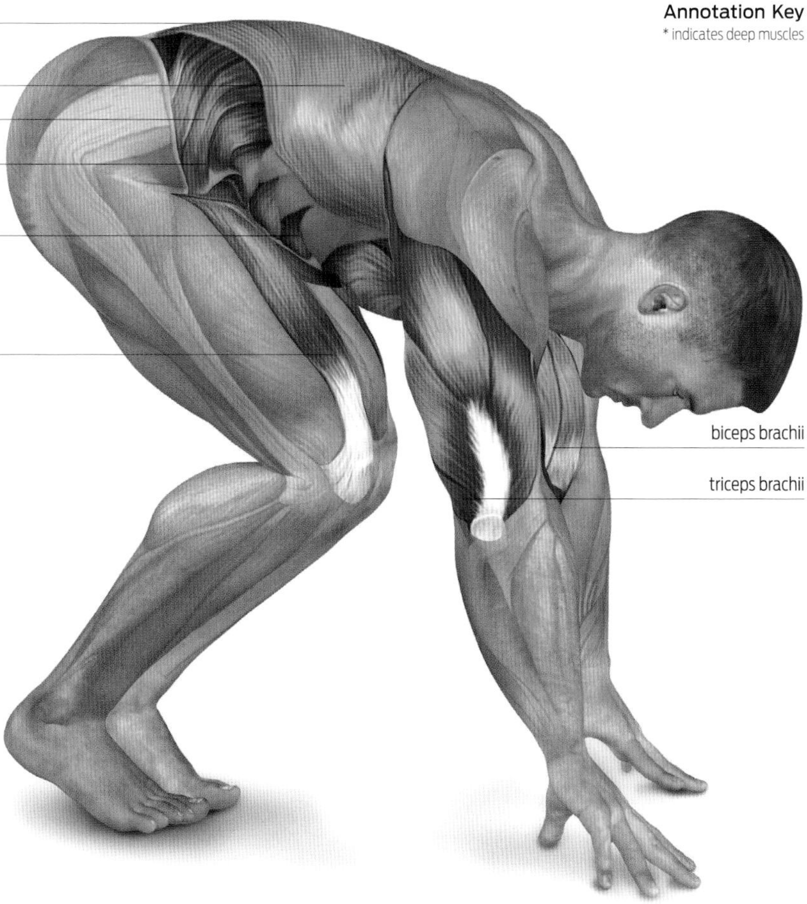

erector spinae*

latissimus dorsi

obliquus externus

obliquus internus*

rectus abdominis

rectus femoris

biceps brachii

triceps brachii

**Annotation Key**
* indicates deep muscles

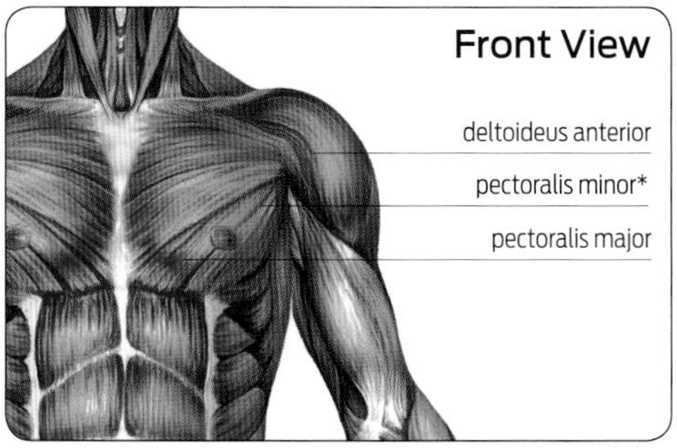

**Front View**

deltoideus anterior

pectoralis minor*

pectoralis major

# Dive Bomber

Performed extensively during special forces training, the Dive Bomber is a great Push-Up variation that places a lot of body weight on the shoulders and arms. The sliding position of the body mimics a bomber aircraft diving toward the ground and then swooping back up.

1 Start in the Drop Position.

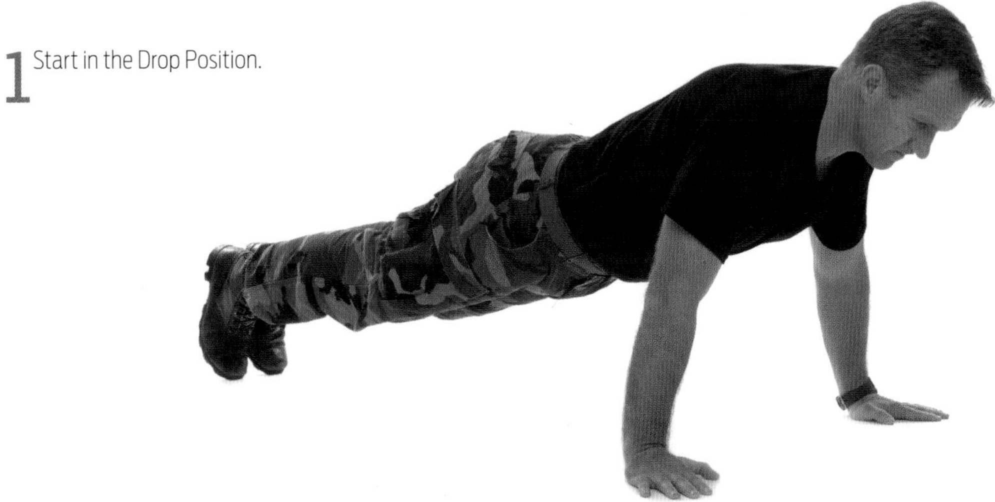

2 Spread your feet, and then walk your hands toward your feet until your butt is up in the air and your shoulders are placed above and slightly behind your hands.

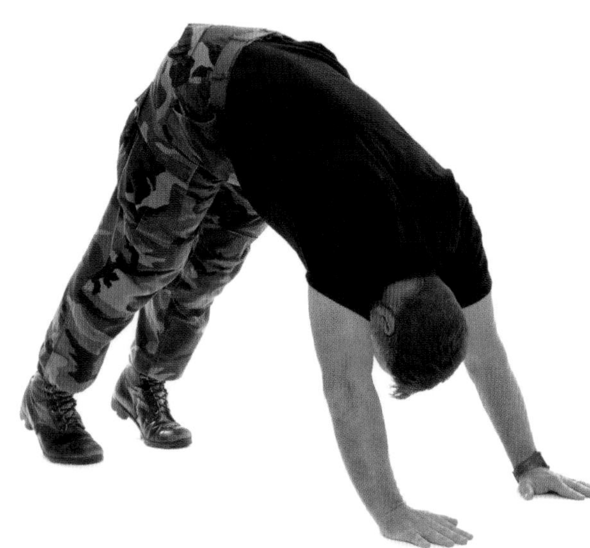

3 Lower your chest in between your hands to the floor while keep your butt in the air.

**Correct form**
- Flex your back forward on the way down, and arch it on the way up.

**Avoid**
- Pausing at the top or bottom of the move—to boost its cardio benefits, make the motion smooth and continuous.

**4** Arch your lower back, and push your body weight out in front of your arms and elevate your chest and straighten your arms. Reverse this movement to the starting position. Perform 25 reps.

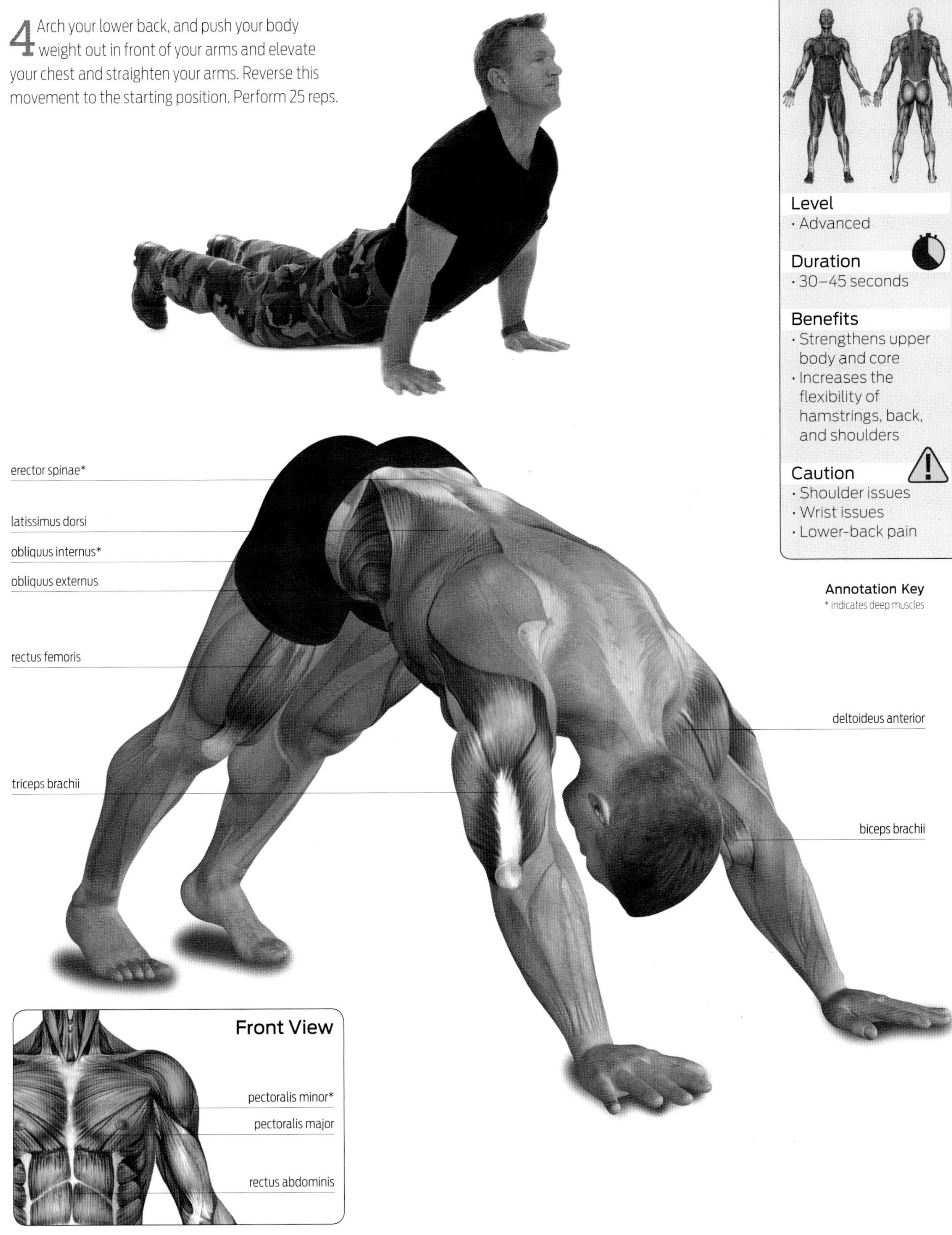


**Level**
- Advanced

**Duration**
- 30–45 seconds

**Benefits**
- Strengthens upper body and core
- Increases the flexibility of hamstrings, back, and shoulders

**Caution**
- Shoulder issues
- Wrist issues
- Lower-back pain

**Annotation Key**
* indicates deep muscles

# Sit–Up

The Sit-Up—often called a Curl-Up in military settings—is a fundamental abdominal and core movement and one of the basic exercises used in military physical fitness tests. Sit-Ups target the rectus abdominis, the paired muscle running vertically on each side of the anterior wall of the abdomen. This "six-pack" muscle is a key postural muscle, as well as one of respiration.

1 Lie on your back with your arms crossed over your chest and your hands resting on the front of each shoulder. Keep your knees slightly bent and your heels on the floor.

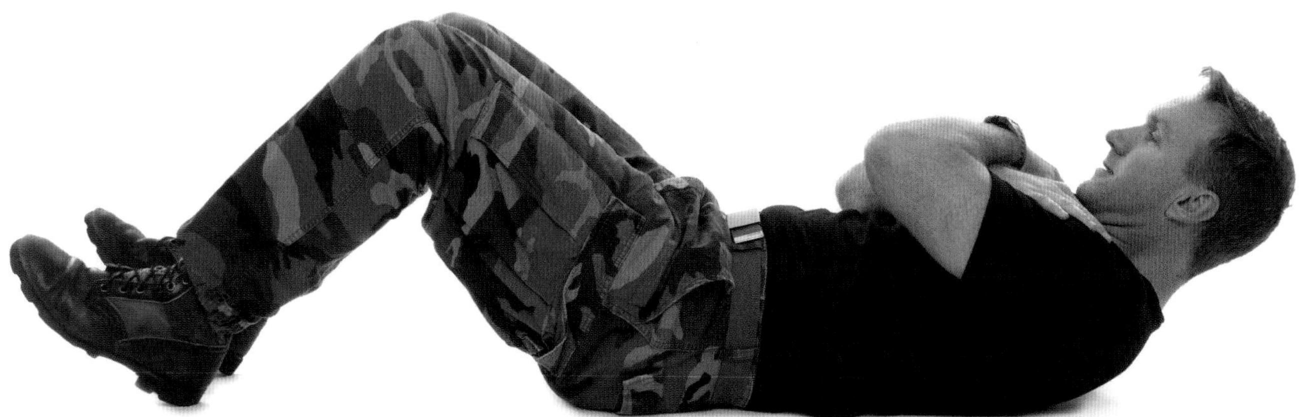

2 Raise your upper body off the floor by contracting your abdominal muscles.

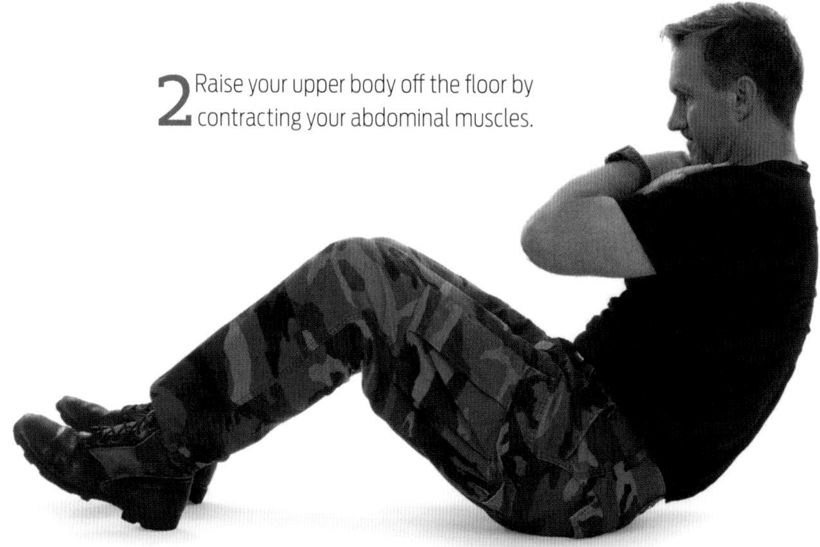

**Correct form**

- Lead with your abdominal muscles, not with your neck.
- Keep your chin tucked into your chest and shoulders rolled forward.
- Keep your heels on the floor.
- Keep your arms folded over your chest.

**Avoid**

- Resting on your back.
- Arching your lower back.
- Move slowly through the range of motion—don't bounce off the floor.

3 Touch your elbows to your mid thighs, and repeat. Touch each shoulder blade to the floor upon each repetition. Perform 10 reps.

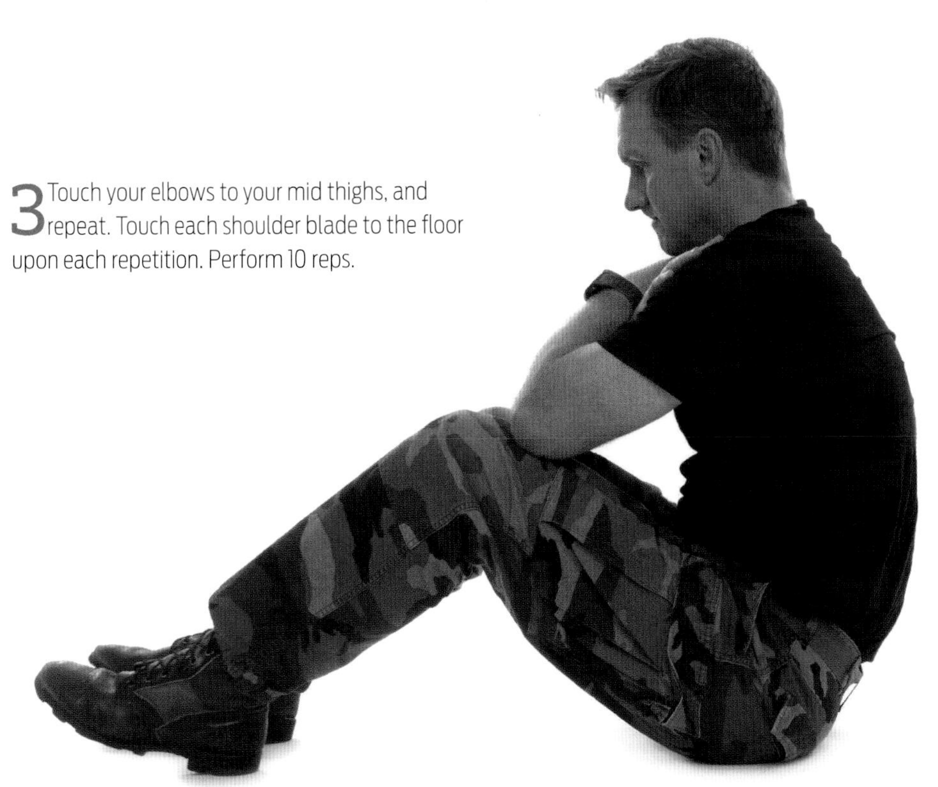

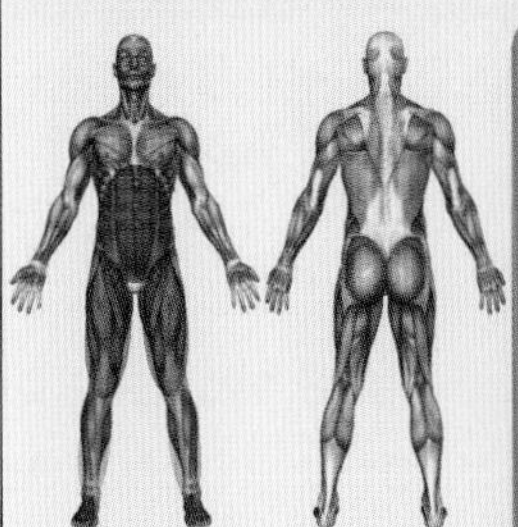

**Level**
· Beginner

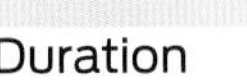

**Duration**
· 45–60 seconds

**Benefits**
· Strengthens upper abdominals

**Caution**
· Neck issues
· Lower-back pain

**Annotation Key**
* indicates deep muscles

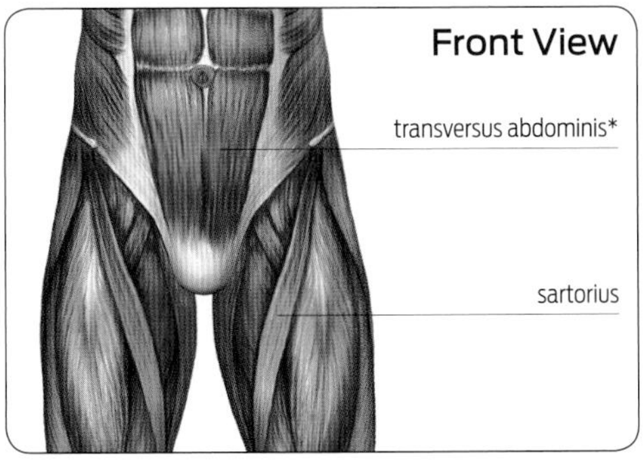

**Front View**

transversus abdominis*

sartorius

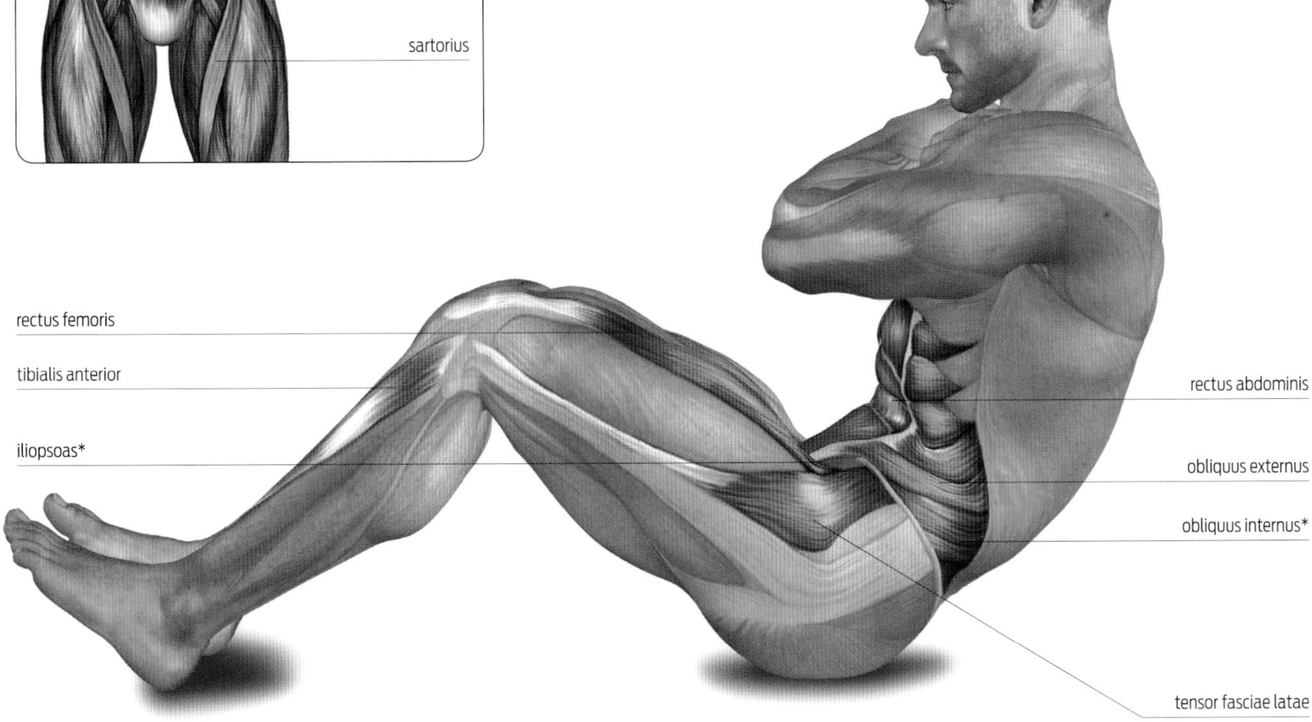

rectus femoris

tibialis anterior

iliopsoas*

rectus abdominis

obliquus externus

obliquus internus*

tensor fasciae latae

# V–Up

The V-Up is both an upper- and lower-abdominal exercise. It takes some practice to learn how to balance on your butt so that you can perform this move well; however, once you have mastered the movement, it can quickly become a favorite.

1 Lie flat on your back with your arms extended overhead and your feet raised slightly above the floor.

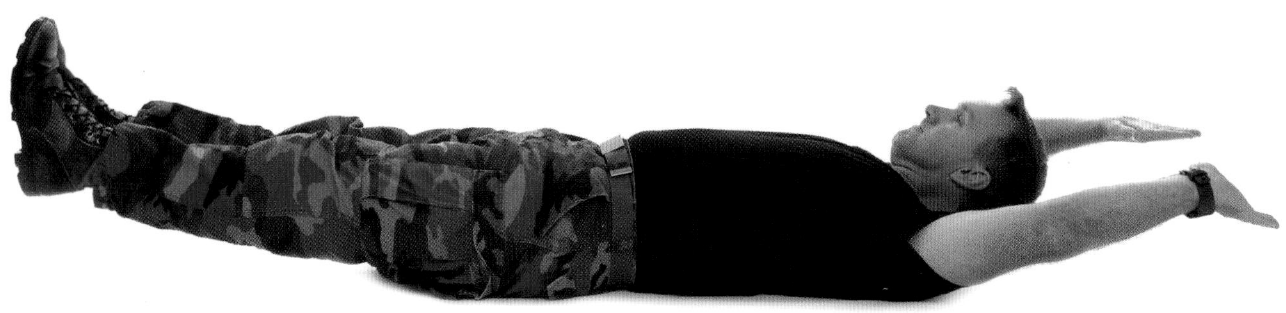

2 Slowly bring your straight arms toward your hips, and lift your upper torso off the floor. While lifting your torso, also lift your legs, making sure to keep them straight.

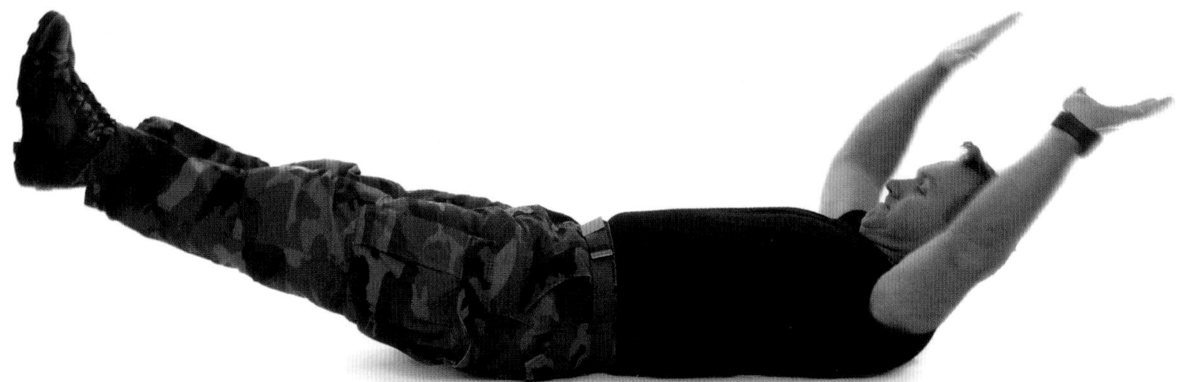

**Correct form**

- Keep your arms and legs straight.

**Avoid**

- Using momentum to get into the V position—engage your abdominals, and keep your movements smooth and controlled.

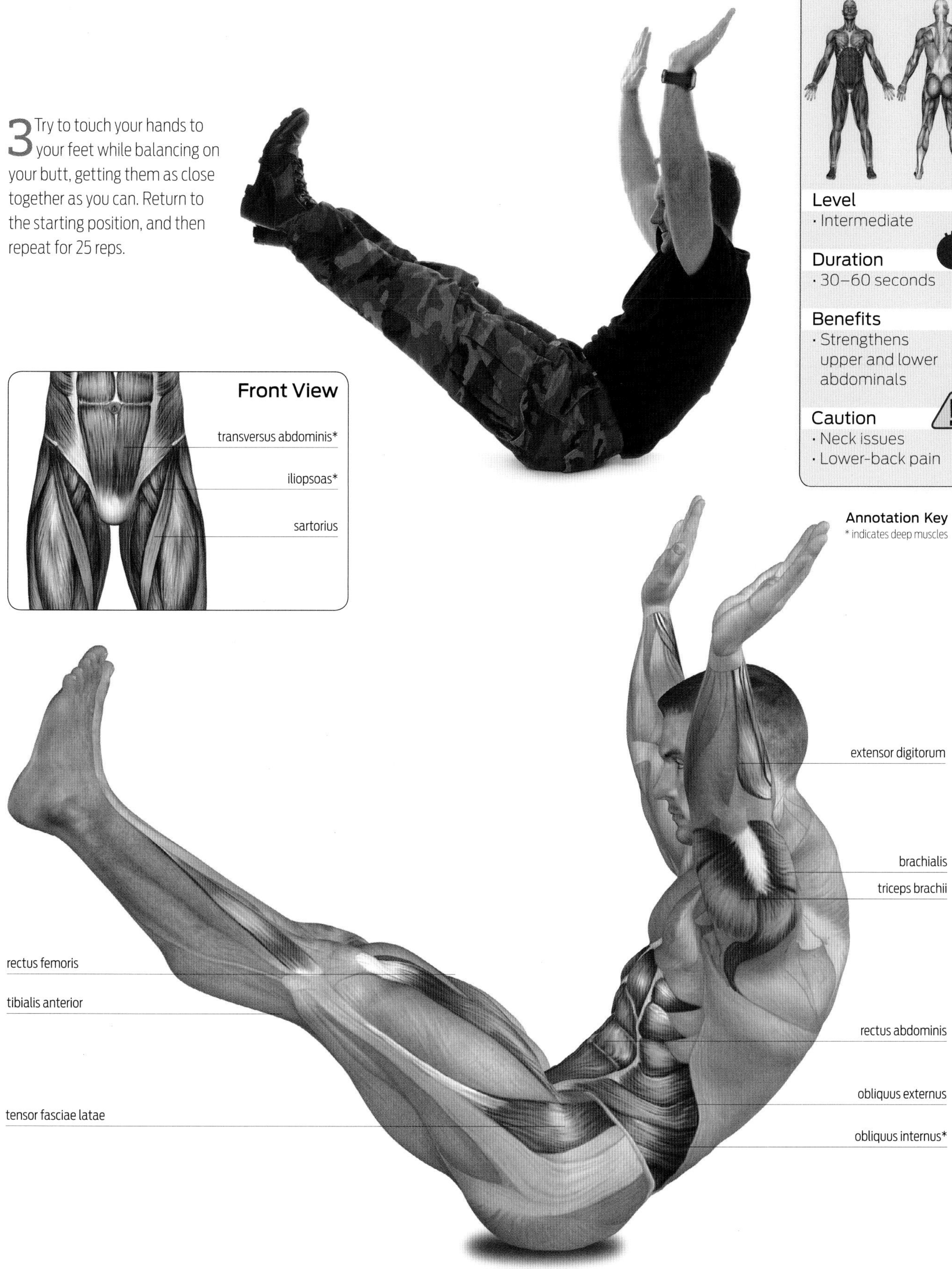


3 Try to touch your hands to your feet while balancing on your butt, getting them as close together as you can. Return to the starting position, and then repeat for 25 reps.

**Level**
- Intermediate

**Duration**
- 30–60 seconds

**Benefits**
- Strengthens upper and lower abdominals

**Caution**
- Neck issues
- Lower-back pain

# Bicycle Crunch

The Bicycle Crunch is so called because the movement of bringing your elbow to the opposite knee resembles pedaling a bicycle. It is a full abdominal exercise that trains both your abs and obliques. It is also an effective cardiovascular movement, engaging multiple muscle groups.

1 Lie on your back with your knees bent, and lift your feet off the floor. Place your hands behind your head. Bring your right elbow to your left knee while twisting at the waist.

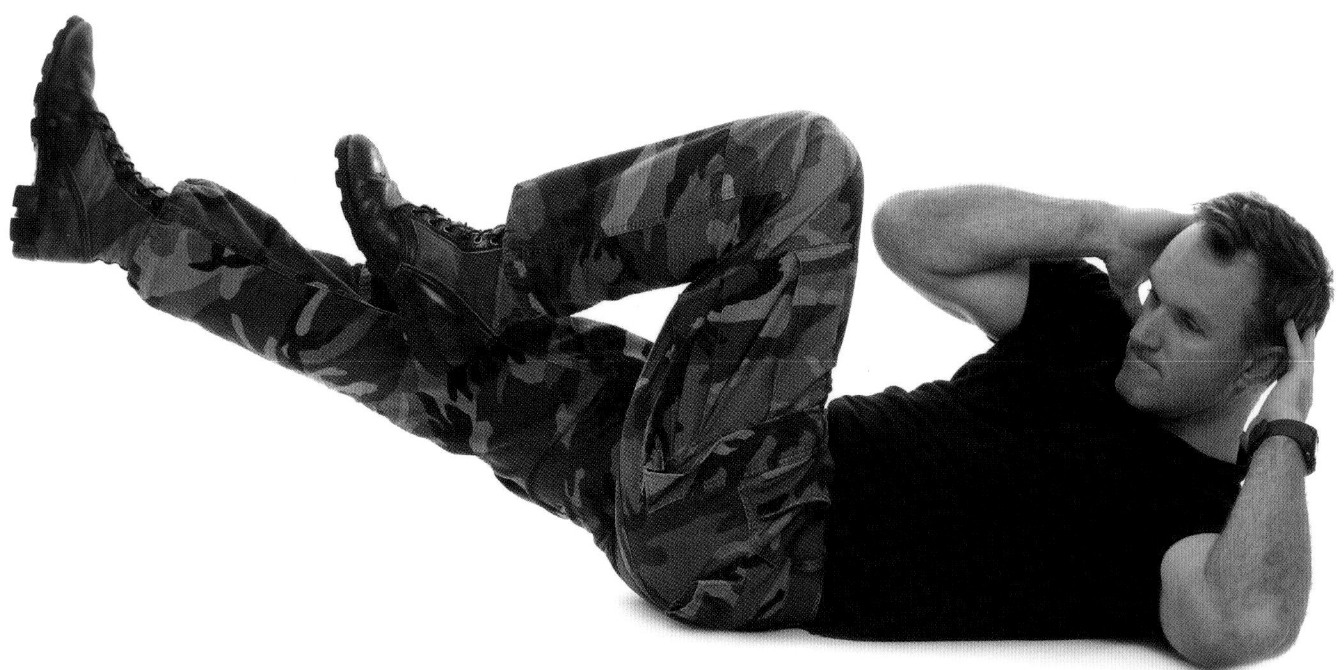

**Correct form**

- Raise your elbow and opposite knee equally, so that they meet in the middle.

**Avoid**

- Raising your lower back off the floor.
- Pulling your head with your hands, which can result in neck pain.

2 Untwist, then bring your left elbow and right knee together, twisting to the opposite side. Repeat, performing as many reps as you can in 60 seconds.

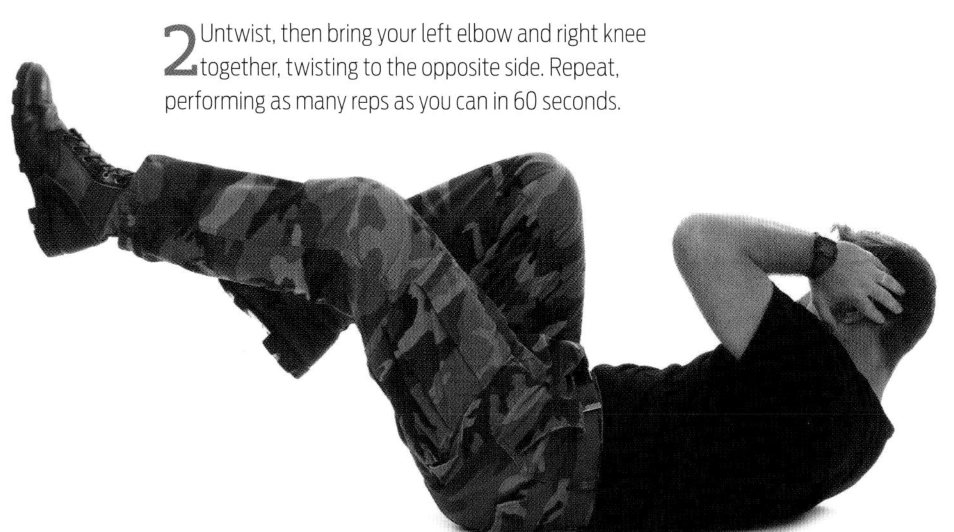

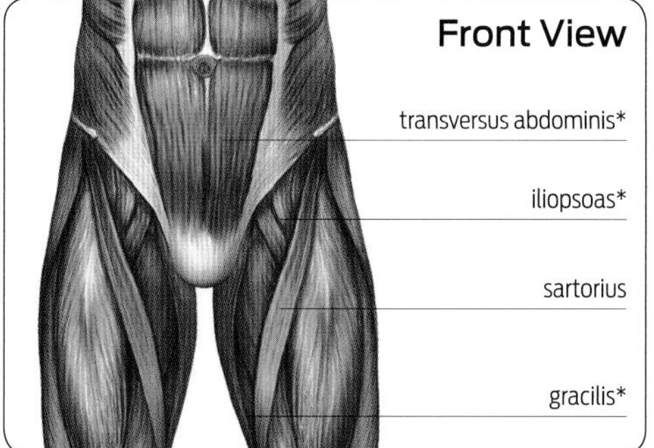


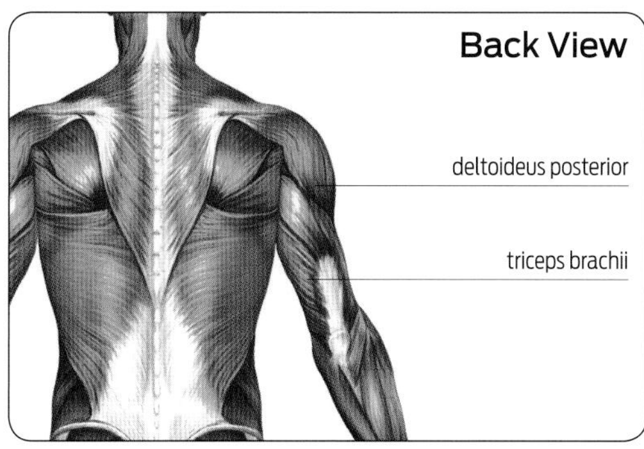


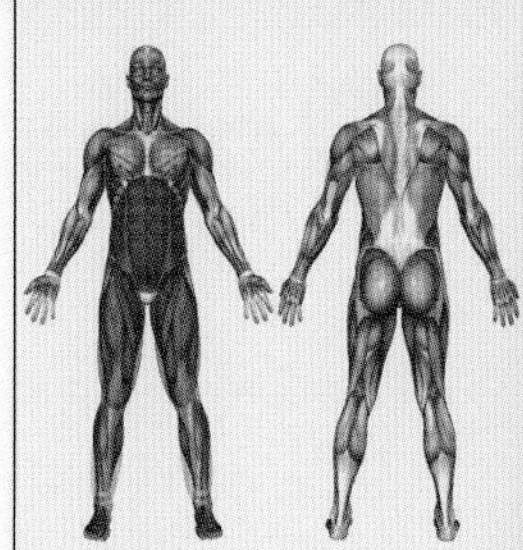

**Level**
- Beginner

**Duration**
- 60 seconds

**Benefits**
- Strengthens abs
- Stabilizes core
- Tones midsection
- Increases cardiovascular endurance

**Caution**
- Lower-back issues
- Neck issues

**Annotation Key**
* indicates deep muscles

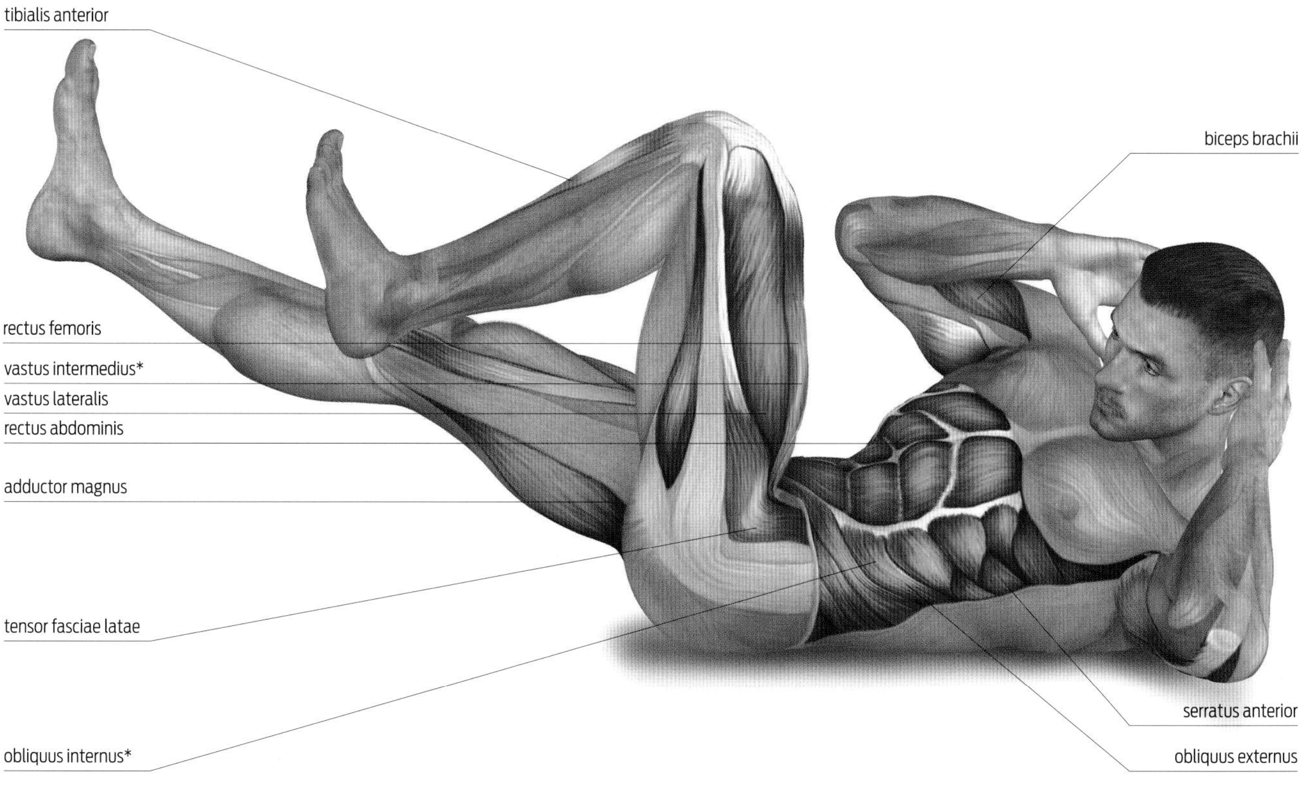

tibialis anterior
biceps brachii
rectus femoris
vastus intermedius*
vastus lateralis
rectus abdominis
adductor magnus
tensor fasciae latae
serratus anterior
obliquus internus*
obliquus externus

# Penguin Crunch

The Penguin Crunch targets your obliques and upper abdominals and will even work the back of your neck. Because it incorporates lateral movement of the abdominals, it is a great exercise to prepare you for any sport that requires rotational movement, such as swimming. It is also a good one to use as a rest between tougher exercises.

1 Lie on your back with your head elevated and your arms straight at your sides and raised off the floor. Bend your knees.

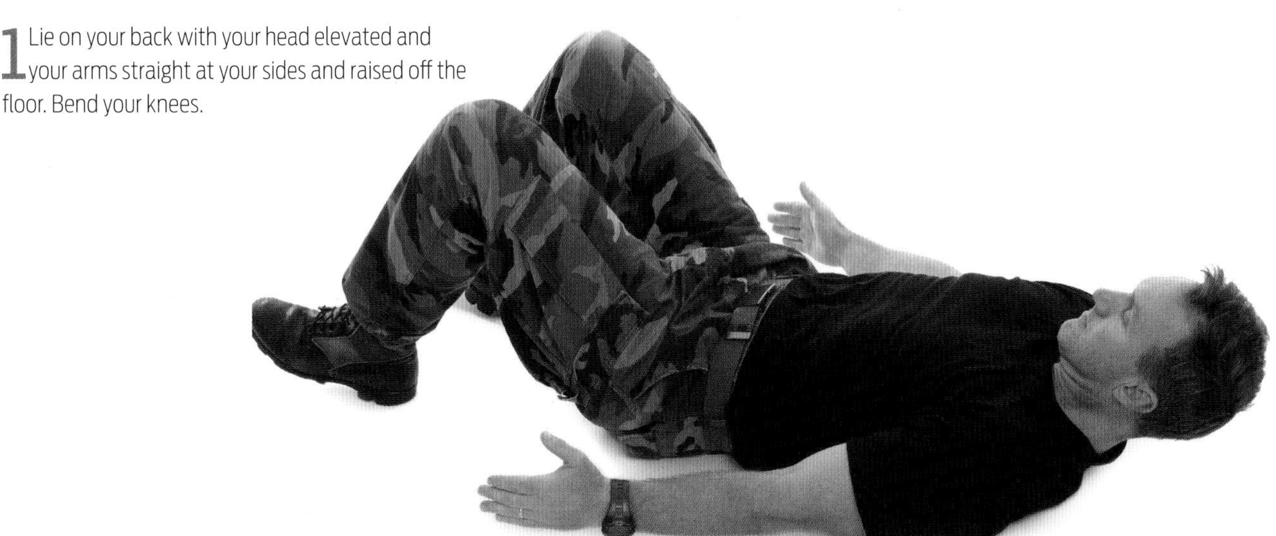

2 Holding your torso in a flexed position, lean to the right, and reach your right hand forward. Hold for one count, and then pull it back.

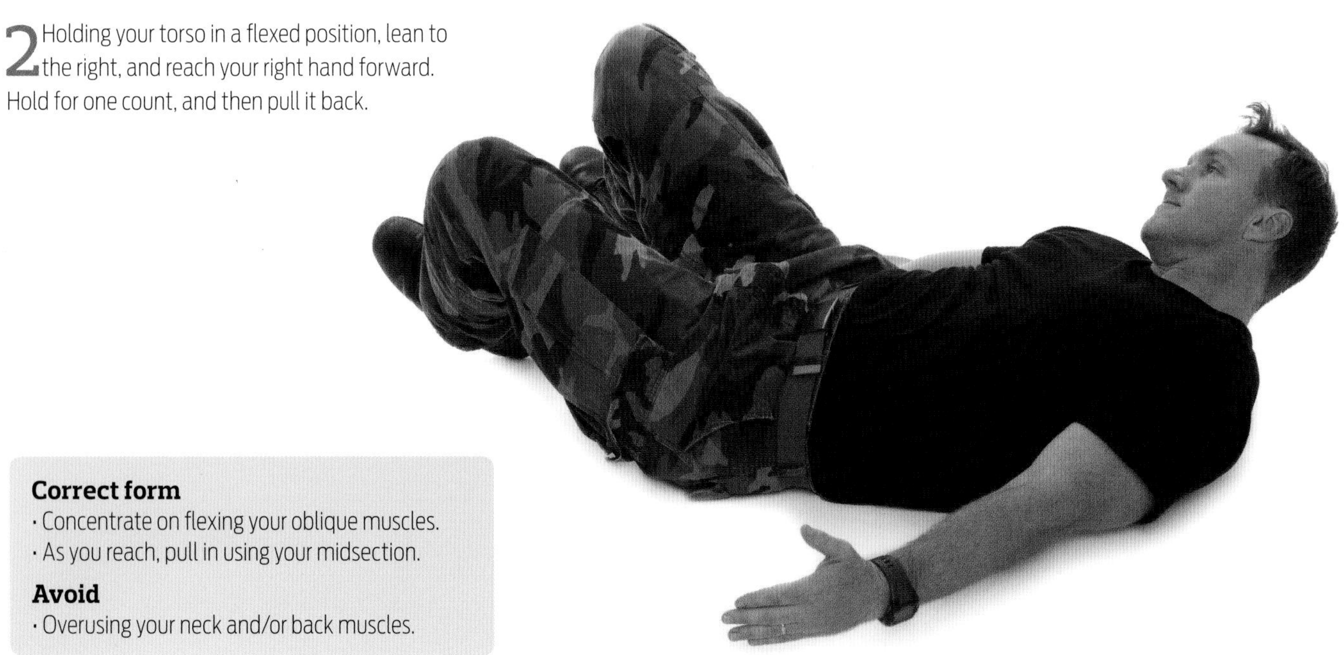

**Correct form**
- Concentrate on flexing your oblique muscles.
- As you reach, pull in using your midsection.

**Avoid**
- Overusing your neck and/or back muscles.

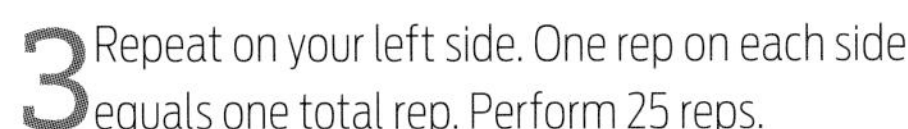

3 Repeat on your left side. One rep on each side equals one total rep. Perform 25 reps.

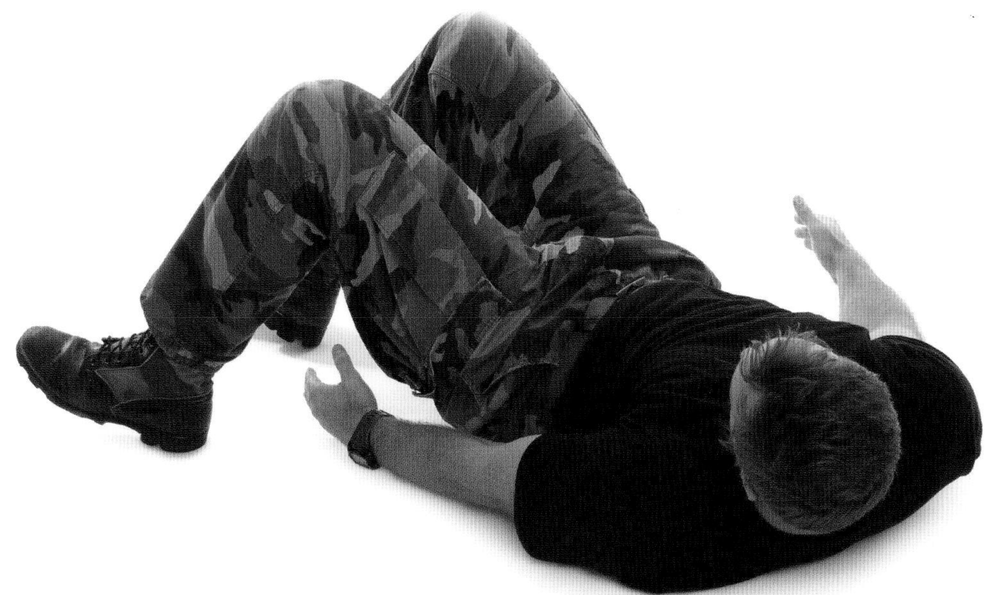

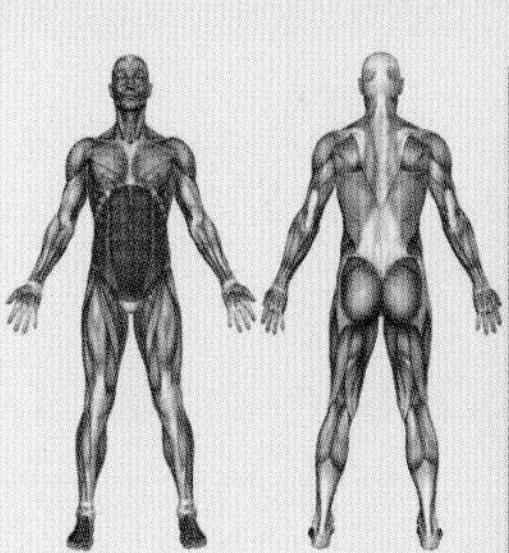

**Level**
- Beginner

**Duration** 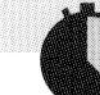
- 30–60 seconds

**Benefits**
- Strengthens core
- Streamlines the abdominals, especially the obliques

**Caution** 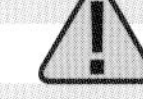
- Lower-back issues

**Annotation Key**
* indicates deep muscles

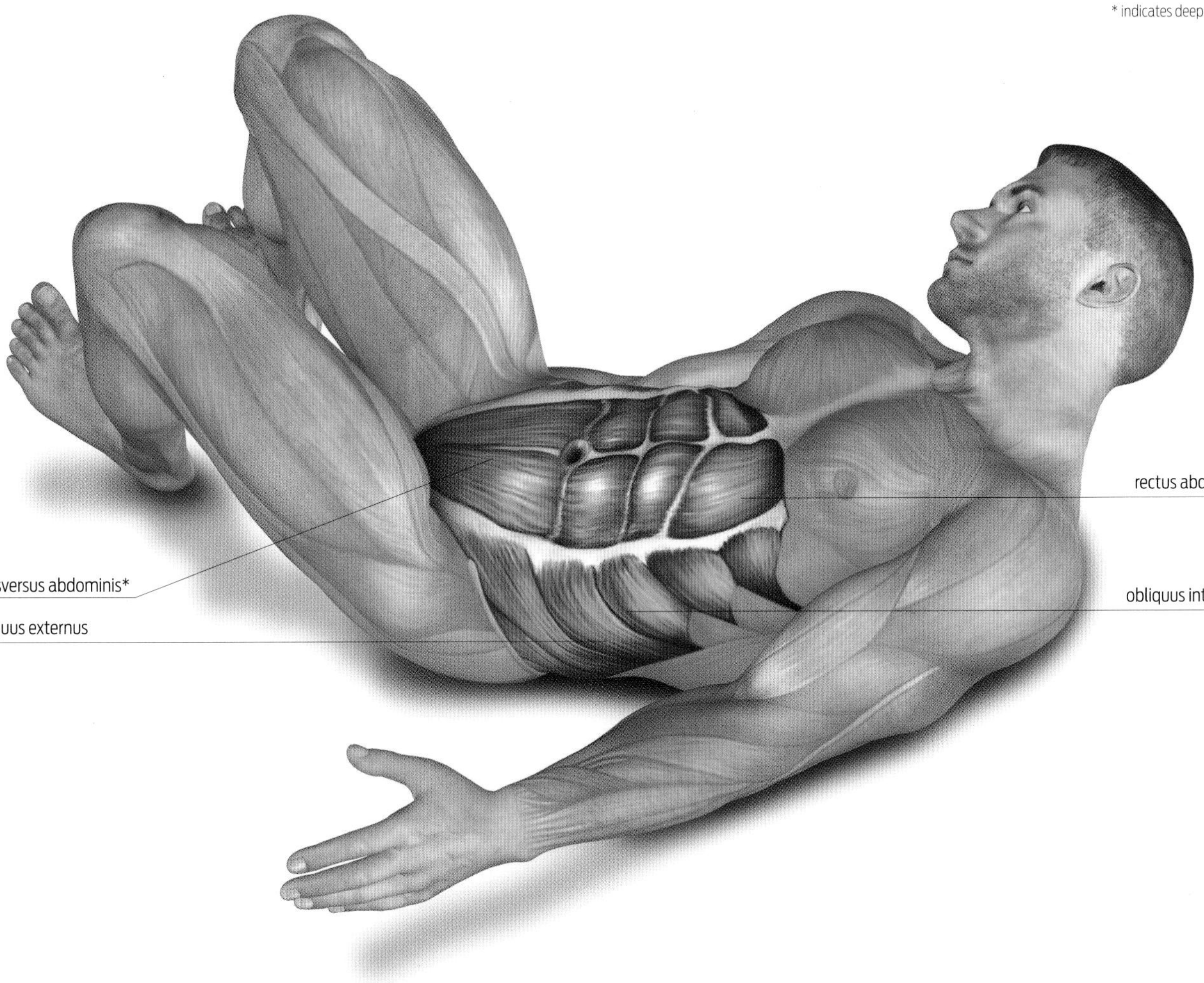

rectus abdominis
transversus abdominis*
obliquus internus*
obliquus externus

# Turtle Shell

The Turtle Shell exercise is so named because it resembles an upturned turtle. Known as a resting position, it is anything but restful, forcing you to fully engage your abdominals and other core muscles.

1 Lie on your back, with your arms outstretched and your legs spread wide.

2 Bring your head, arms, and legs off the floor, so that you are only resting on your back. Hold this position for 60 seconds.

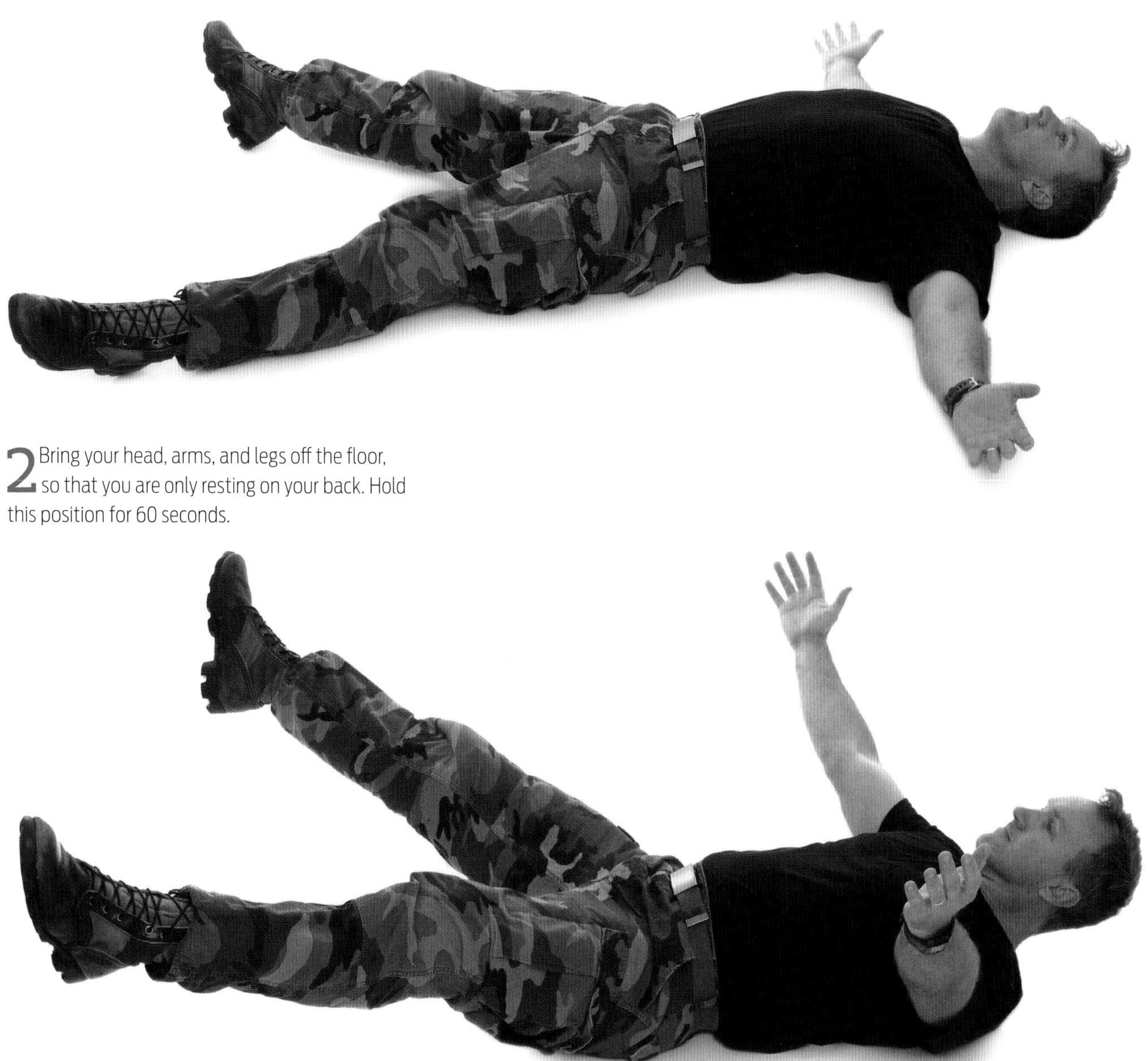

3 Release your abdominals, and slowly return to the starting position.

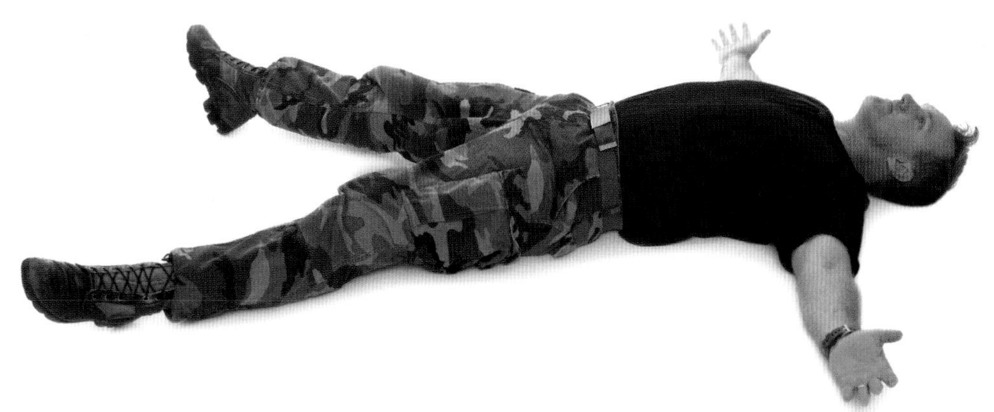

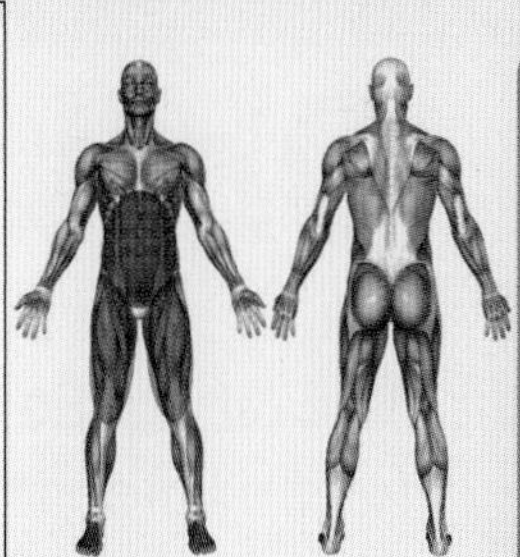

Level
· Beginner

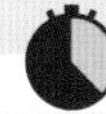

Duration
· 60 seconds

Benefits
· Strengthens abdominals
· Isometrically stabilizes core

Caution
· Lower-back issues

**Correct form**
· Keep your abdominals tight.

**Avoid**
· Allowing any body part other than your back to touch the floor.

Annotation Key
* indicates deep muscles

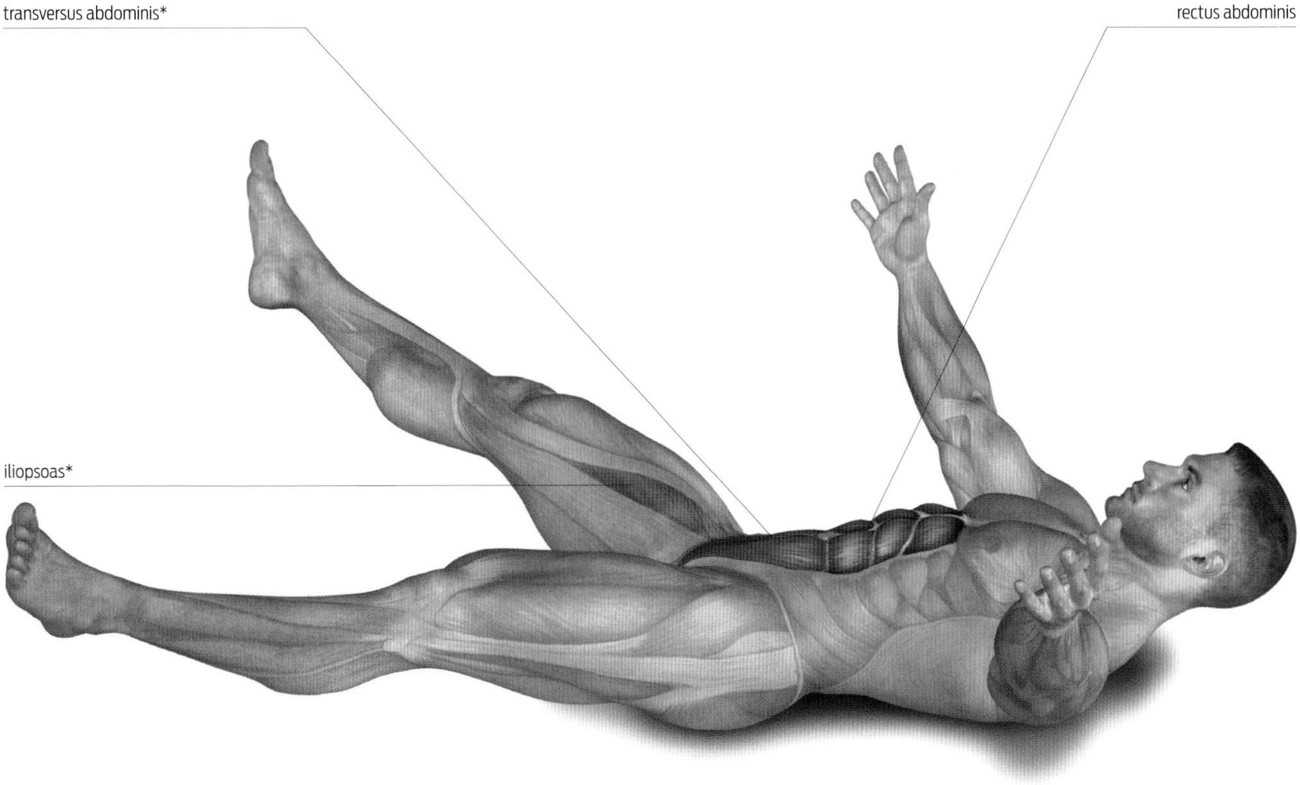

transversus abdominis*

rectus abdominis

iliopsoas*

# Obliques

The Obliques exercise targets the serratus anterior and obliquus muscles, which lie on the sides of your torso. It is the opposite movement of the Bicycle Crunch in that there is no twisting torso movement.

1 Lie on your back with your knees bent and your right hand behind your head and your left hand over the top of your right rib cage. Raise your right knee to rest your right foot on your left knee, bringing your hip to a 90-degree angle.

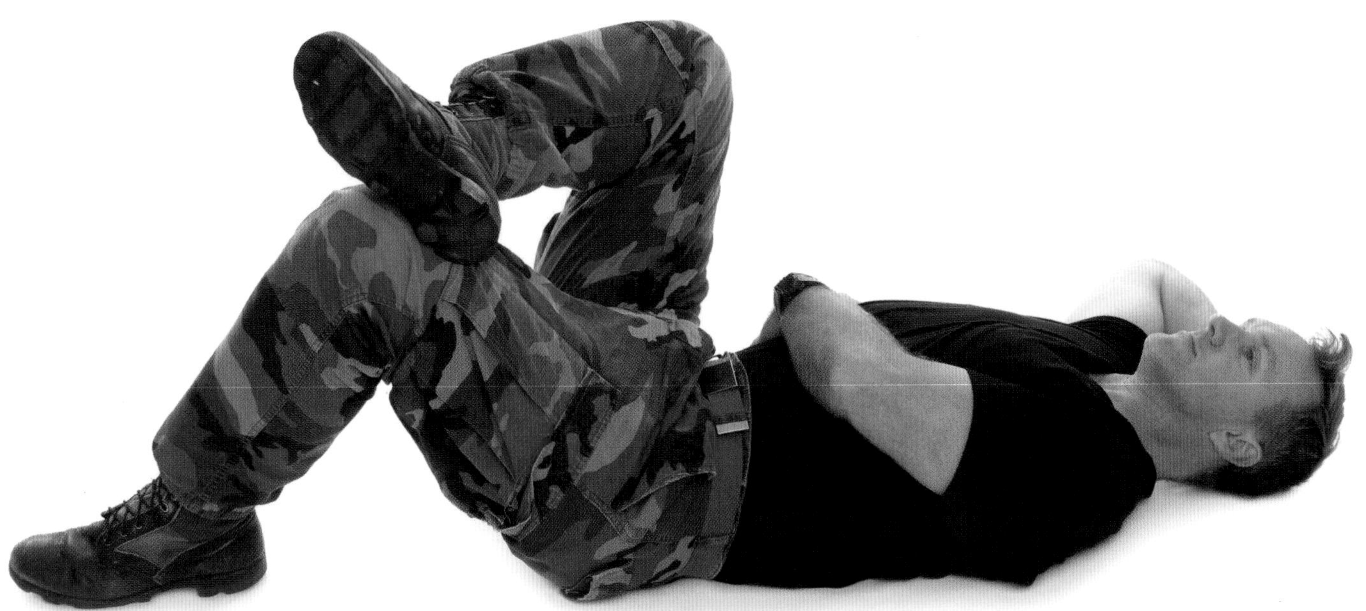

**Correct form**

- Bring your elbow back to the floor upon completion of each rep to get a full stretch of the serratus anterior and latissimus dorsi muscles.

**Avoid**

- Fast or jerky movements—keep your movements slow and controlled, making sure to contract the muscles of your rib cage.

2 Bring your right elbow to your right knee, contracting the serratus anterior and oblique muscles on your right side. Hold for one count, and then bring your right elbow back to the floor next to your head while you lie back. Switch your arm and leg positions, and repeat on the other side. Perform 50 times on each side.

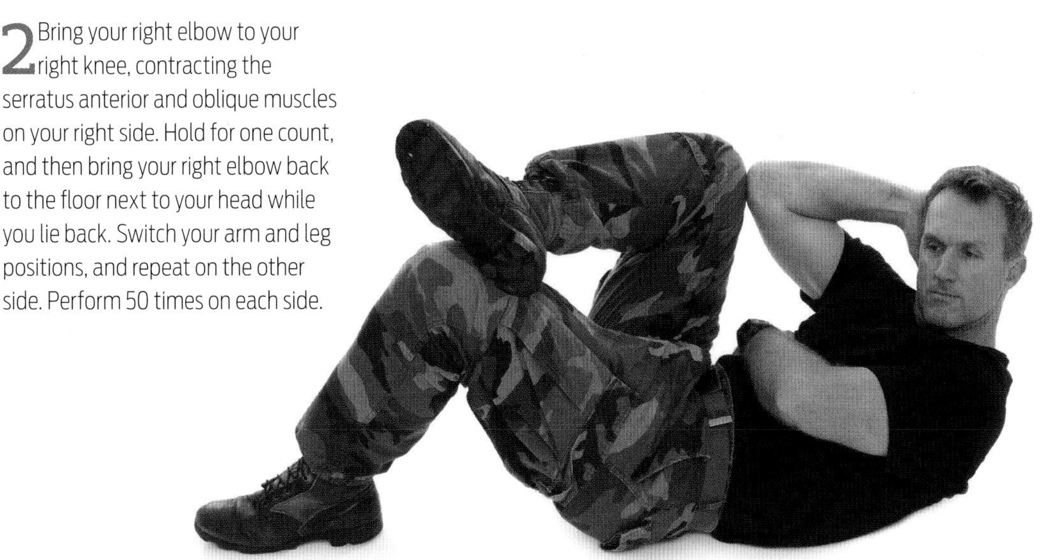

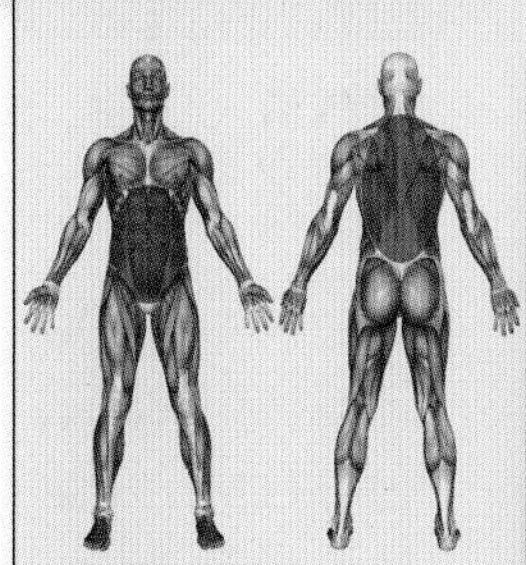

**Level**
· Intermediate

**Duration**

· 1½–2 minutes

**Benefits**
· Strengthens muscles of the rib cage
· Defines serratus anterior muscle

**Caution**
· Lower-back pain

**Annotation Key**
* indicates deep muscles

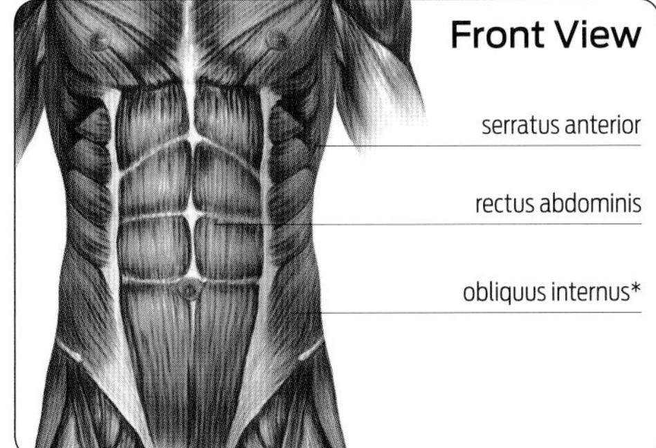


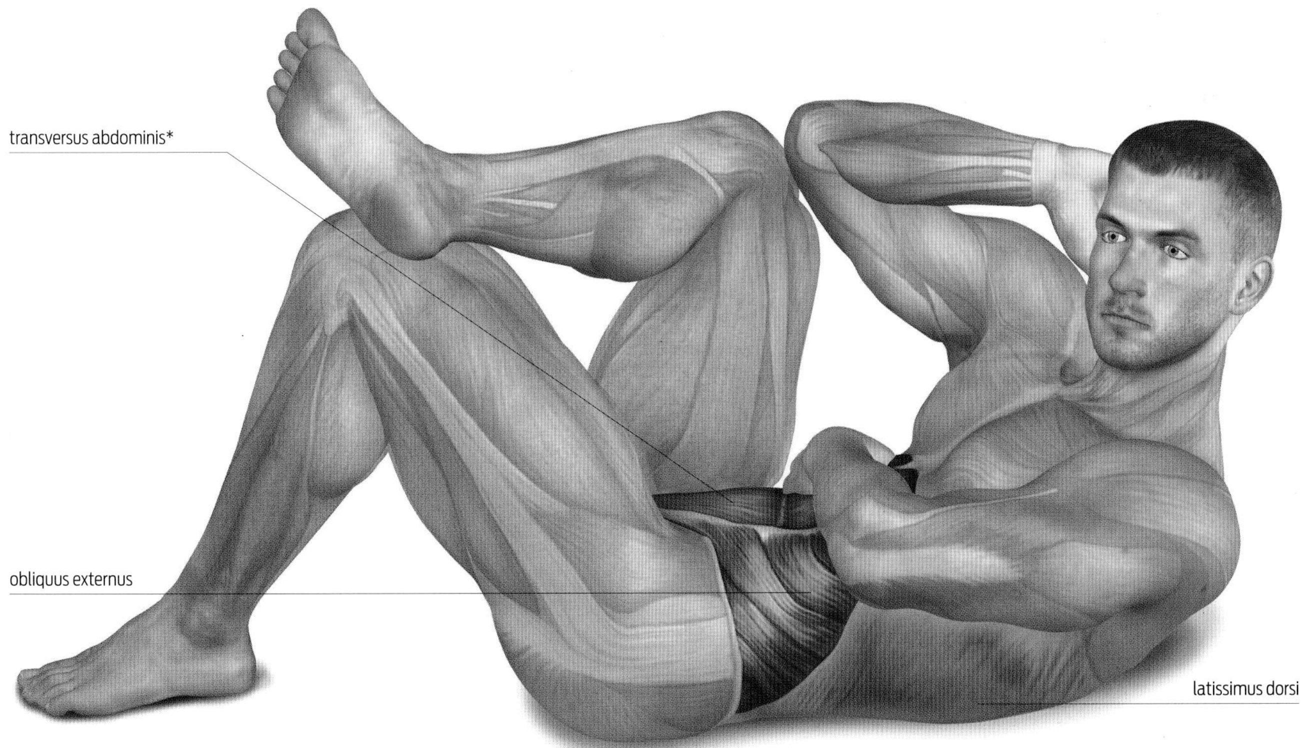

# Flutter Kick

Flutter Kick is a fundamental exercise for special operations training, especially for members of maritime units, such as the SEALs. This exercise strengthens your swimming muscles because it mimics the kind of kick used in a backstroke.

1 Lie on your back with legs straight and your head raised off the floor. Place both hands under your butt to straighten the lumbar spine, and then lift both legs so that your feet are about 6 inches off the floor. Your knees should be bent slightly and your toes pointed away from you.

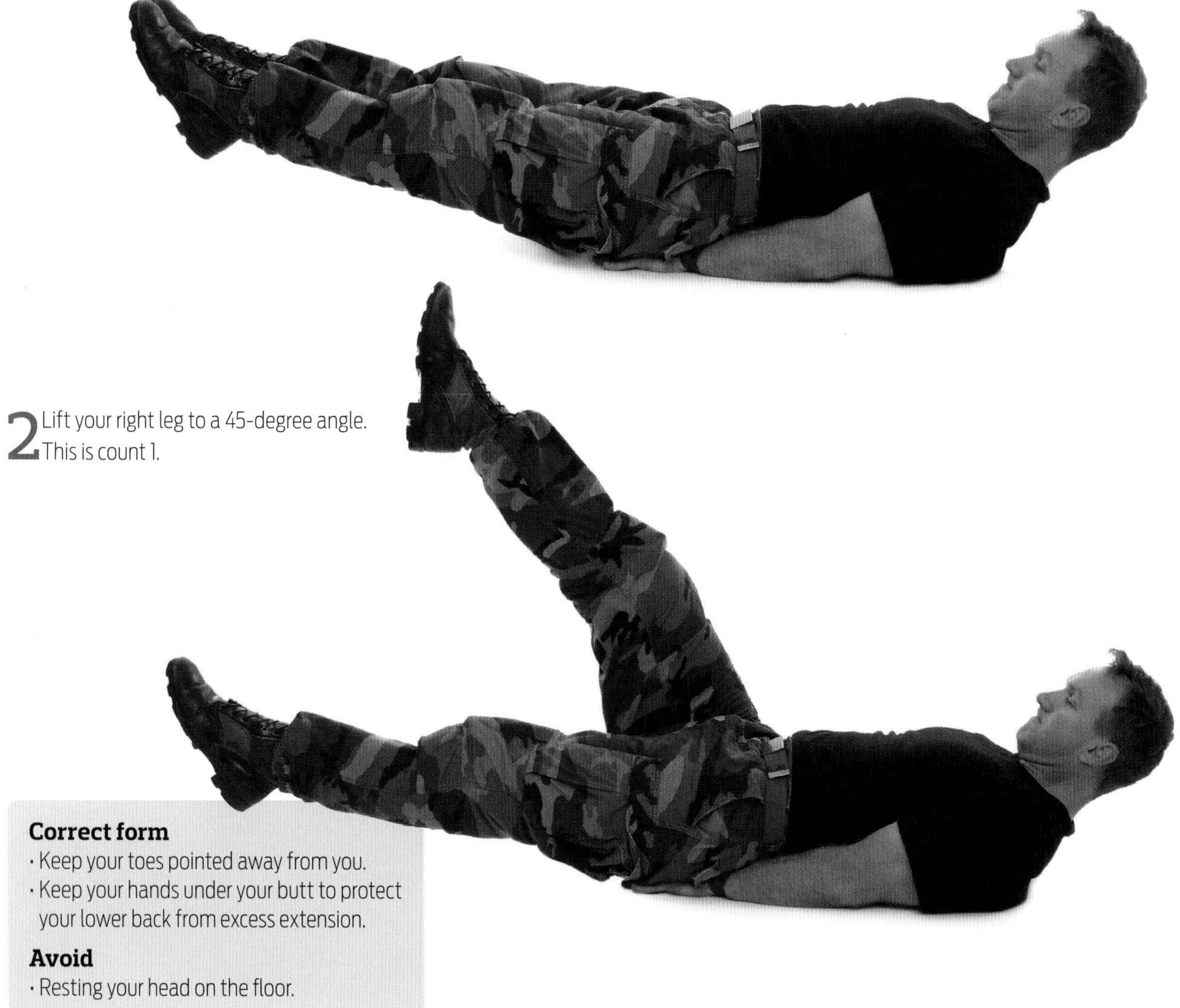

2 Lift your right leg to a 45-degree angle. This is count 1.

**Correct form**

- Keep your toes pointed away from you.
- Keep your hands under your butt to protect your lower back from excess extension.

**Avoid**

- Resting your head on the floor.

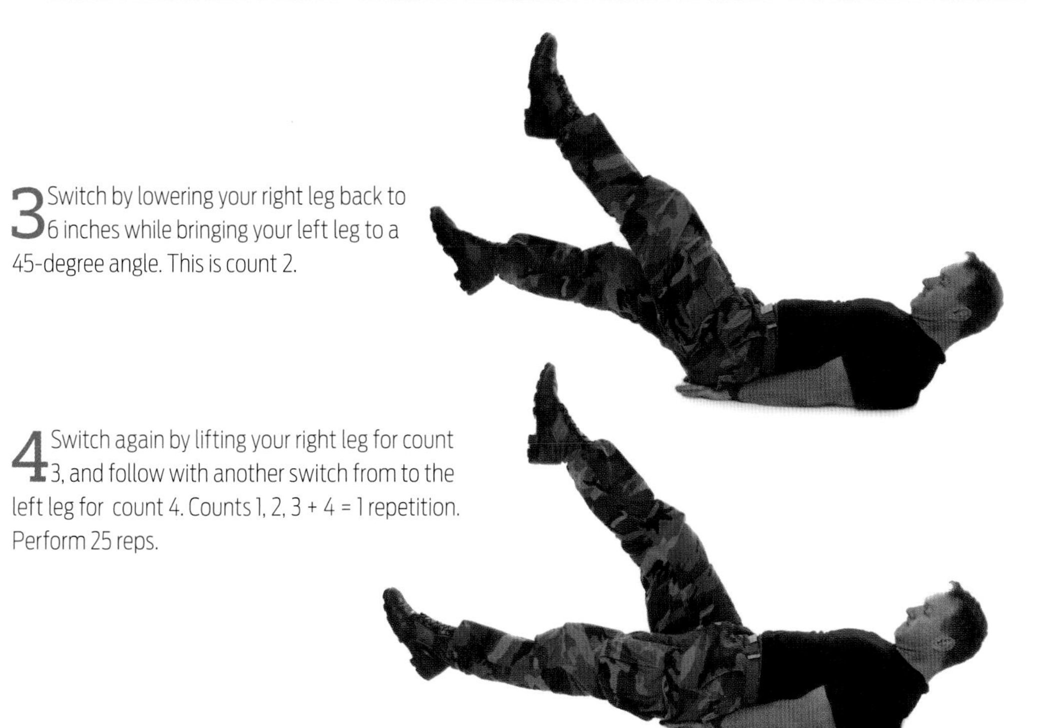

3 Switch by lowering your right leg back to 6 inches while bringing your left leg to a 45-degree angle. This is count 2.

4 Switch again by lifting your right leg for count 3, and follow with another switch from to the left leg for count 4. Counts 1, 2, 3 + 4 = 1 repetition. Perform 25 reps.

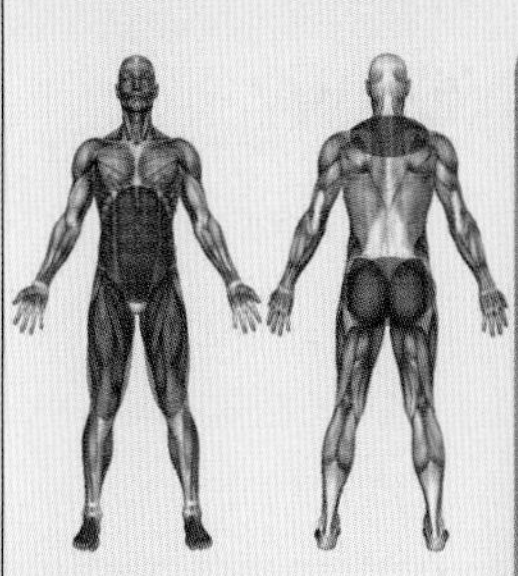

**Level**
- Intermediate

**Duration**
- 30–45 seconds

**Benefits**
- Strengthens abdominals and hip flexors
- Increases running and swimming endurance

**Caution**
- Lower-back pain

**Annotation Key**
* indicates deep muscles

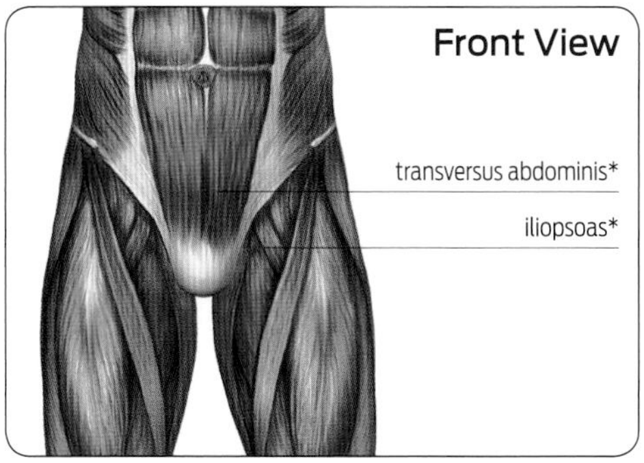

Front View

transversus abdominis*

iliopsoas*

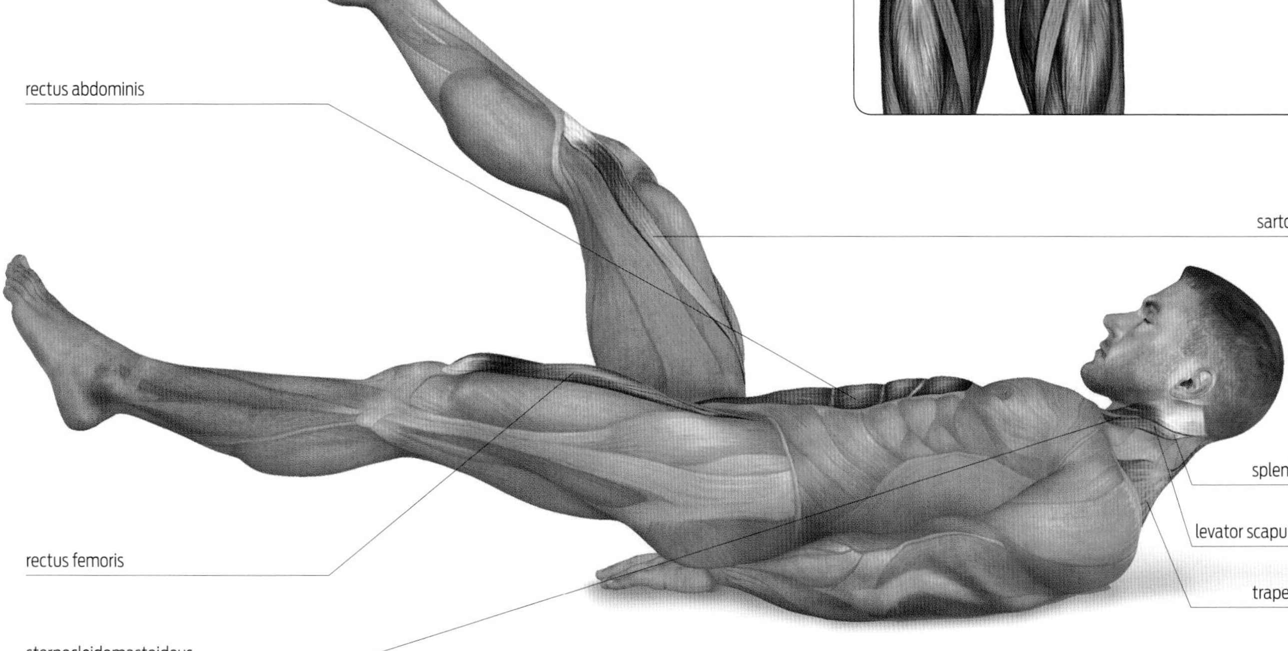

rectus abdominis

sartorius

splenius*

levator scapulae*

trapezius

rectus femoris

sternocleidomastoideus

# Knees to Chest

Knees to Chest targets your lower abs and hip flexors. This exercise is similar to the Flutter Kick (pages 66–67) and the three exercises that follow (see exercise 6-90 on pages 70–71; Good Morning, Darling on pages 72–73; and Leg Levelers on pages 74–75), and it works well in conjunction with them. Knees to Chest is a multiphase exercise featuring four movements performed to a counting beat.

1 Lie on your back with your legs straight and your head raised off the floor. Place both hands under your butt to straighten the lumbar spine, and then lift both legs so that your feet are about 6 inches off the floor. Your knees should be bent slightly.

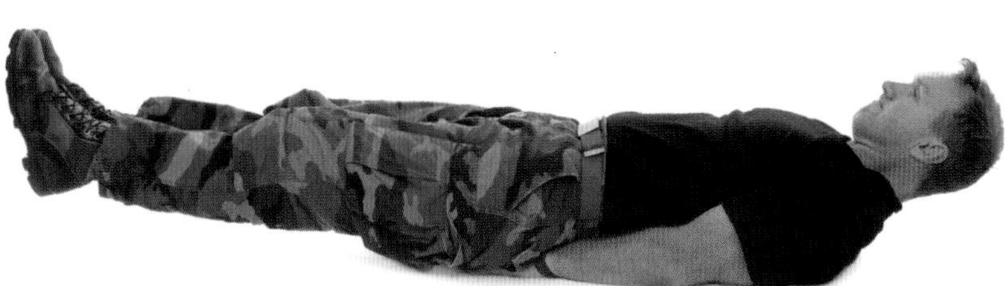

2 Keeping your feet together, bring both knees to your chest for count 1, and then straighten your legs for count 2. Repeat this movement for counts 3 and 4. Counts 1, 2, 3 + 4 = 1 repetition. Perform 25 reps.

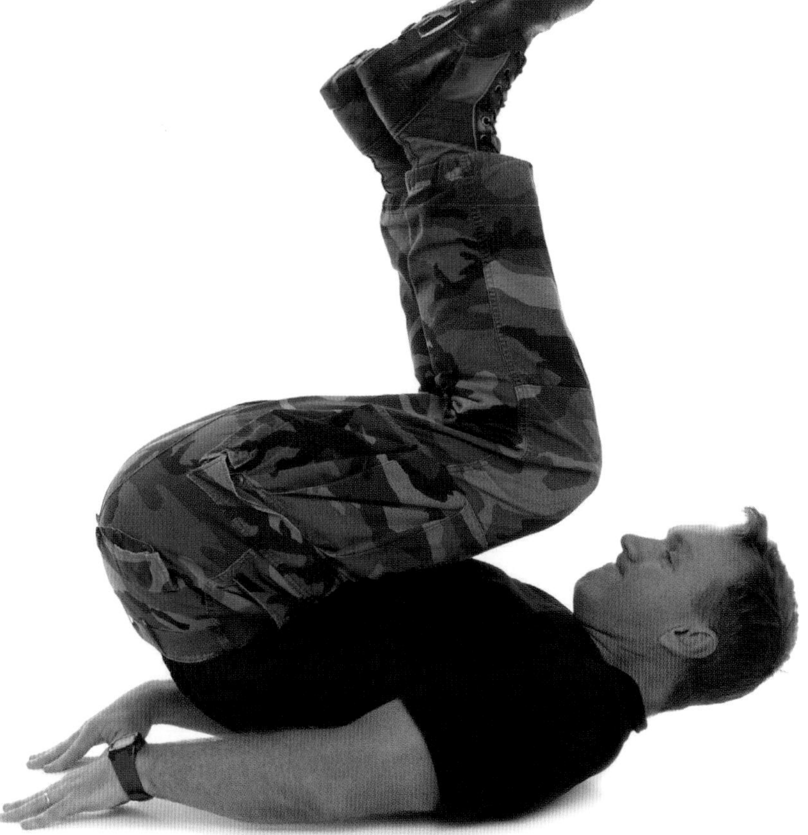

**Correct form**

- Keep your hands under your butt to protect your lower back from excess extension.

**Avoid**

- Resting your head on the floor.

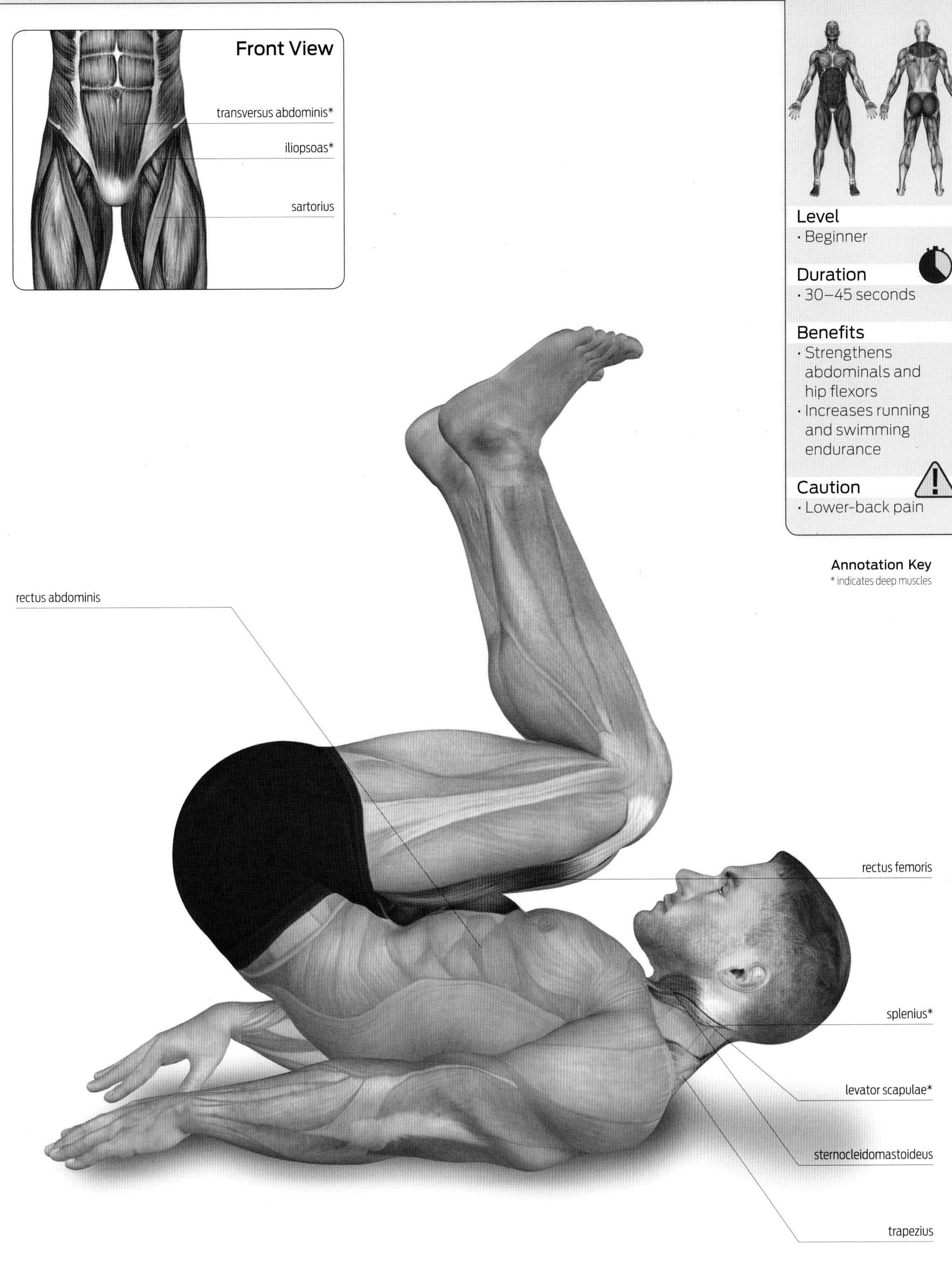


## Level
- Beginner

## Duration
- 30–45 seconds

## Benefits
- Strengthens abdominals and hip flexors
- Increases running and swimming endurance

## Caution
- Lower-back pain

**Annotation Key**
* indicates deep muscles

# 6–90

Like Knees to Chest (see pages 68–69), the 6-90 is a multiphase exercise featuring four movements performed to a counting beat. The "6" in its title stands for "6 inches," and the "90" stands for "90 degrees"—which describes the movement of starting with your feet 6 inches from the floor and raising them until your hips and legs form a 90-degree angle. This exercise works the hip flexors and lower-abdominal muscles, which makes it a great addition to a workout for swimmers and runners.

1 Lie on your back with legs straight and your head raised off the floor. Place both hands under your butt to straighten the lumbar spine, and then lift both legs so that your feet are about 6 inches off the floor.

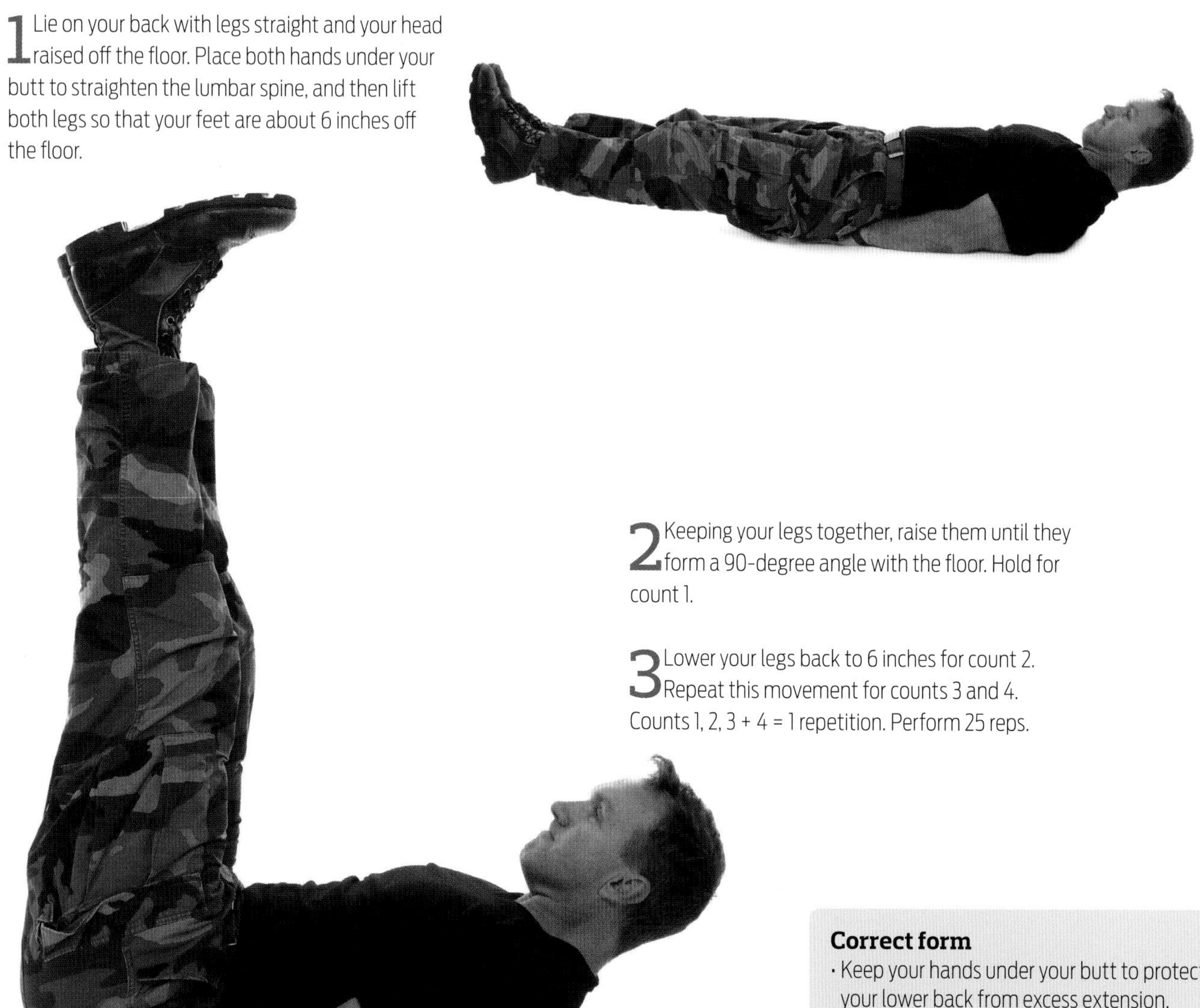

2 Keeping your legs together, raise them until they form a 90-degree angle with the floor. Hold for count 1.

3 Lower your legs back to 6 inches for count 2. Repeat this movement for counts 3 and 4. Counts 1, 2, 3 + 4 = 1 repetition. Perform 25 reps.

**Correct form**

- Keep your hands under your butt to protect your lower back from excess extension.
- Keep your legs as straight as possible.

**Avoid**

- Resting your head on the floor.

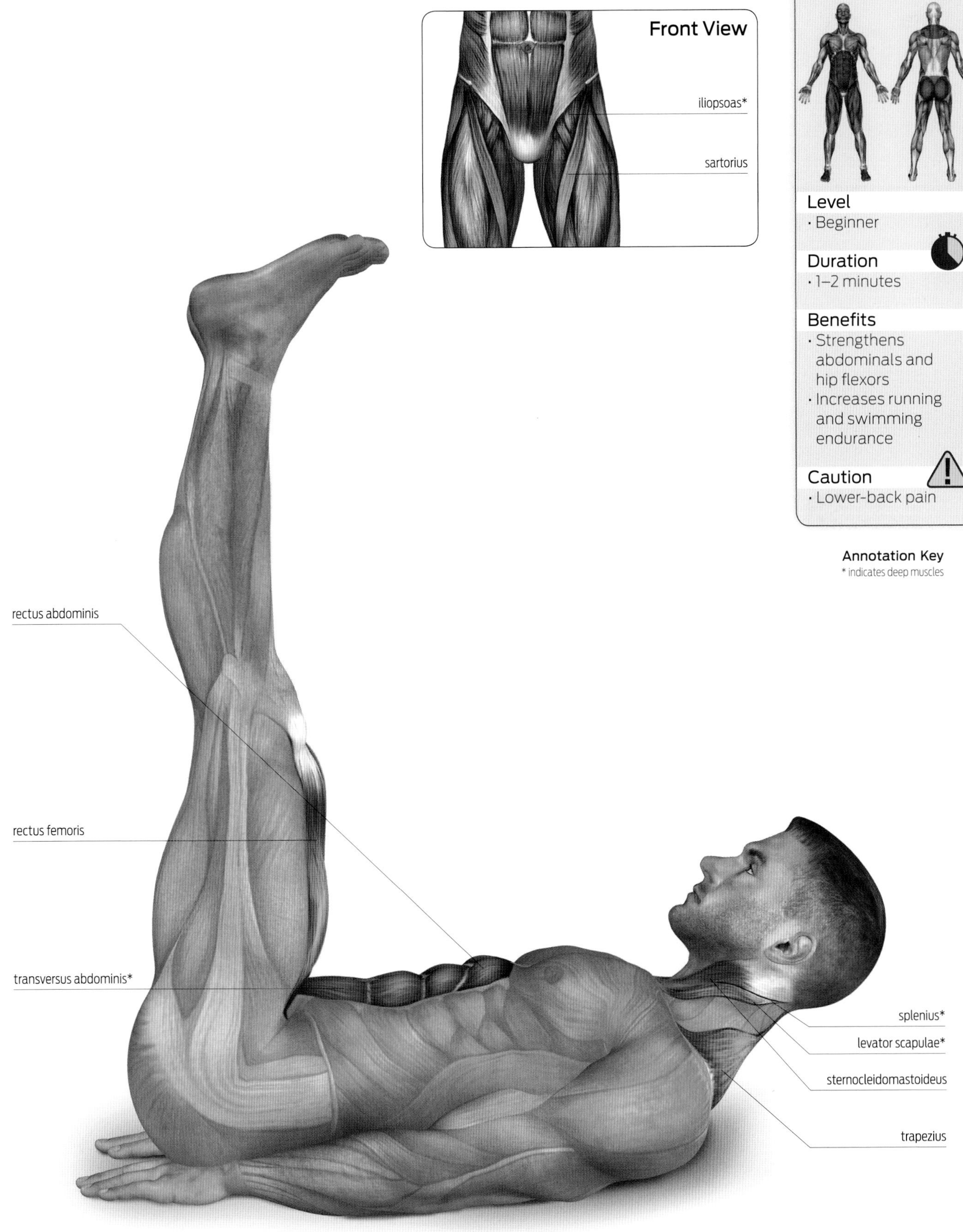


**Level**
- Beginner

**Duration**
- 1–2 minutes

**Benefits**
- Strengthens abdominals and hip flexors
- Increases running and swimming endurance

**Caution**
- Lower-back pain

**Annotation Key**
* indicates deep muscles

# Good Morning, Darling

A movement for the inner and outer thighs, as well as the hip flexors and lower-abdominal muscles, Good Morning, Darling is a must for runners. Running is a hip flexion and extension exercise that neglects the inner and outer thighs, which creates muscular imbalances. Performing this exercise will help keep both the inner and outer thigh muscles strong. It also helps stabilize the knees for people who run on soft surfaces like sand.

1 Lie on your back with legs straight and your head raised off the floor. Place both hands under your butt to straighten the lumbar spine, and then lift both legs so that your feet are about 6 inches off the floor. Your knees should be bent slightly.

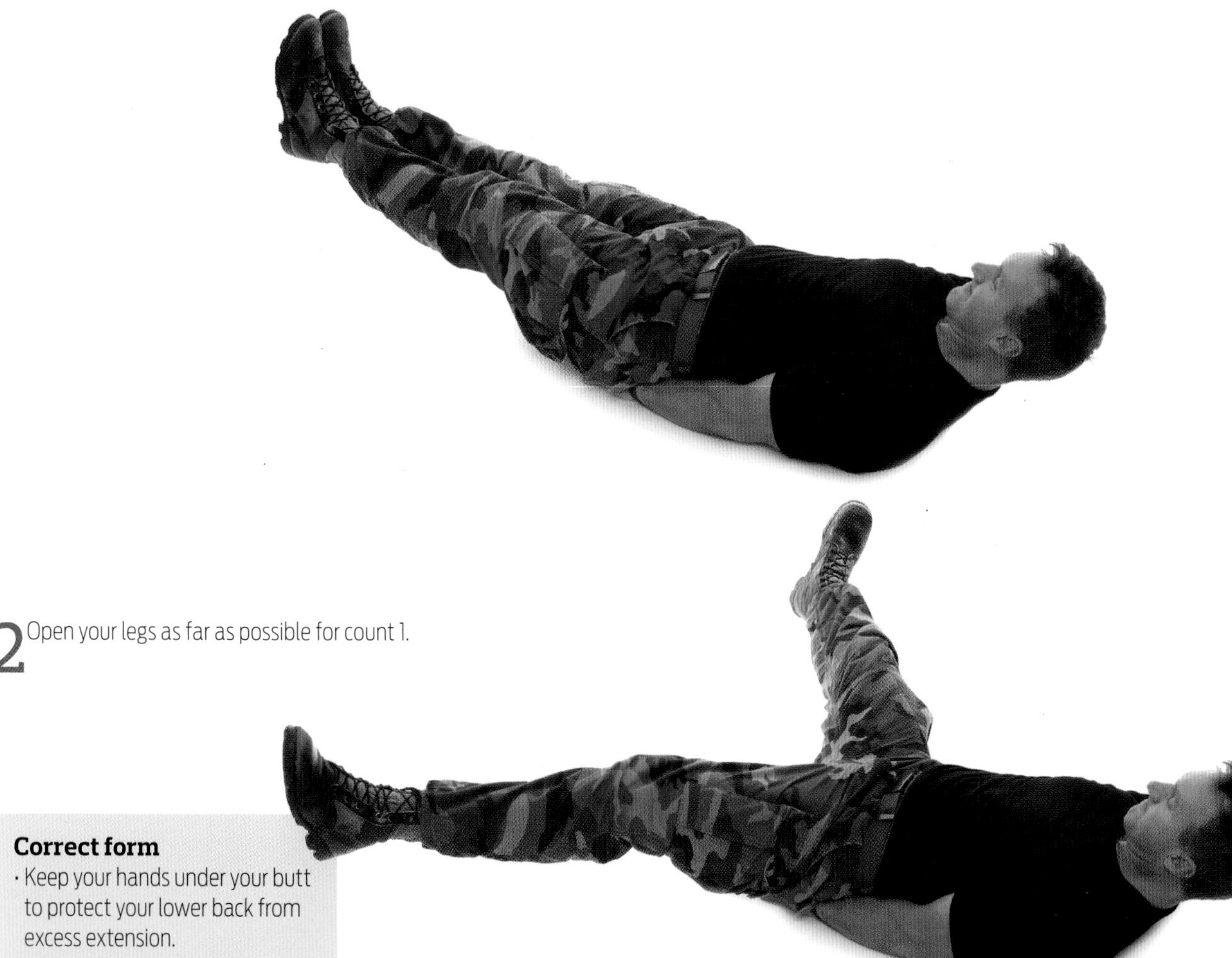

2 Open your legs as far as possible for count 1.

**Correct form**
- Keep your hands under your butt to protect your lower back from excess extension.

**Avoid**
- Resting your head on the floor.

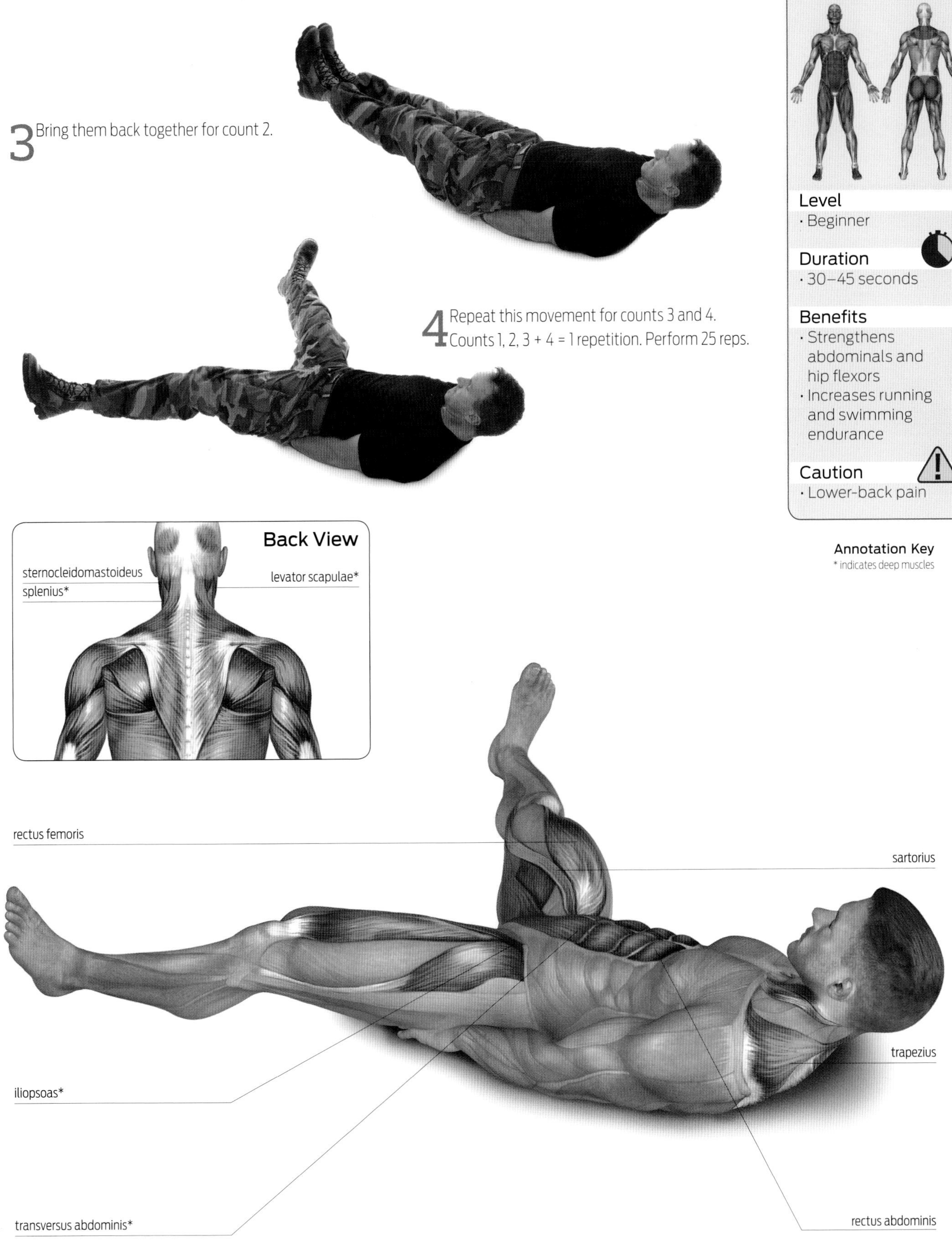


3 Bring them back together for count 2.

4 Repeat this movement for counts 3 and 4. Counts 1, 2, 3 + 4 = 1 repetition. Perform 25 reps.

**Level**
- Beginner

**Duration**
- 30–45 seconds

**Benefits**
- Strengthens abdominals and hip flexors
- Increases running and swimming endurance

**Caution**
- Lower-back pain

**Annotation Key**
* indicates deep muscles

# Leg Levelers

Leg Levelers is similar to the 6-90 exercise (pages 70–71), but instead of raising your legs to 90 degrees, you will only lift them to 45 degrees. This exercise is a quick movement, similar to performing the Flutter Kick (pages 66–67) while keeping your legs together.

1 Lie on your back with legs straight and your head raised off the floor. Place both hands under your butt to straighten the lumbar spine, and then lift both legs so that your feet are about 6 inches off the floor. Your knees should be bent slightly.

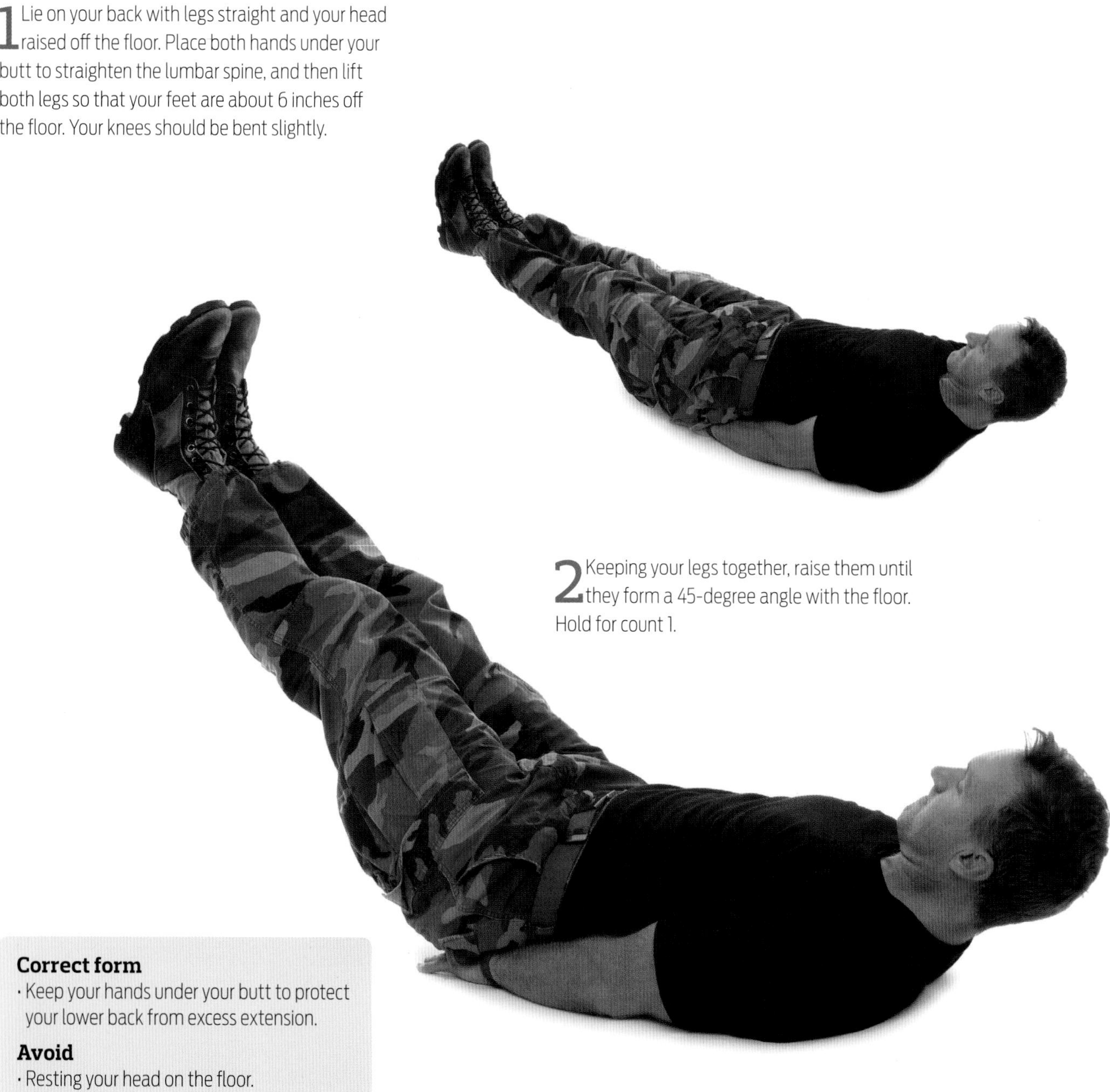

2 Keeping your legs together, raise them until they form a 45-degree angle with the floor. Hold for count 1.

**Correct form**

- Keep your hands under your butt to protect your lower back from excess extension.

**Avoid**

- Resting your head on the floor.

3 Lower your legs back to 6 inches for count 2. Repeat this movement for counts 3 and 4. Counts 1, 2, 3 + 4 = 1 repetition. Perform 25 reps.

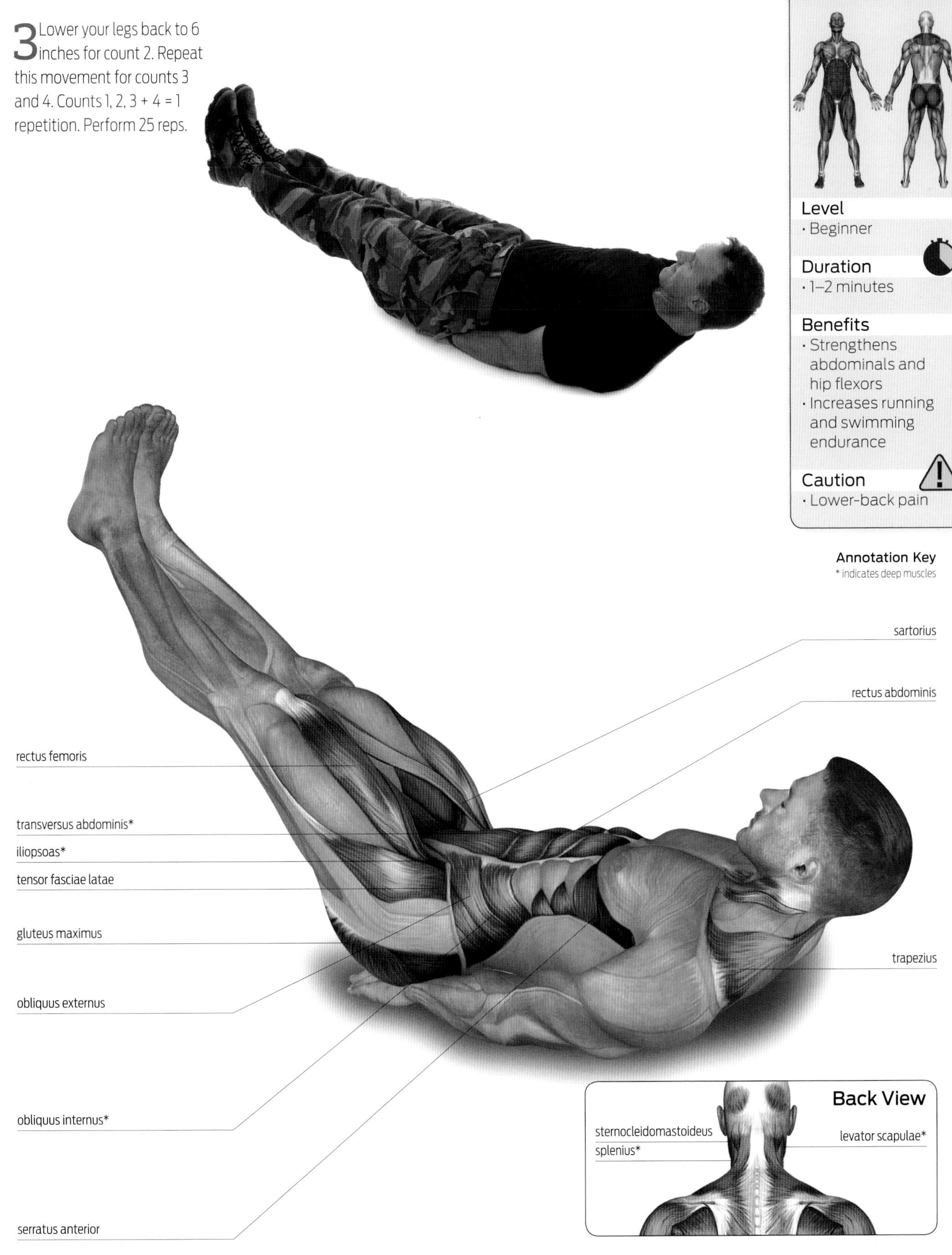


**Level**
- Beginner

**Duration**
- 1–2 minutes

**Benefits**
- Strengthens abdominals and hip flexors
- Increases running and swimming endurance

**Caution**
- Lower-back pain

**Annotation Key**
* indicates deep muscles

# Pull–Up: Neutral Grip

One of the exercises used in special forces qualifying tests, the Pull-Up is a fundamental upper-body-strength movement that targets your latissimus dorsi. It calls for you to pull your own body weight, so heavier people tend to have more trouble performing this exercise. Adjustable pull-up bars that can be installed in a home doorway are readily available.

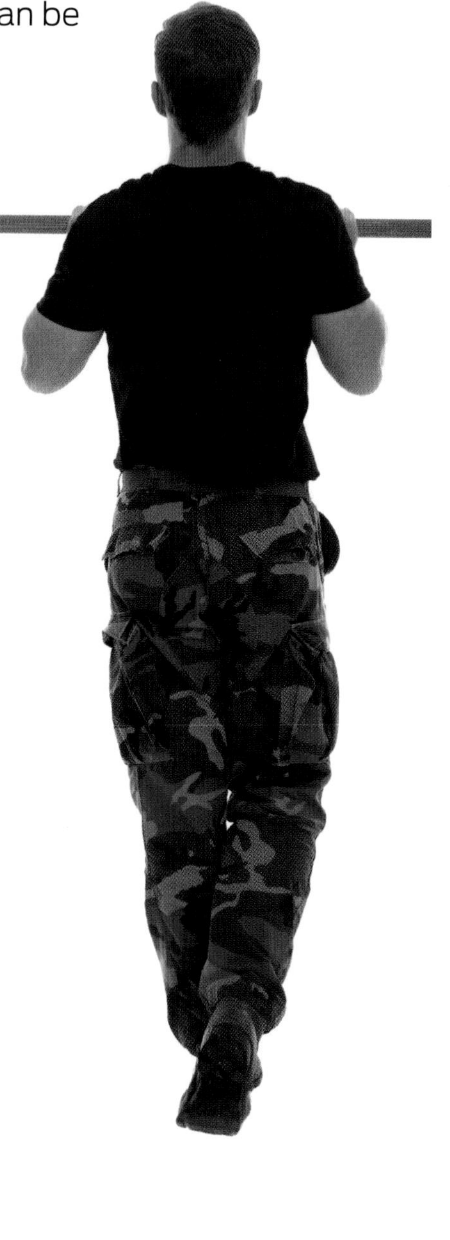

1 Place your hands shoulder-width apart on a bar, and hang until your arms are straight.

2 Pull yourself up until your chest touches the bar. Hold yourself in this position for one second, and then lower yourself slowly to the hanging position.

3 Repeat, performing 10 reps in total.

**Correct form**
- Be sure your arms are straight in the hanging position, or the rep does not count.
- To strengthen your grip while performing pull-ups, grip your thumb over the top of the bar rather than wrapping it around the bar.

**Avoid**
- Kipping, or swinging, your body during the pull-up—a kipping movement can injure your rotator cuffs.

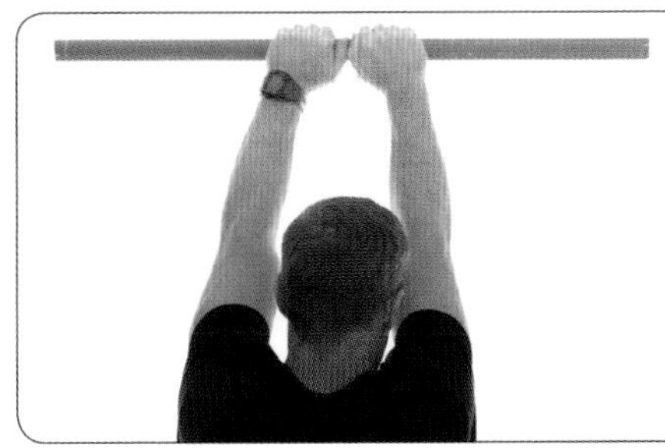

## Modification

**Same difficulty:** To perform Pull-Up: Close Grip, grasp the bar with a firm overhand grip with your hands touching or separated by no more than 6 inches. Continue as you would for Pull-Up: Neutral Grip. The narrow separation between your hands in this variation of the Pull-Up ensures greater emphasis on your lower lats.

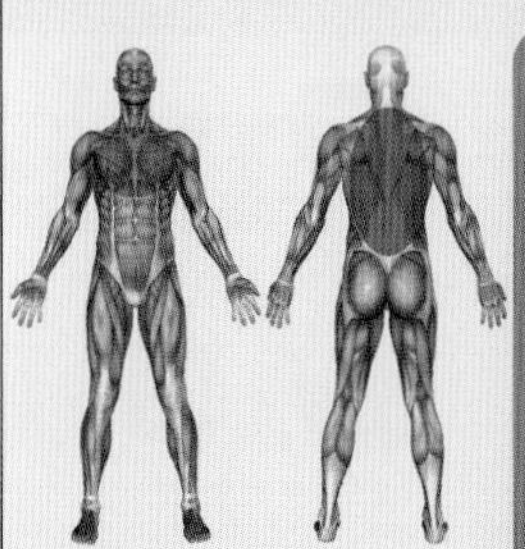

**Level**
· Intermediate

**Duration**
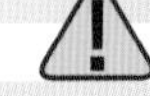
· 15–30 seconds

**Benefits**
· Strengthens upper body

**Caution**
· Shoulder issues
· Wrist issues

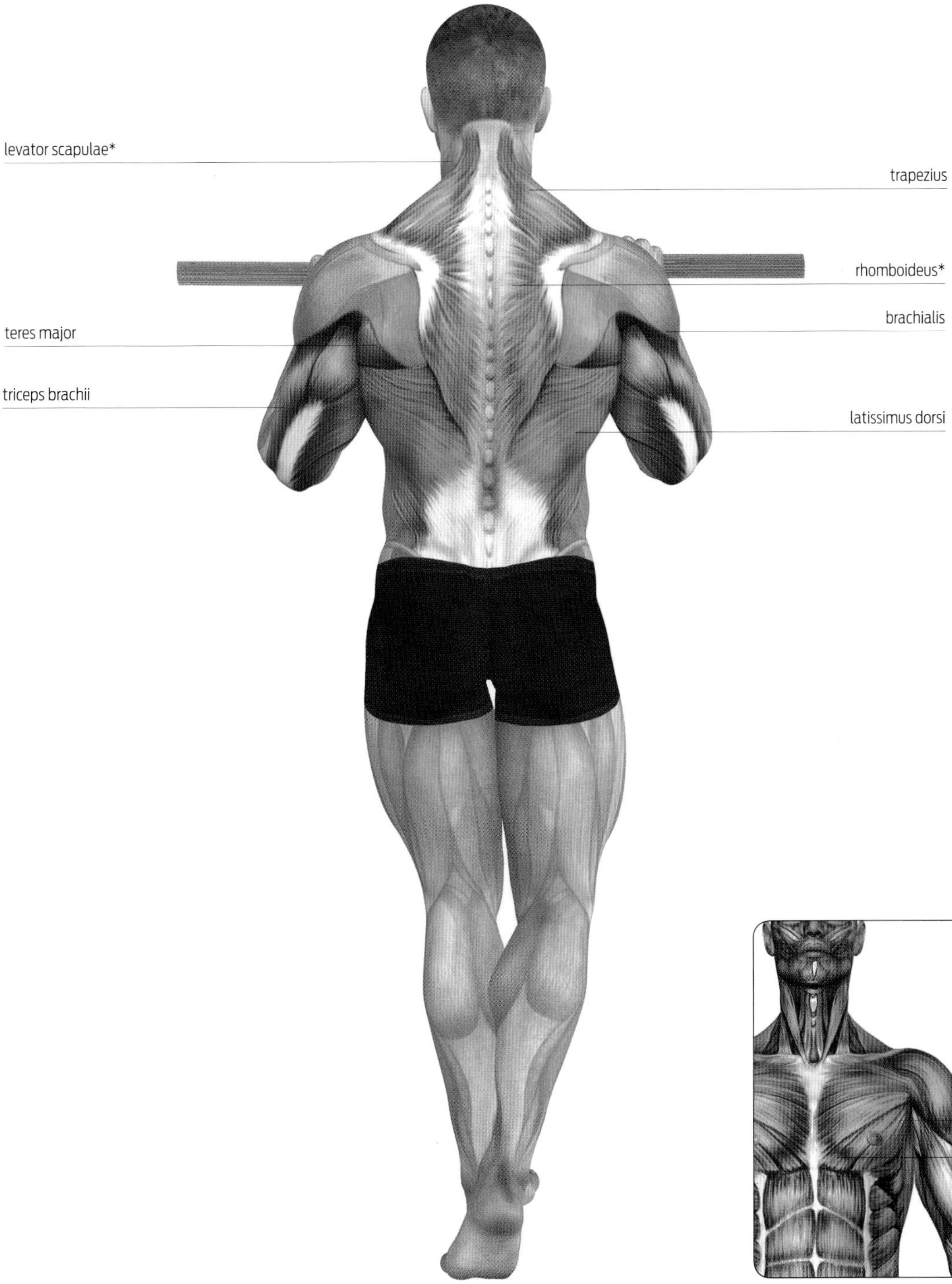

levator scapulae*

trapezius

rhomboideus*

brachialis

teres major

triceps brachii

latissimus dorsi

**Annotation Key**
* indicates deep muscles

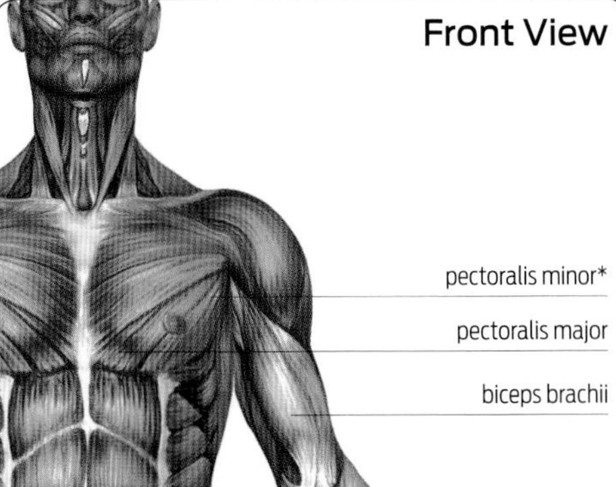

# Pull-Up: Mountain-Climber Grip

Special forces teams perform Pull-Ups with many different grips to simulate situations such as pulling the body into windows or up ropes and climbing mountains. Different grips also work the back and forearms at different angles, adding to your overall fitness ability. In Pull-Up: Mountain-Climber Grip, the bar will be at your side, rather than facing you. This version is also called the Commando Pull-Up.

1 Place one hand in front of the other on the bar with palms facing each other, and wrap your fingers around the bar.

2 Pull yourself up until your chin is over the bar. Hold yourself in this position for one second, and then lower yourself slowly, stopping just before your arms are completely straight.

3 Repeat, performing 20 reps in total.

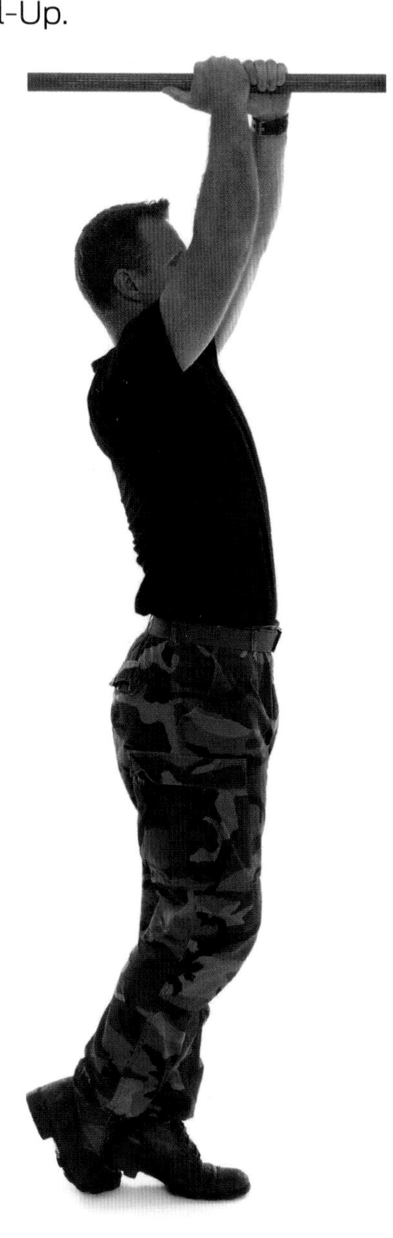

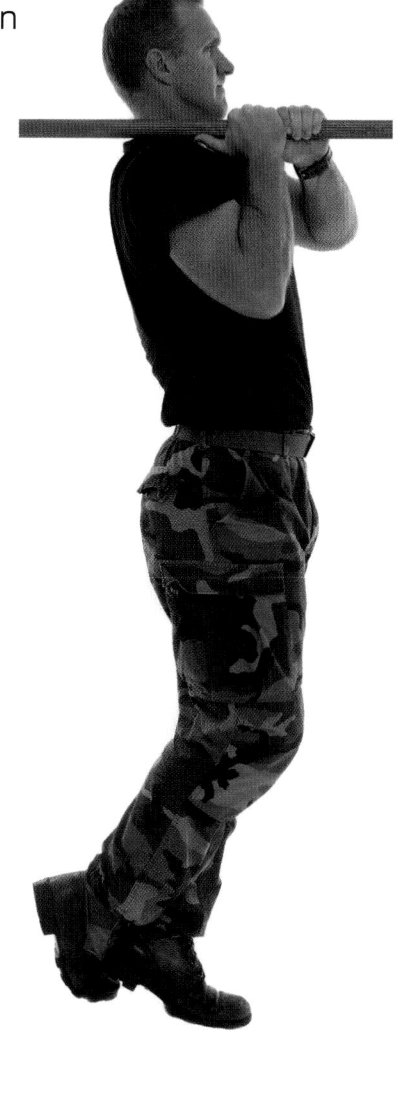

**Correct form**
- Place whichever hand feels the most comfortable closest to your head.
- Pull your body as high onto the bar as possible.

**Avoid**
- Kipping, or swinging, your body—a kipping movement can injure your rotator cuffs.
- Lowering yourself until your arms are perfectly straight—this is called a "dead hang."

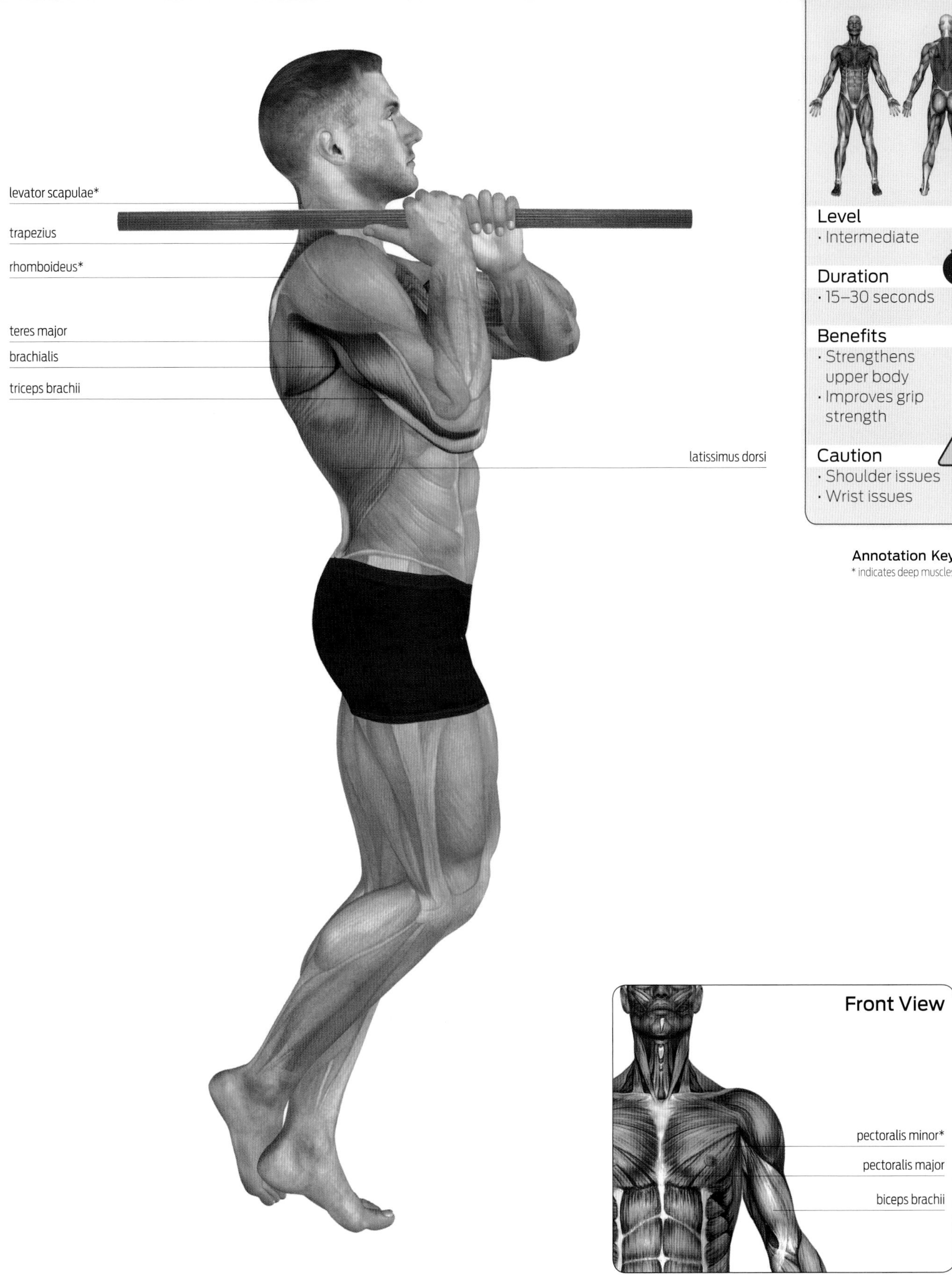


**Level**
· Intermediate

**Duration**
· 15–30 seconds

**Benefits**
· Strengthens upper body
· Improves grip strength

**Caution**
· Shoulder issues
· Wrist issues

**Annotation Key**
* indicates deep muscles

# Pull–Up: Reverse Grip

Sometimes referred to as "Chin-Ups for Chins," Pull-Up: Reverse Grip has you grasp the bar with your palms facing you, which places more focus on the biceps than other Pull-Ups. It is a great variation to add to your upper-body workout routine.

1 Place both hands on the bar with palms facing your head, and hang until your arms are straight.

2 Pull yourself up until your chin is over the bar. Hold yourself in this position for one second, and then lower yourself slowly, stopping just before your arms are completely straight.

3 Repeat, performing 20 reps in total.

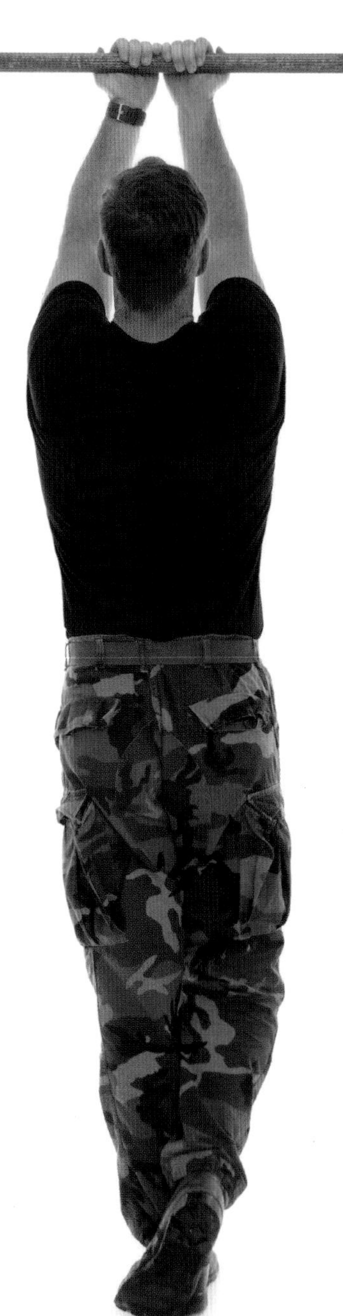

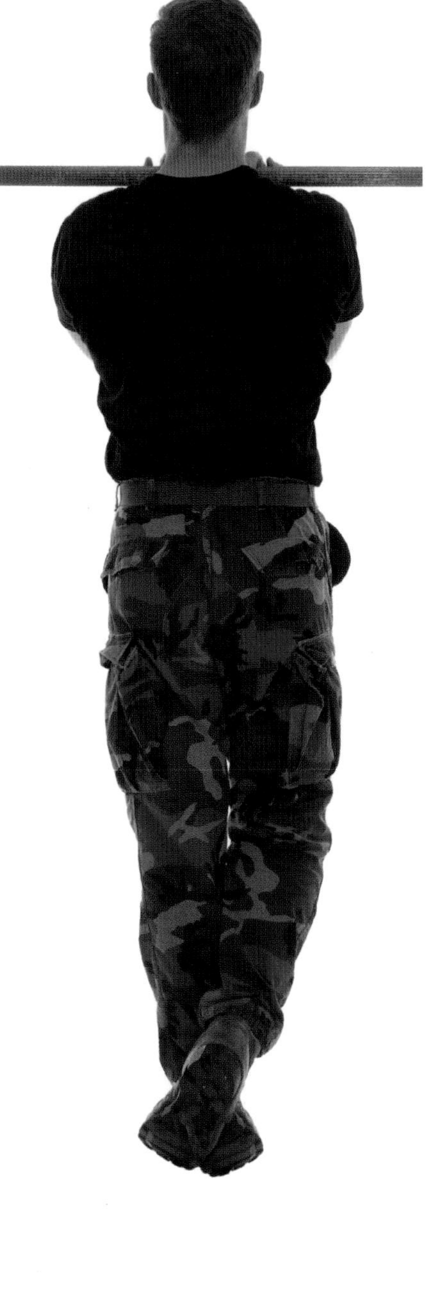

**Correct form**

- Pull your body as high onto the bar as possible—your chin over the bar is the minimum height.

**Avoid**

- Kipping, or swinging, your body—a kipping movement can injure your rotator cuffs.

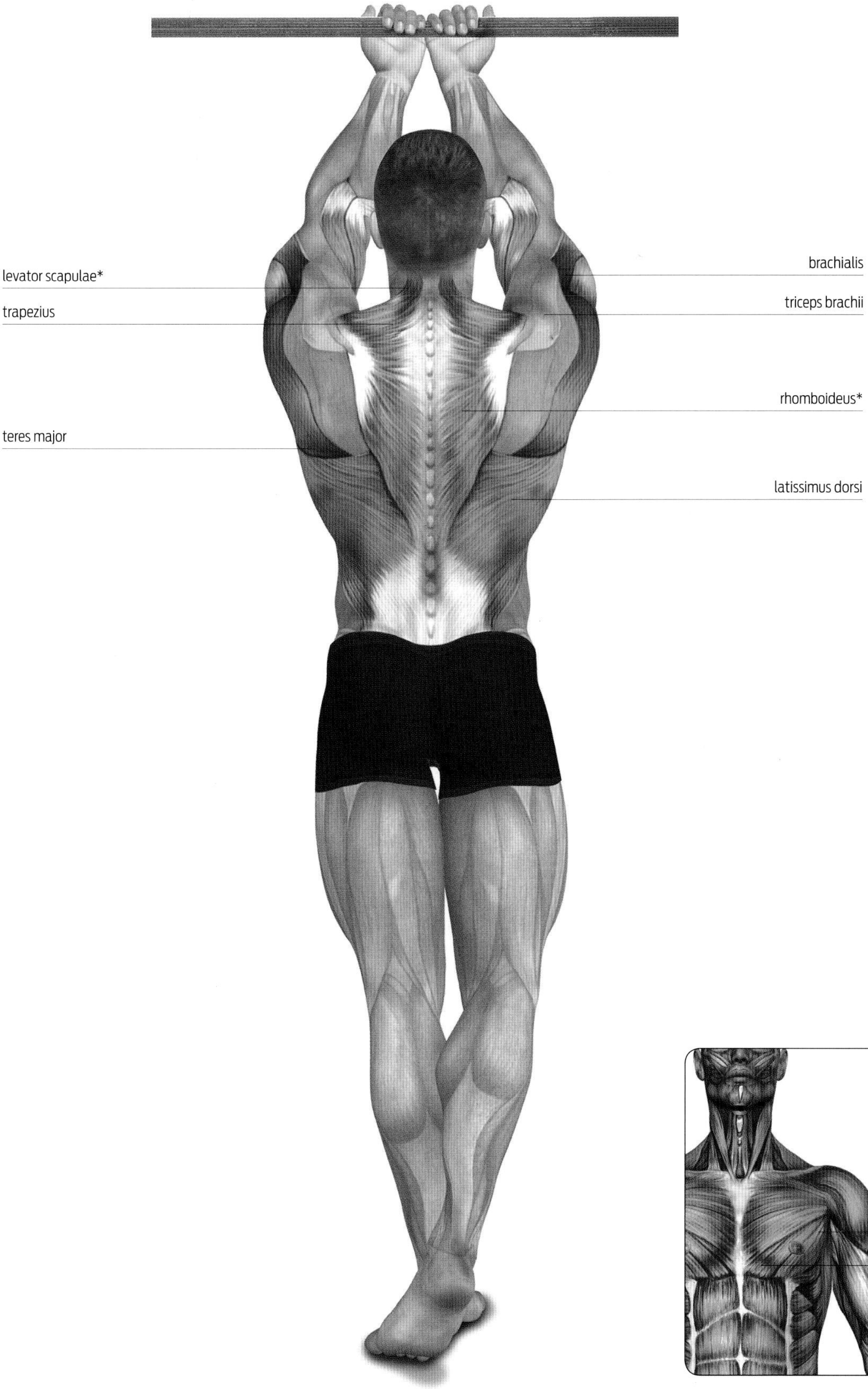

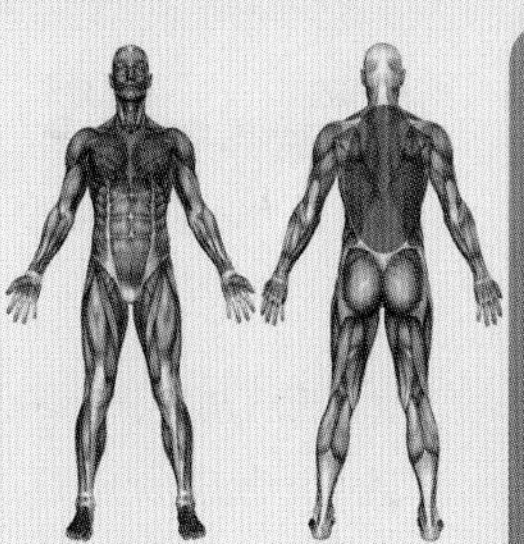

**Level**
- Beginner

**Duration**
- 15–30 seconds

**Benefits**
- Strengthens upper body
- Strengthens biceps

**Caution**
- Shoulder issues
- Wrist issues

**Annotation Key**
* indicates deep muscles

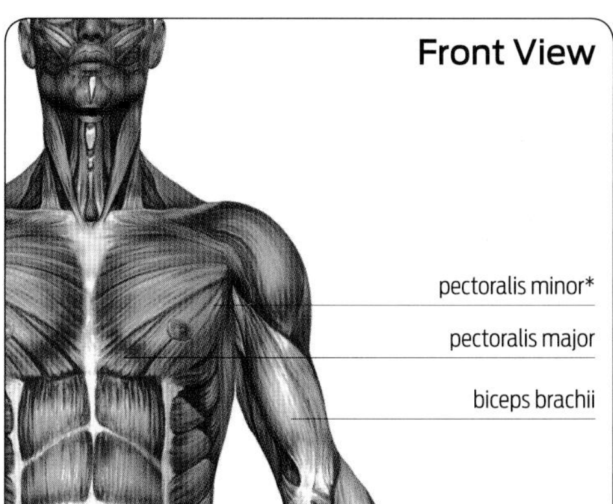

# Pull–Up: Wide Grip

Pull-Up: Wide Grip is a challenging exercise. It calls for you to engage your latissimus dorsi more than the rhomboids, as you would in closer-grip versions of the Pull-Up. Lifting your entire body weight in this position may be hard to master, but your practice will be well worth the effort, paying off with greater back strength and development.

1 Place your hands on the bar with your palms facing away from you, spacing them as wide as possible.

2 Pull yourself up until y our chest touches the bar. Hold yourself in this position for one second, and then lower yourself slowly to the hanging position.

3 Repeat, performing 20 reps in total.

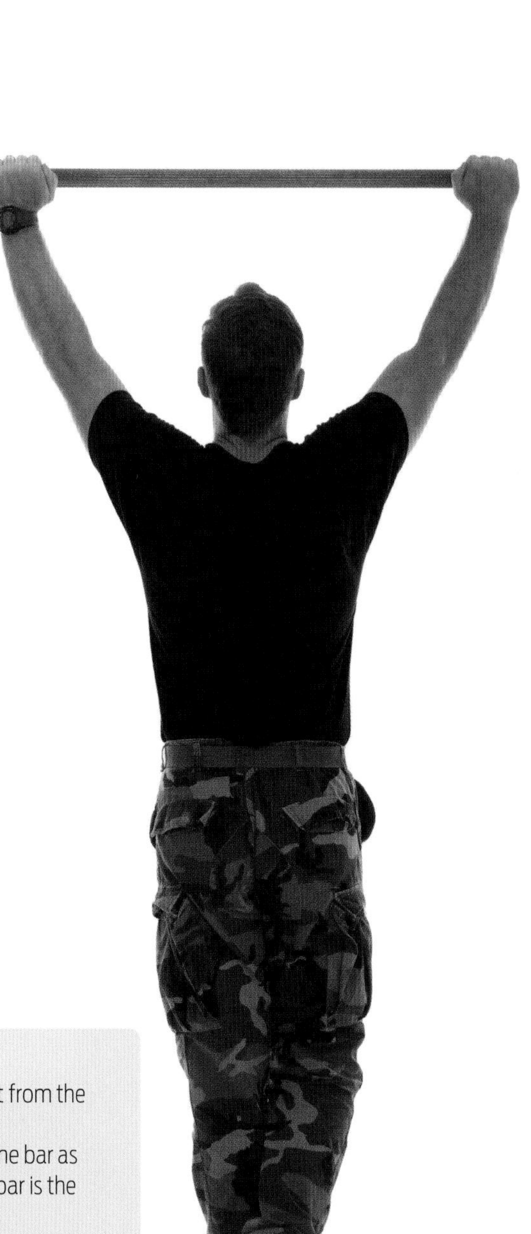

**Correct form**

- Start and end the movement from the dead hang position.
- Pull your body as high onto the bar as possible—your chin over the bar is the minimum height.

**Avoid**

- Kipping, or swinging, your body—a kipping movement can injure your rotator cuffs.

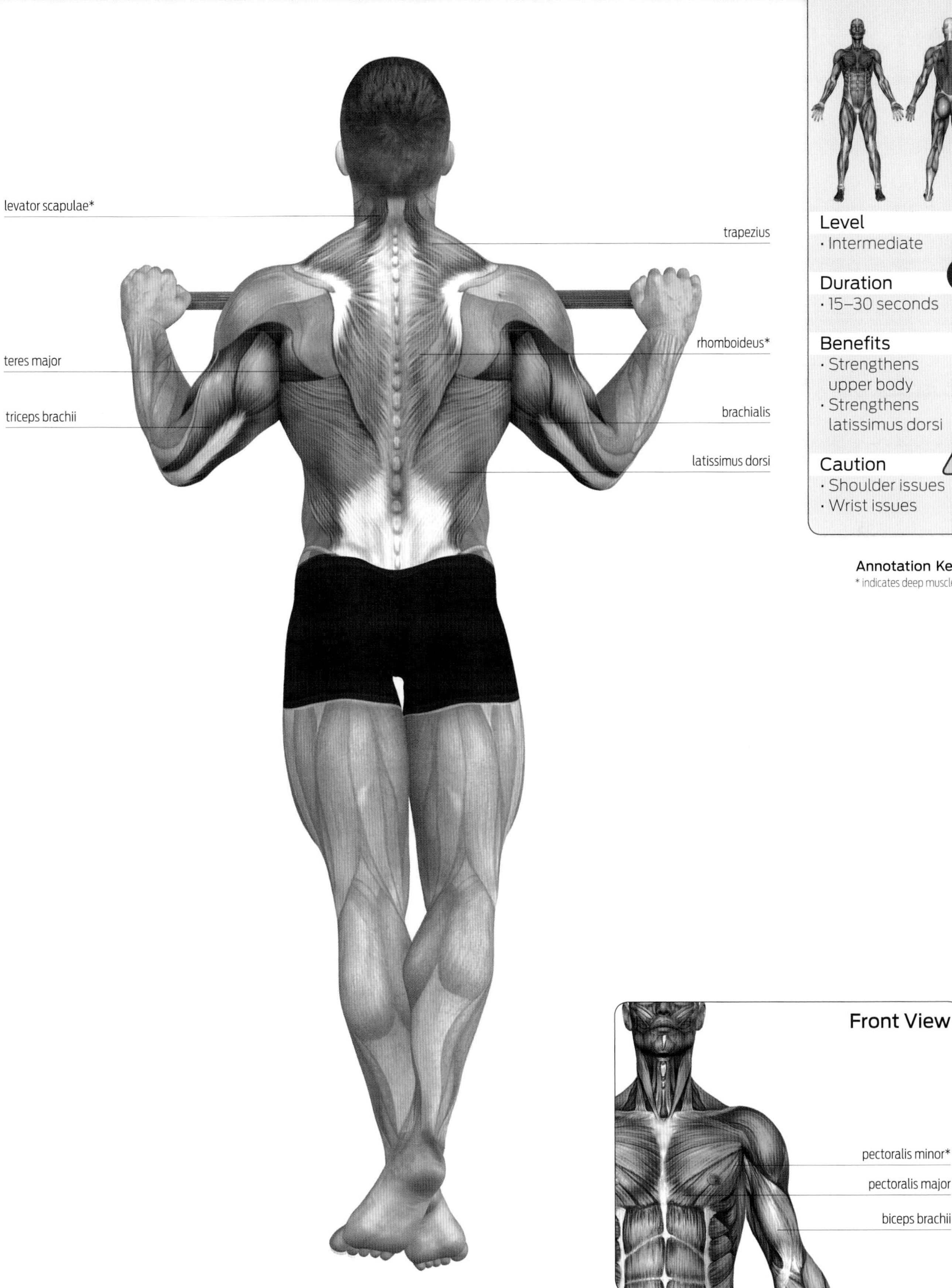


## Level
· Intermediate

## Duration
· 15–30 seconds

## Benefits
· Strengthens upper body
· Strengthens latissimus dorsi

## Caution
· Shoulder issues
· Wrist issues

**Annotation Key**
* indicates deep muscles

# Chair Dip

Any dip exercise targets the triceps brachii, the three-headed muscle at the back of your upper arm. In training, special forces candidates perform this exercise on parallel bars, but you can easily perform the Chair Dip version at home on a sturdy chair, sofa, or bench. Much like a Pull-Up, you are lifting your own body weight, so heavier people may find this a challenge at first.

1 Sit up tall on the front edge of a sturdy chair or bench. Place your hands beside your hips, wrapping your fingers over the front edge of the chair. Extend your legs, flexing your feet upward so that just your heels touch the floor.

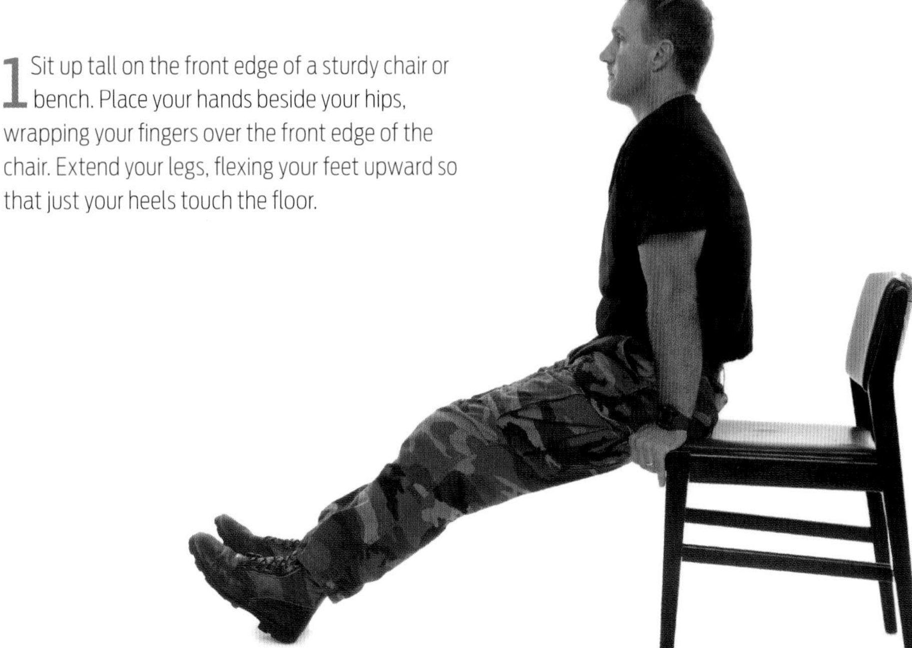

2 Scoot off the edge so that your torso will be able to clear the chair as you dip down.

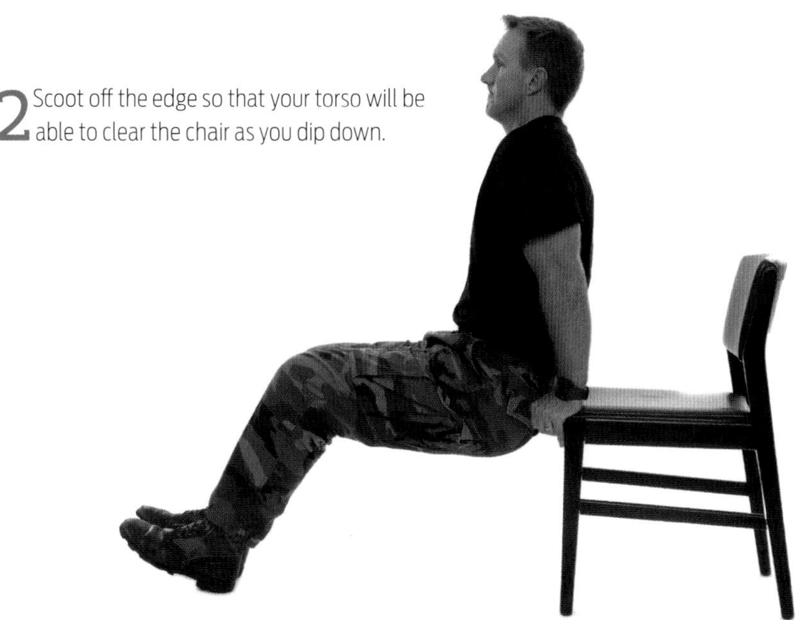

**Correct form**

- Keep your body close to the chair.
- Keep your spine in neutral position throughout the movement.
- Keep your feet in the same position throughout the movement.

**Avoid**

- Pushing up solely with your feet, rather than using your arm strength.
- Dipping below a 90-degree angle; this places stress on the shoulder and elbow joints.
- Splaying your elbows outward as you dip.

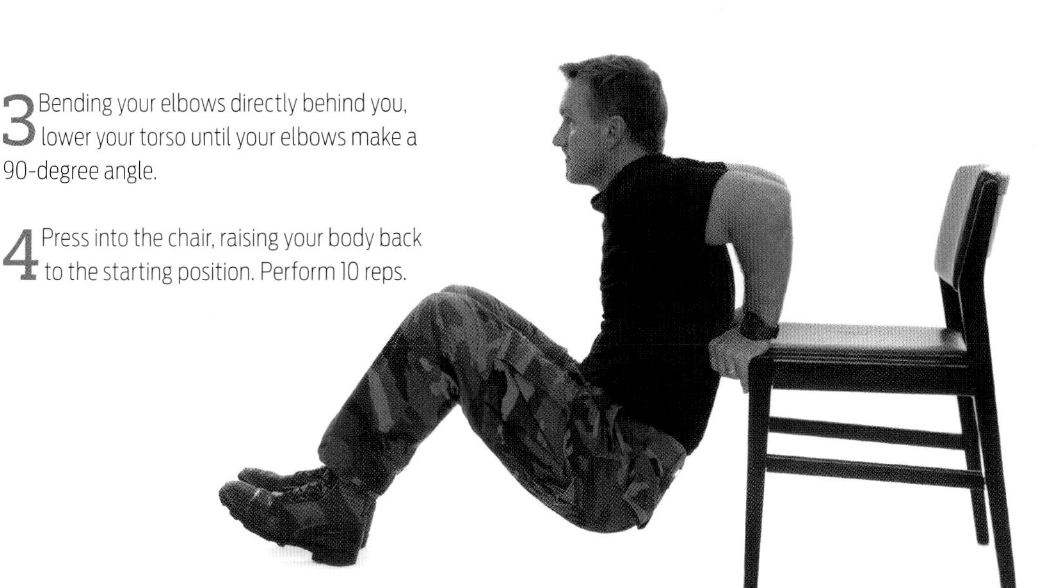

3 Bending your elbows directly behind you, lower your torso until your elbows make a 90-degree angle.

4 Press into the chair, raising your body back to the starting position. Perform 10 reps.

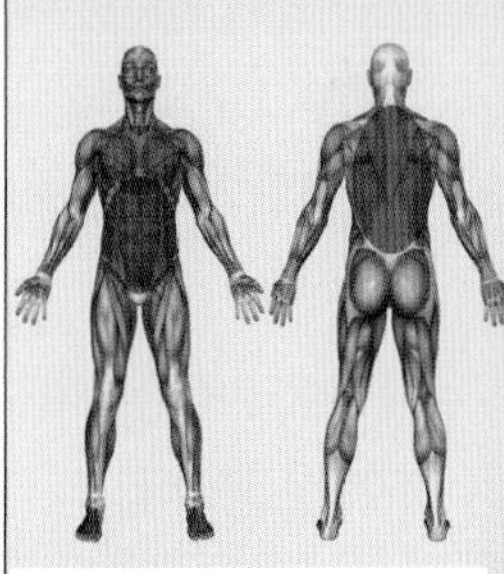

**Level**
· Beginner

**Duration**
· 45–60 seconds

**Benefits**
· Strengthens triceps

**Caution**

· Shoulder issues
· Wrist issues
· Elbow pain

**Annotation Key**
* indicates deep muscles

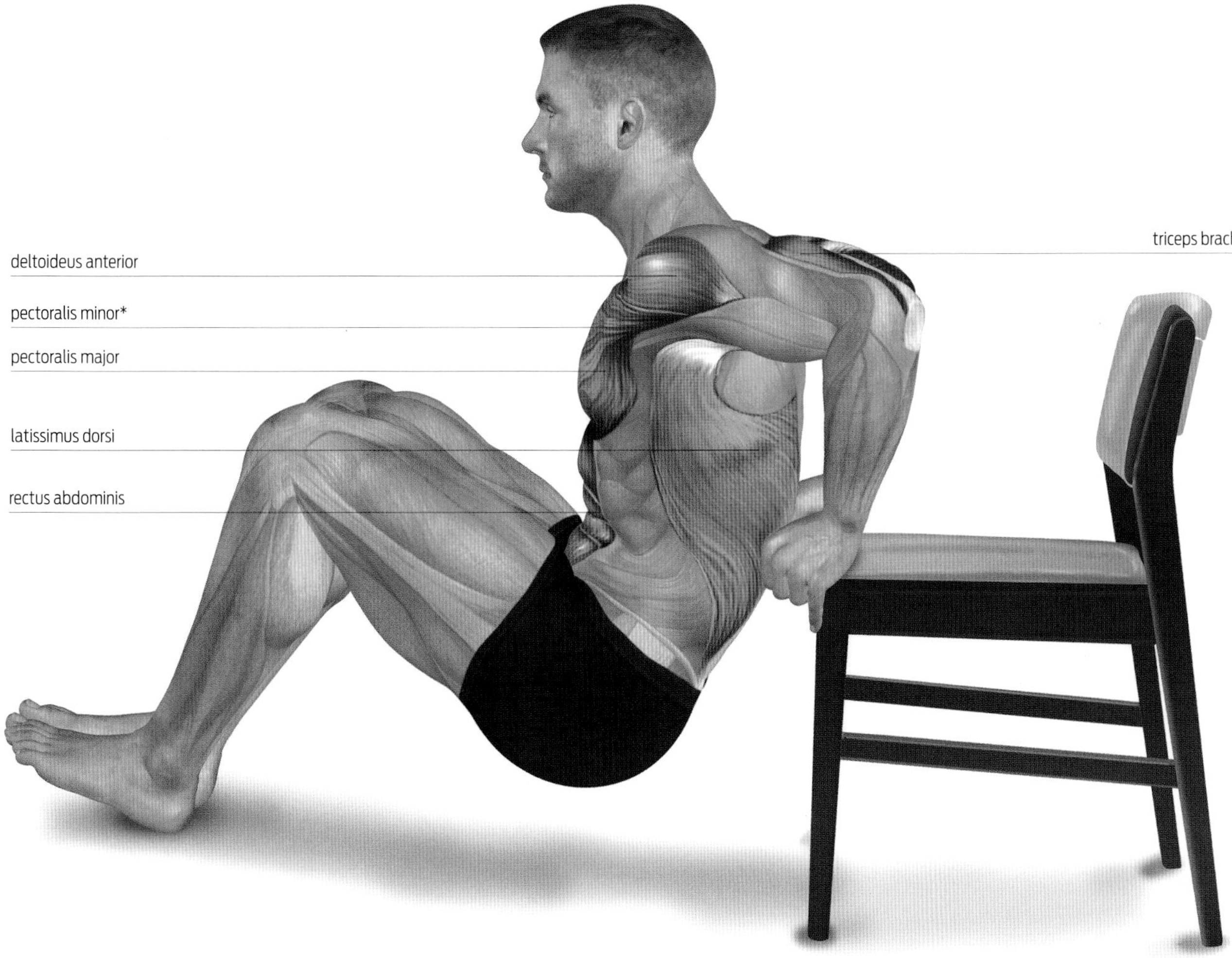

deltoideus anterior

pectoralis minor*

pectoralis major

latissimus dorsi

rectus abdominis

triceps brachii

# 8-Count Body Builder

The 8-Count Body Builder is a multiphase exercise featuring eight movements performed to a counting beat. This combination of Push-Ups with Squats will really put you through your paces, offering a mix of intense cardio and resistance training. Devised to train military recruits as effectively as possible, this exercise promotes weight loss and builds lean muscles. Each 1-to-8 count equals one rep.

1 For the number 1 count, assume a full squat with your torso folded over your bent knees and your hands flat on the floor. Rest lightly on the balls of your feet.

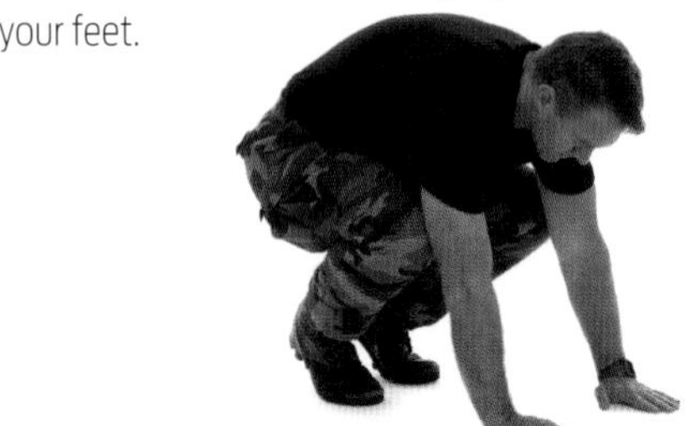

2 Kick your legs backward into Drop Position for count 2.

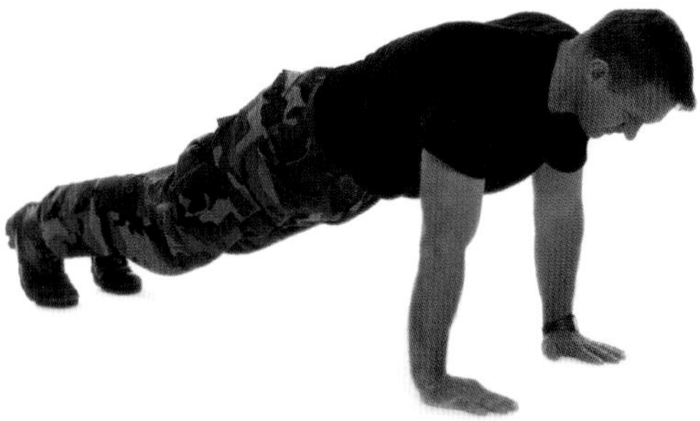

3 Push downwards for a Push-Up until your chest touches the floor for count 3.

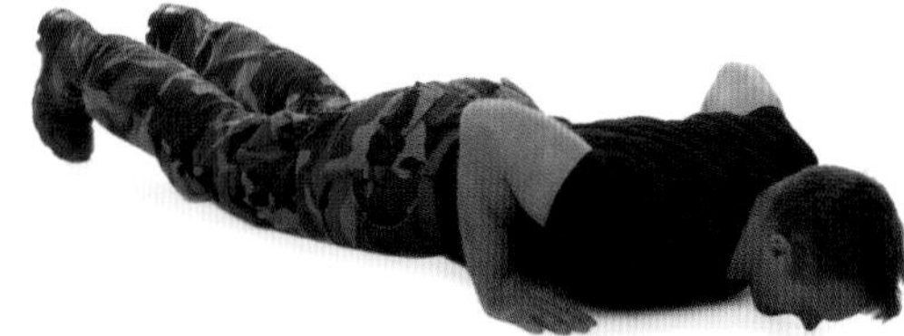

**Correct form**

- Keep your hands close to your chest in the Push-Up position.

**Avoid**

- Resting your chest on the floor on count 3.

4 Press back up to straighten your arms for count 4.

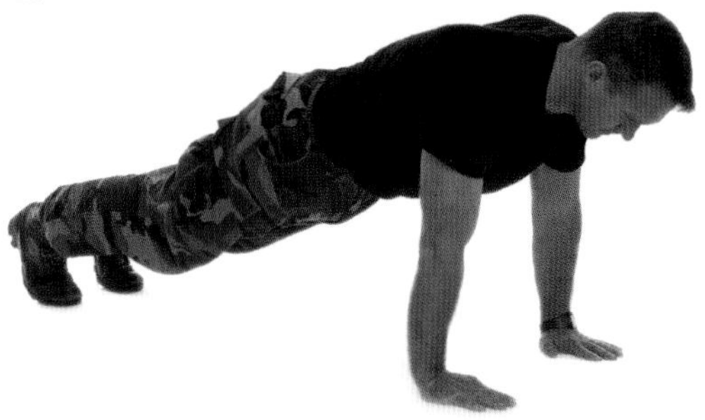

5 Spread your legs for count 5.

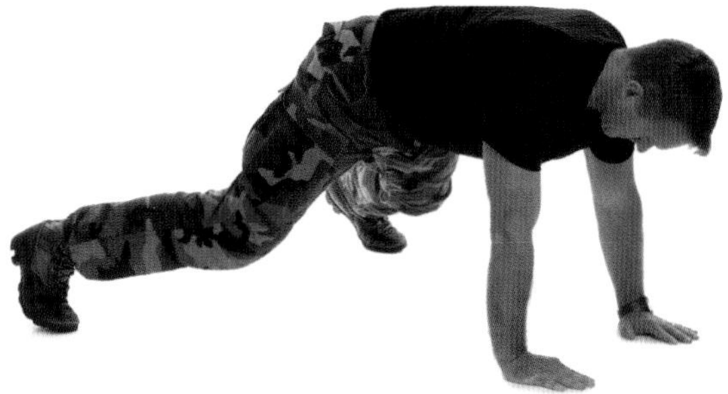

6 Close your legs for count 6.

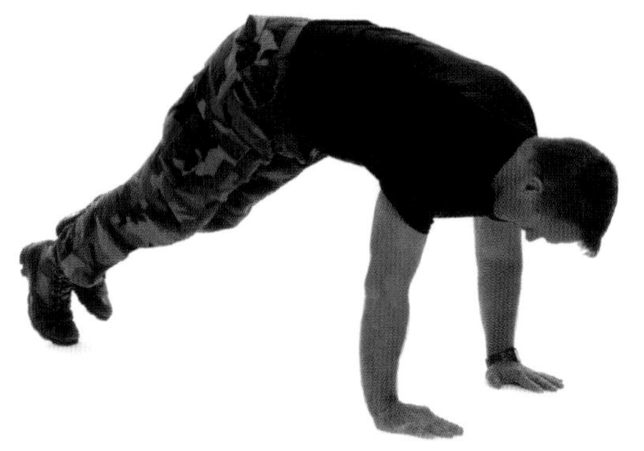

7 Jump both knees to your chest for count 7.

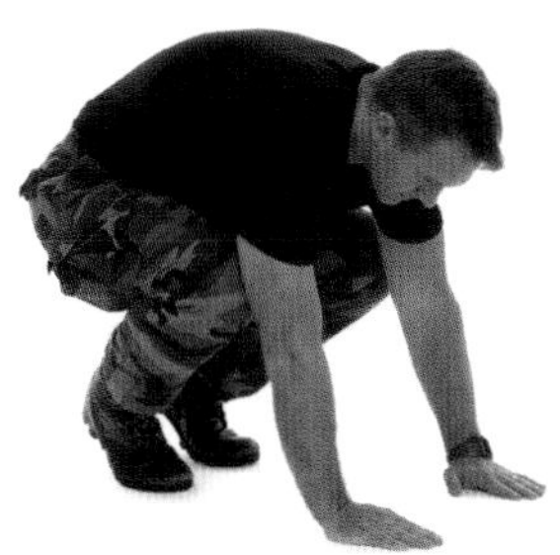

8 Stand for count 8. Each 1-to-8 count equals one repetition. Perform 10 reps.

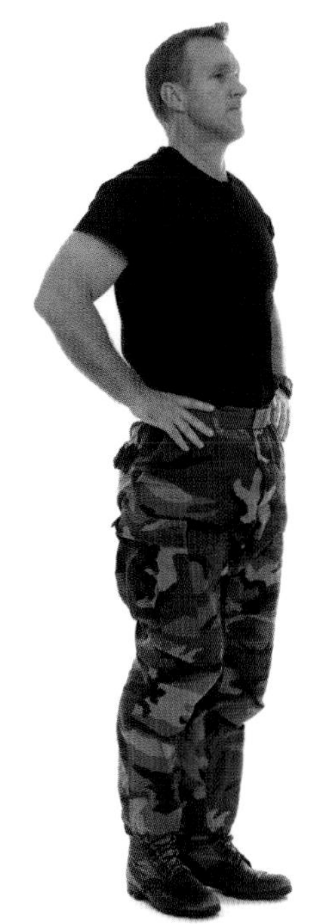

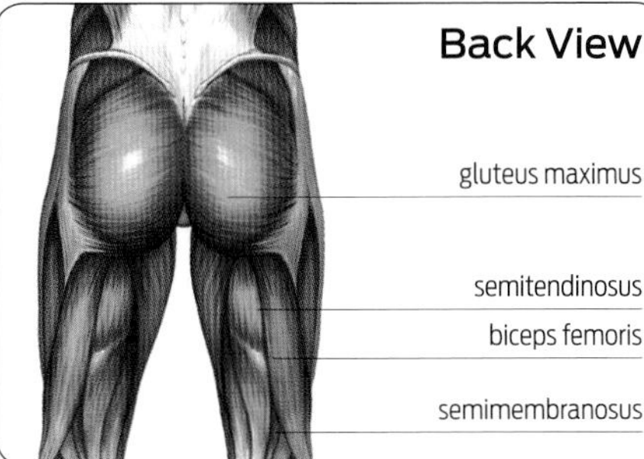


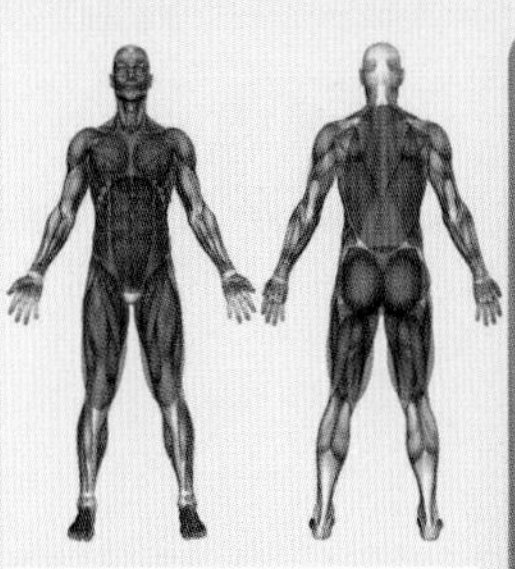

**Level**
- Advanced

**Duration**
- 45–90 seconds

**Benefits**
- Works the entire body
- Increases cardiovascular endurance

**Caution**
- Shoulder issues
- Wrist issues
- Lower-back pain

**Annotation Key**
* indicates deep muscles

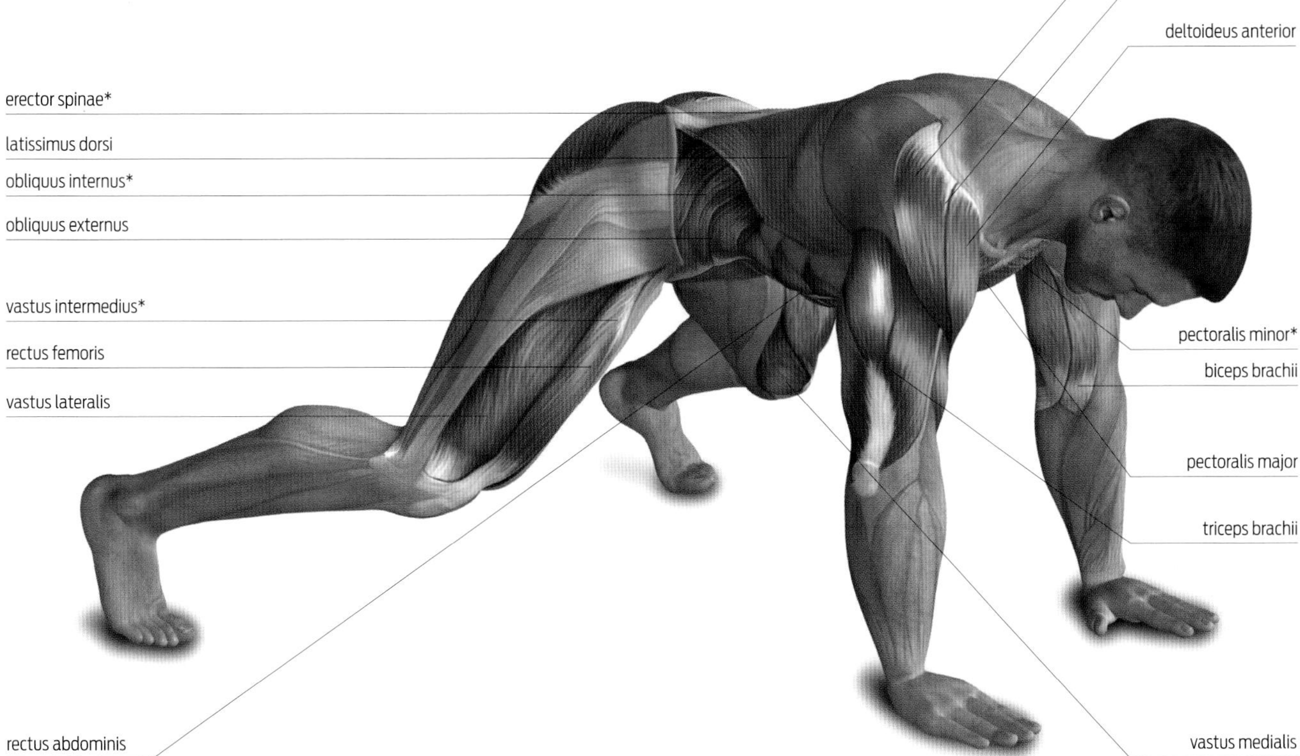

# 10-Count Body Builder

The 10-Count Body Builder adds the resistance of weights to challenge you even further. Along with the Push-Ups and Squats found in the 8-Count Body Builder (pages 86–87), this version of the exercise includes a Biceps Curl, which will tone your upper arms. Until you have built up sufficient strength and balance, make sure to use weights with a flat edge so that they don't roll to the side when you jump to the Drop Position.

1 For count 1, with your palms facing each other, start with a set of dumbbells in your hands. Bend down and place the dumbbells on the floor in front of you.

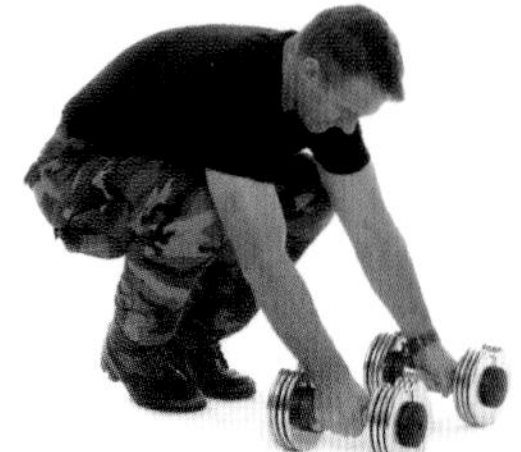

2 Kick your feet backward into Drop Position while keeping your hands on the weights. This is count 2.

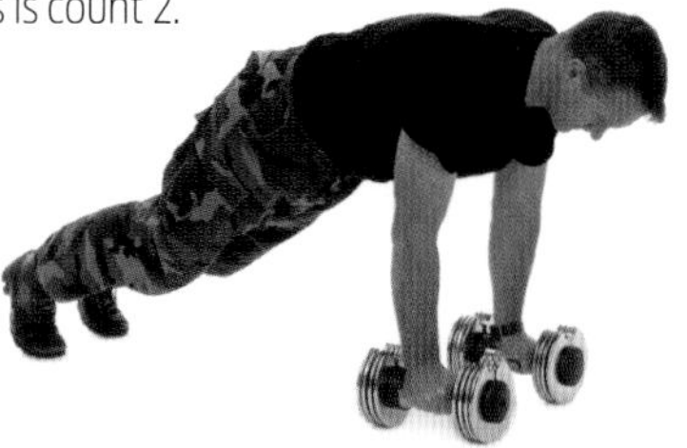

3 Push downward for a Push-Up until your chest touches the dumbbells for count 3.

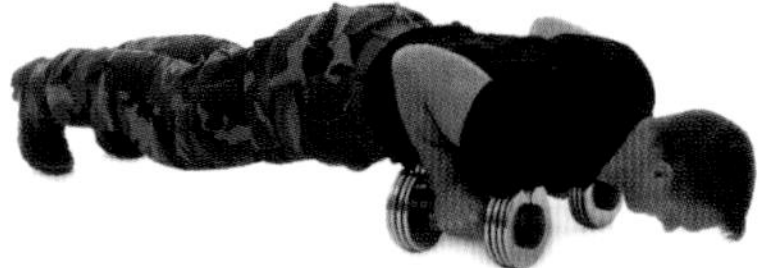

4 Press back up to straighten your arms for count 4.

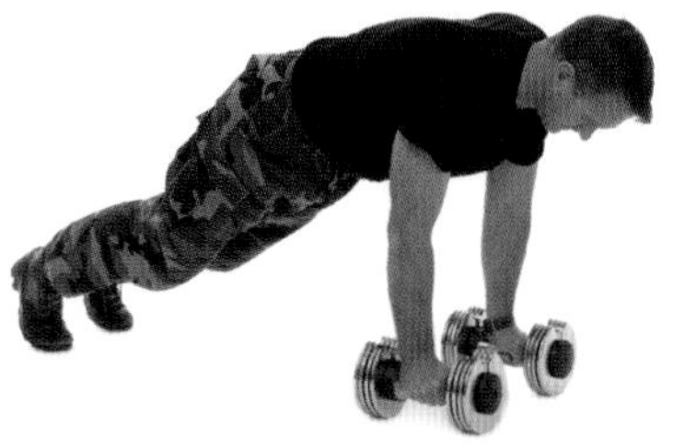

5 Spread your legs for count 5.

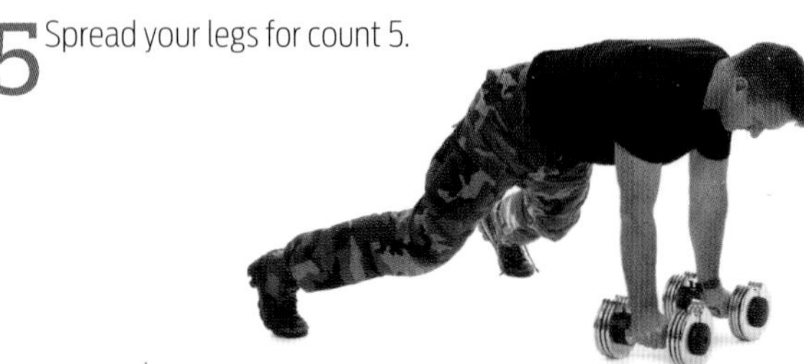

6 Close your legs for count 6.

7 Jump both knees to your chest for count 7.

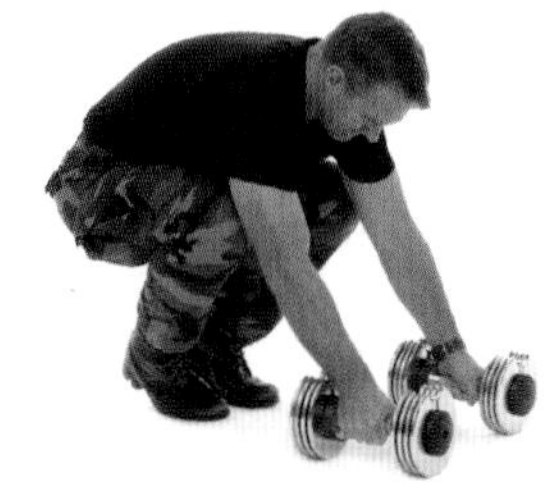

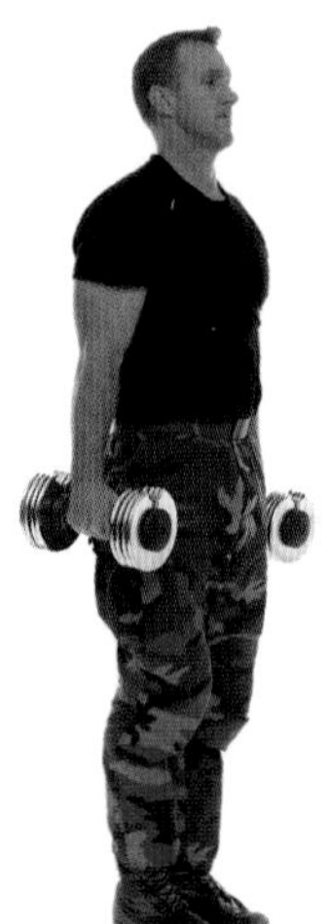

8 Stand for count 8.

**Correct form**
- Keep your hands close to your chest in the Push-Up position.

**Avoid**
- Resting your chest on the dumbbells on count 3.

**9** Lift the weights to your shoulders to perform a Biceps Curl for count 9.

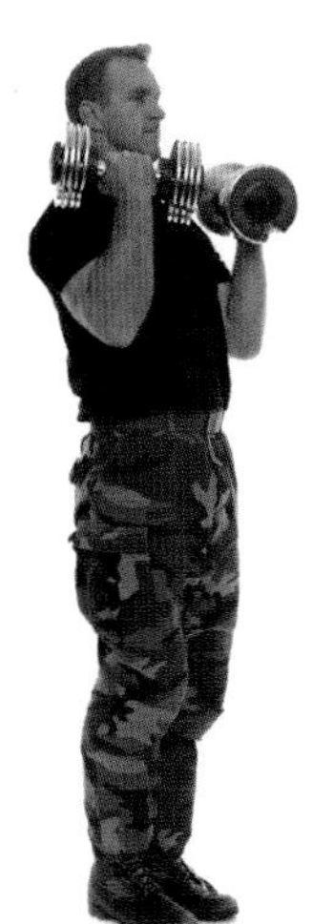

**10** Lower the weights to your sides for count 10. Each 1-to-10 count equals one repetition. Perform 10 reps.

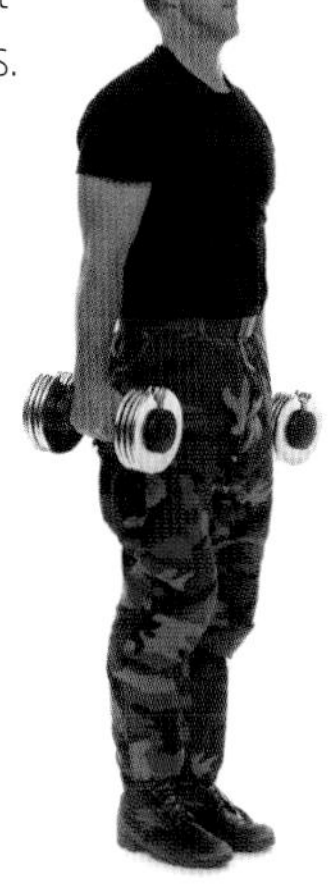

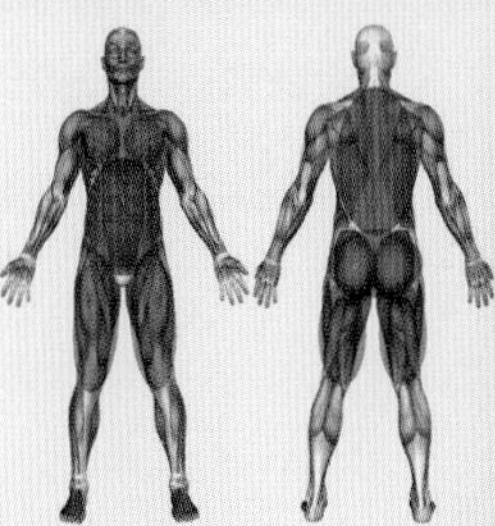

**Level**
- Advanced

**Duration**

- 60–90 seconds

**Benefits**
- Works the entire body
- Increases cardiovascular endurance

**Caution**

- Shoulder issues
- Wrist issues
- Lower-back pain

deltoideus posterior

deltoideus medialis

brachialis

triceps brachii

latissimus dorsi

erector spinae*

obliquus externus

vastus intermedius*

rectus femoris

vastus lateralis

deltoideus anterior

**Annotation Key**
* indicates deep muscles

rectus abdominis

obliquus internus*

vastus medialis

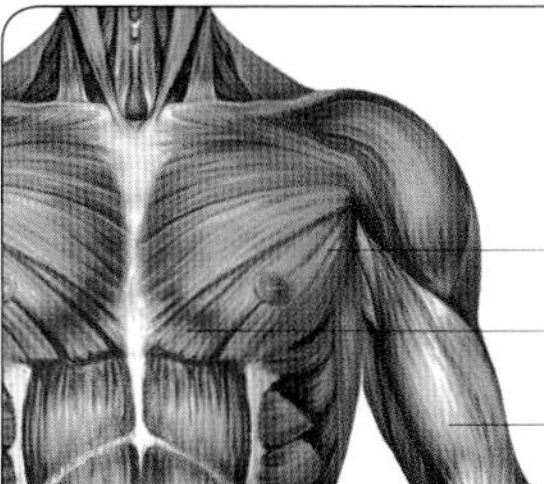
**Front View**

pectoralis minor*

pectoralis major

biceps brachii

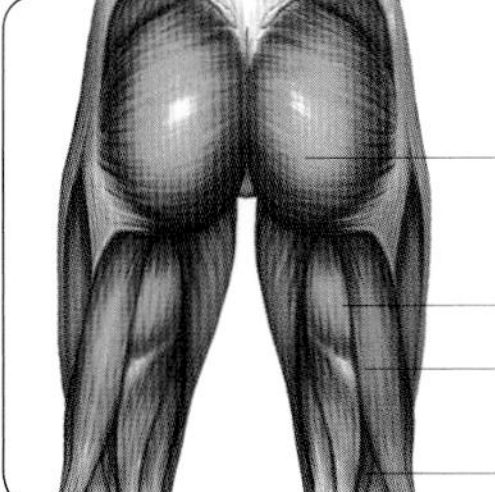
**Back View**

gluteus maximus

semitendinosus

biceps femoris

semimembranosus

# 12–Count Body Builder

The 12-Count Body Builder takes the Body Builder exercise to yet another level, adding a Shoulder Press to the movement. It effectively works the cardiovascular system by using multiple muscle systems. It is a great movement for wrestlers, mixed martial arts fighters, and military personnel. As with the 10-Count Body Builder, be sure to use flat-edged weights until you have built up sufficient strength and balance.

1 For count 1, with your palms facing each other, start with a set of dumbbells in your hands. Bend down and place the dumbbells on the floor in front of you.

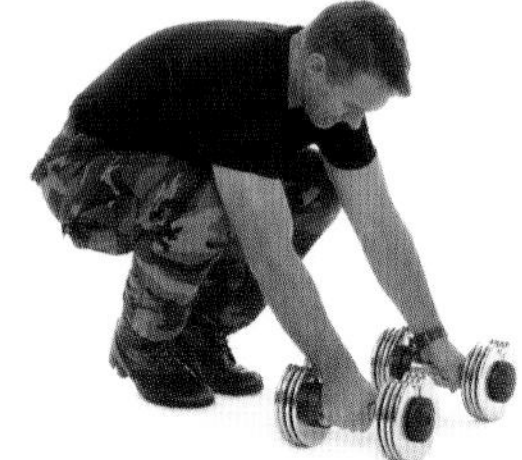

2 Kick your feet backward into Drop Position while keeping your hands on the weights. This is count 2.

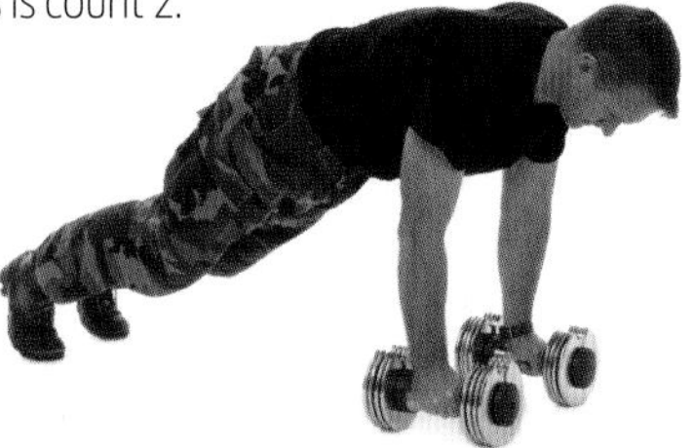

3 Push downward for a Push-Up until your chest touches the dumbbells for count 3.

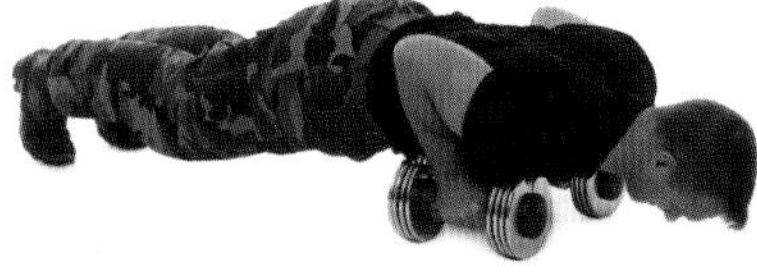

4 Press back up to straighten your arms for count 4.

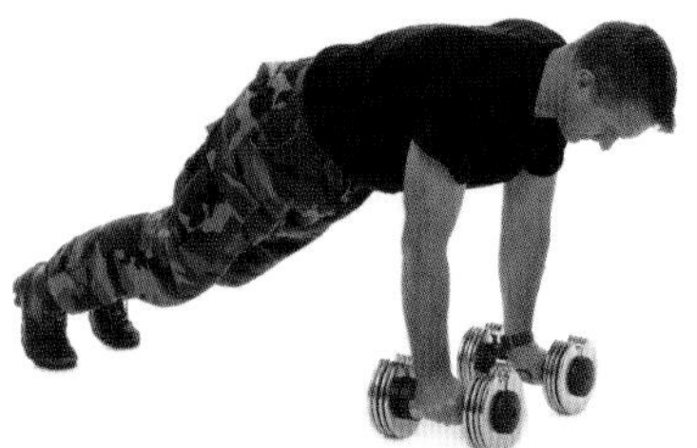

5 Spread your legs for count 5.

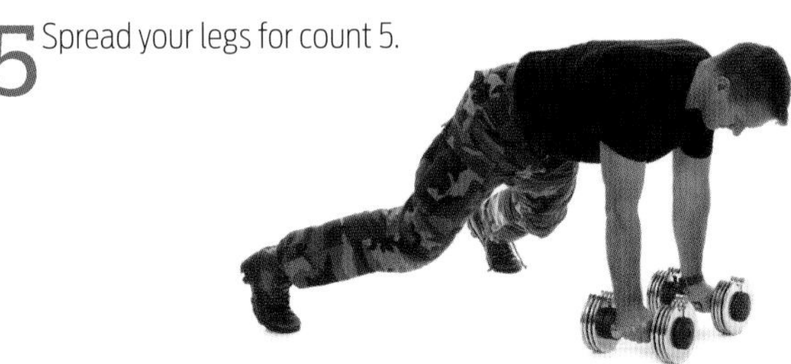

6 Close your legs for count 6.

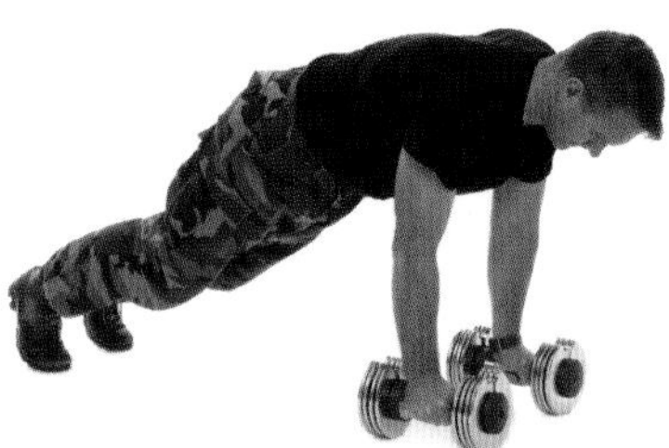

7 Jump both knees to your chest for count 7.

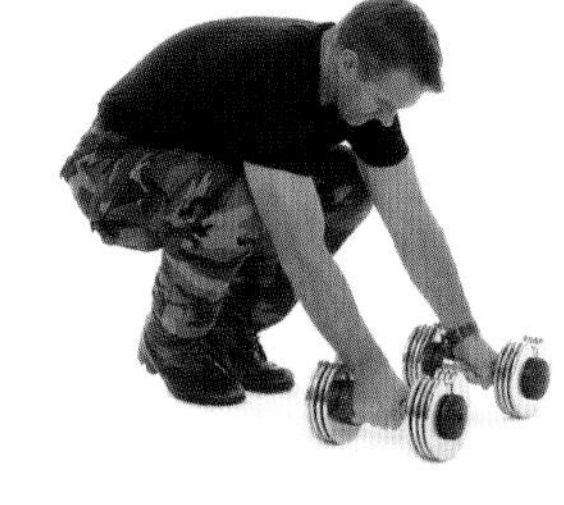

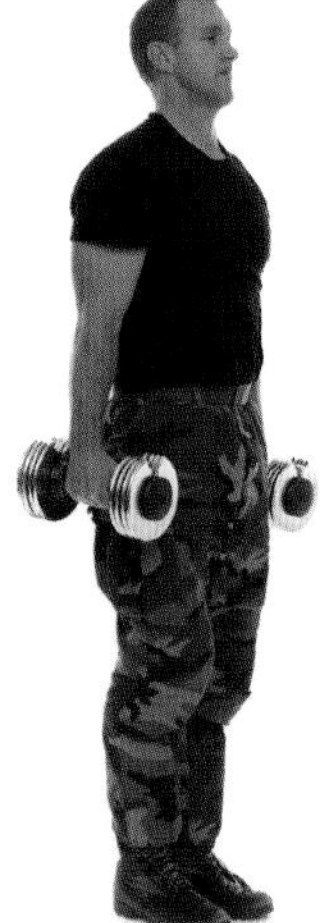

8 Stand for count 8.

**Correct form**
- Keep your hands close to your chest in the Push-Up position.

**Avoid**
- Resting your chest on the dumbbells on count 3.

**9** Lift the weights to your shoulders to perform a Biceps Curl for count 9.

**10** Lower the weights to your sides for count 10. Each 1-to-10 count equals one repetition. Perform 10 reps.

**11** Raise the weights over your head to perform a Shoulder Press for count 11.

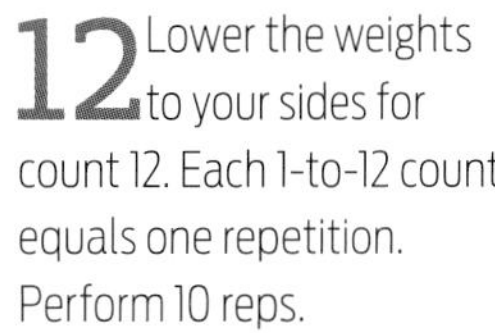

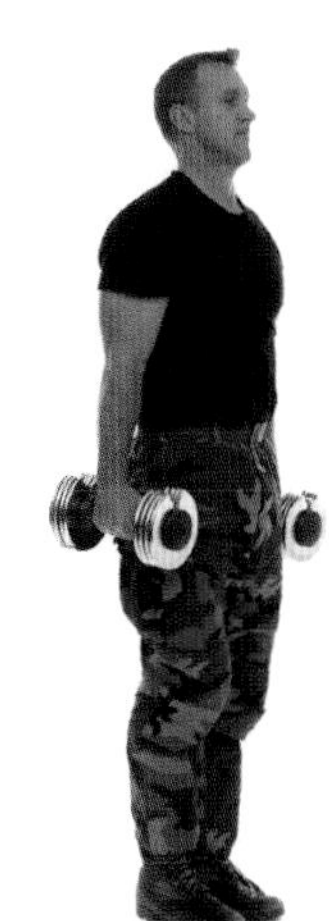

**12** Lower the weights to your sides for count 12. Each 1-to-12 count equals one repetition. Perform 10 reps.

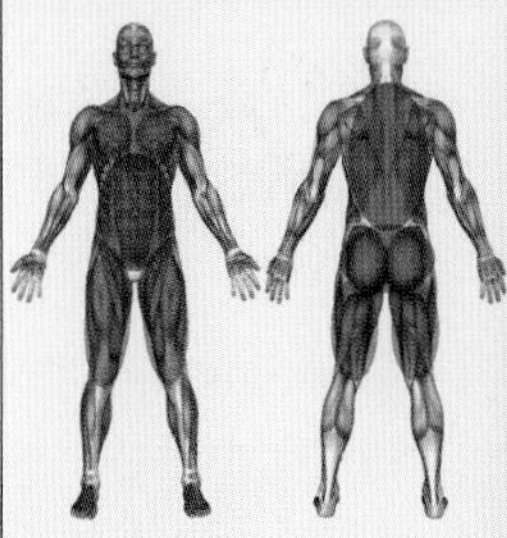

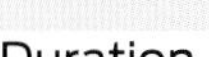

**Level**
**Level**
- Advanced

**Duration**
- 60–90 seconds

**Benefits**
- Works the entire body
- Increases cardiovascular endurance

**Caution**
- Shoulder issues
- Wrist issues
- Lower-back pain

Annotation Key
* indicates deep muscles

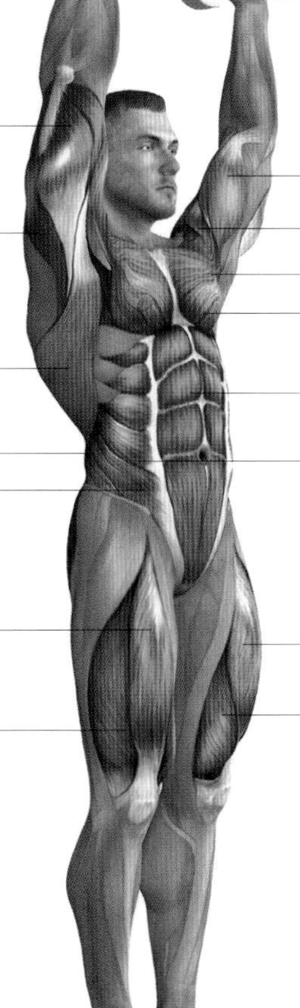


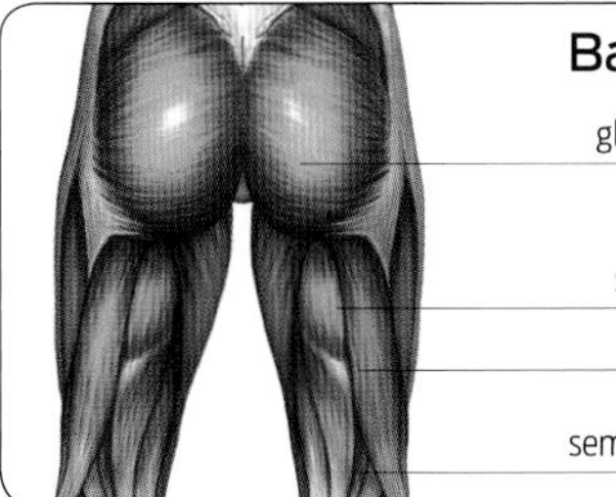


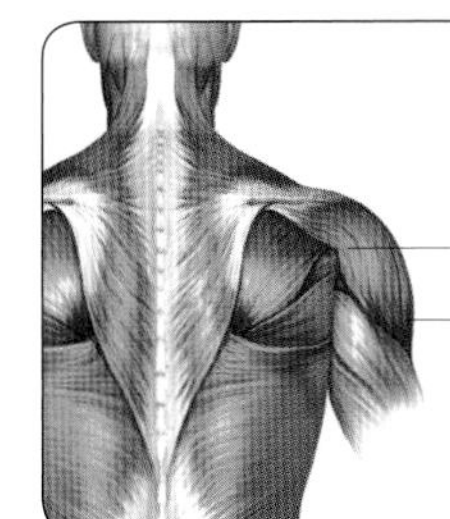

# Lower–Back Extension

The lower back can take a lot of abuse during a workout. To protect your lumbar spinal region, it is smart to include a lower-back isolation exercise as part of any fitness routine. The Lower-Back Extension will help prevent lumbar issues by building strength in your lower-back and gluteal muscles. It also increases the flexibility of your hamstrings, which can help with lower-back movement.

1 Stand, holding a weight in each hand.

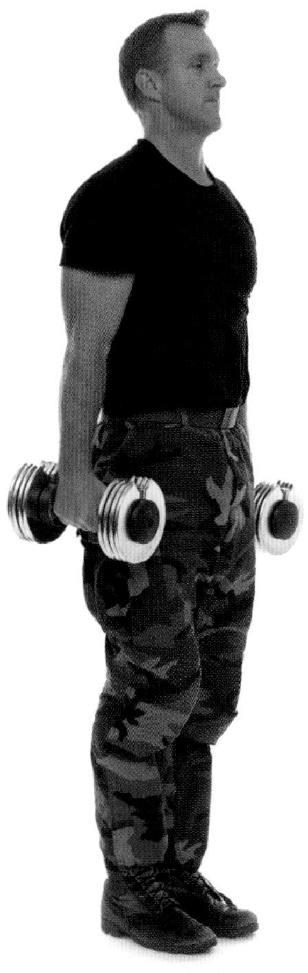

2 While keeping your legs straight, lean forward and reach toward your toes. Try to touch the weights to the floor with your legs straight.

3 Stand back up to neutral position. Perform 10 reps.

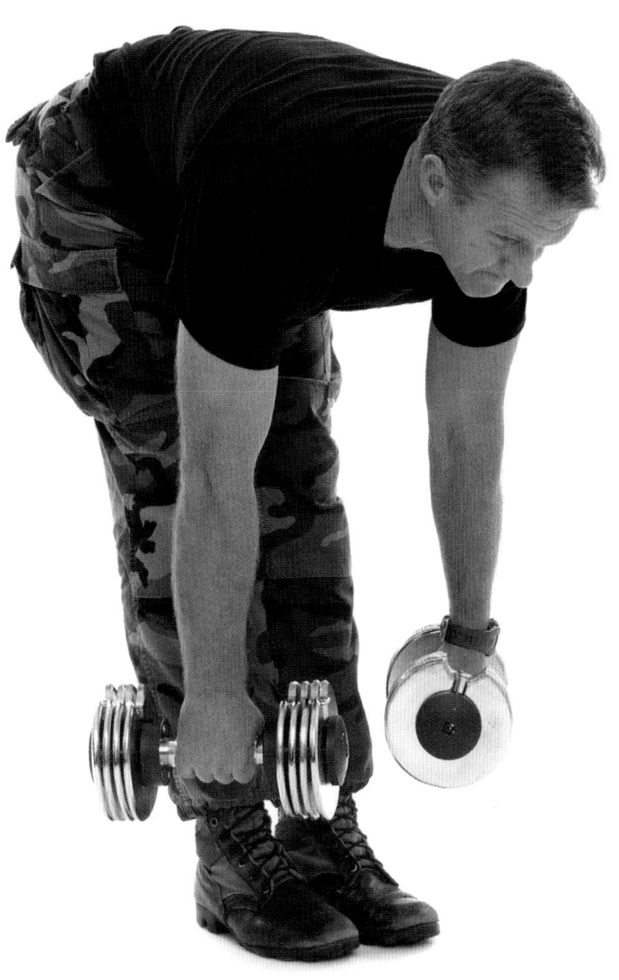

**Correct form**

- As you lean forward, shift your weight to your heels.
- Contract your abdominal muscles as you bend forward and rise back up.

**Avoid**

- Jerky movements—keep your movements smooth and controlled.

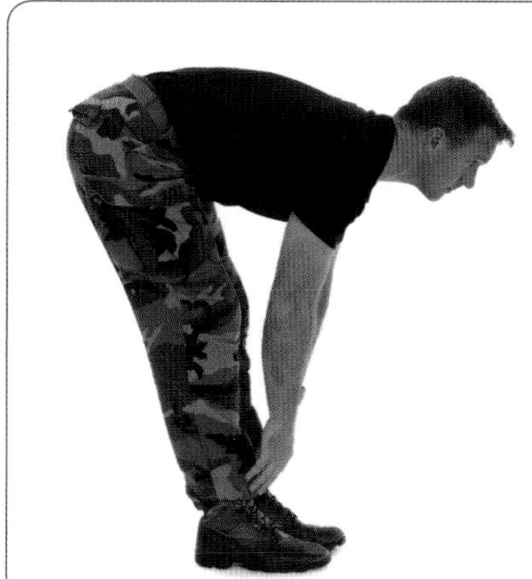

## Modification

**Easier:** Perform the exercise without the weights, trying to touch your fingers to the floor.

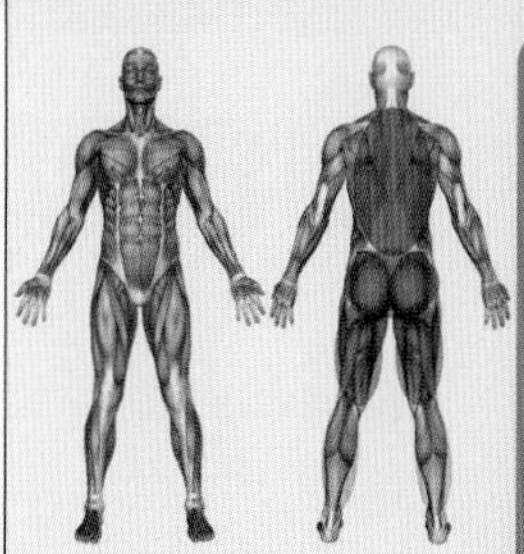

**Level**

- Beginner

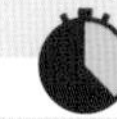

**Duration**

- 30–45 seconds

**Benefits**

- Strengthens lower-back muscles
- Strengthens glutes
- Increases hamstring flexibility

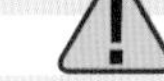

**Caution**

- Lower-back issues

**Annotation Key**

* indicates deep muscles

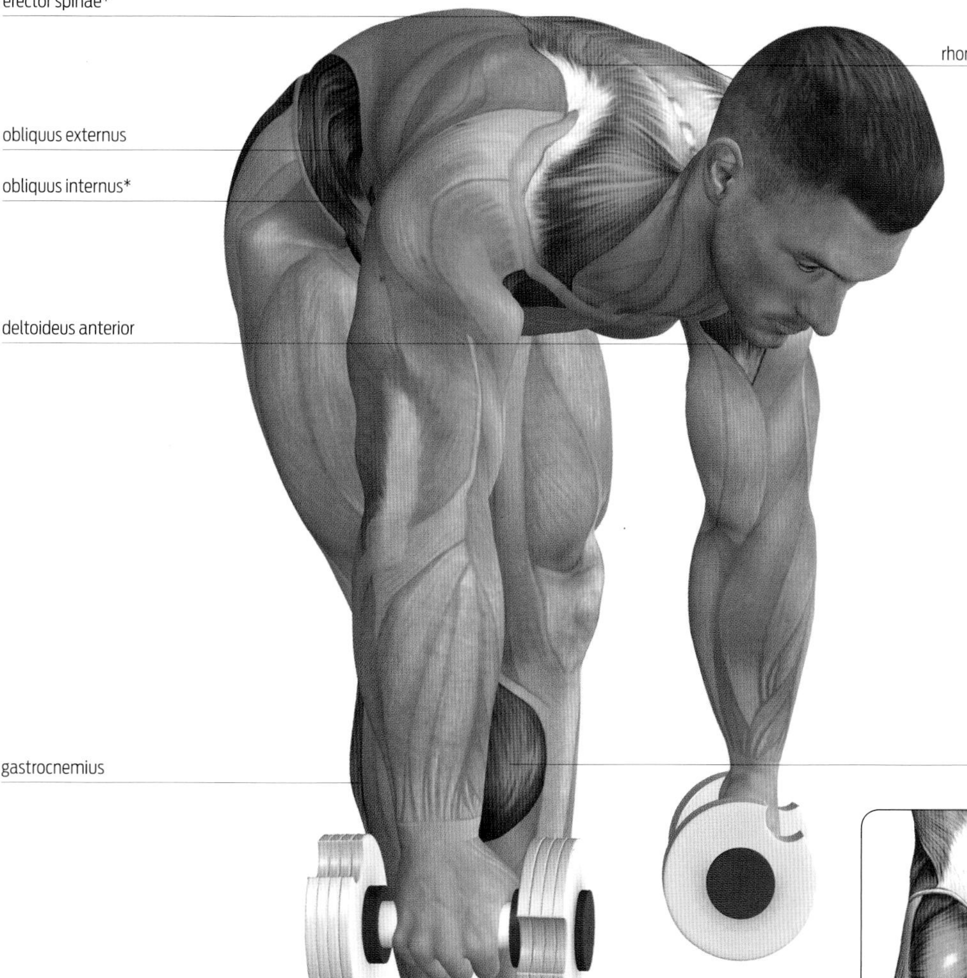


**Back View**

gluteus minimus*
gluteus medius*
gluteus maximus
semitendinosus
biceps femoris
semimembranosus

# Deep Squat

The Deep Squat is one of the best exercises for working the muscles of your thighs, glutes, and core. It is a multipurpose move that integrates balance and coordination training, resistance, and stretching to target your leg muscles. To work on perfecting your form and improving your stability, you can hold a weight in your hands during this exercise to counterbalance your lower body as you squat. This will help to keep your heels firmly grounded and prevent you from tipping backward.

1 Stand with your feet shoulder-width apart, and your toes slightly flared to a 45-degree angle.

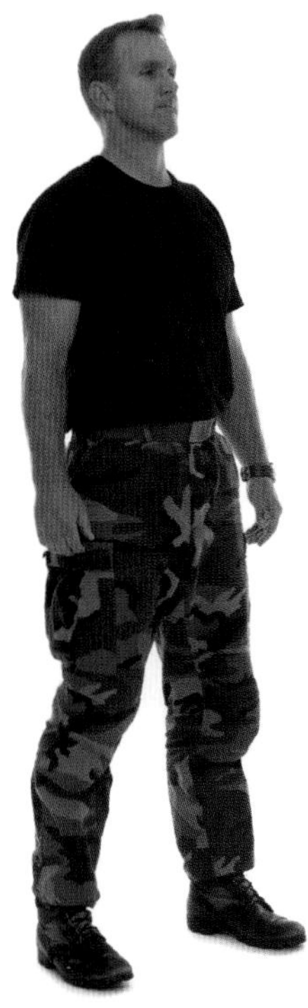

2 Lower your body, and extend your arms forward, palms down. Keep your heels on the floor, your lower back arched and your chest out. Move slowly, sinking deeply until you can no longer keep your heels on the floor.

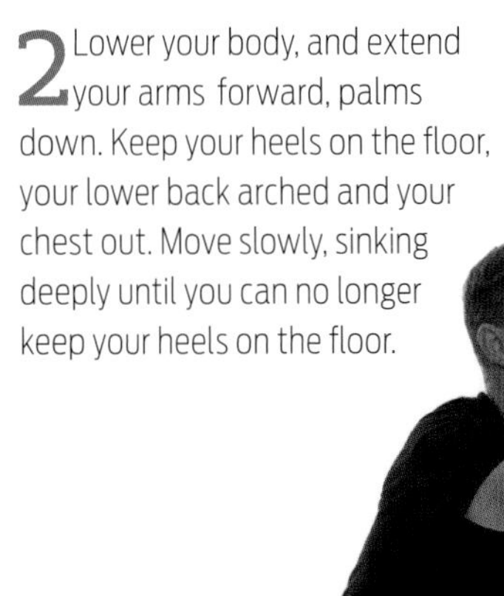

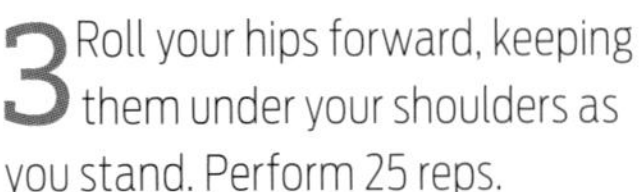

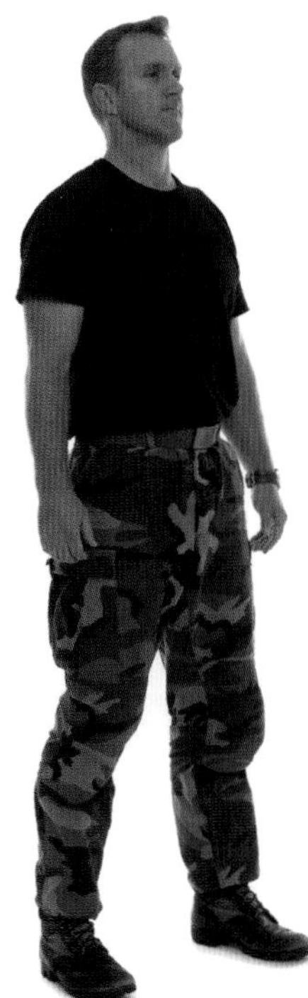

3 Roll your hips forward, keeping them under your shoulders as you stand. Perform 25 reps.

**Correct form**

- Upon squatting, your hips move backward first to help keep your heels on the floor.
- As you squat, point your toes outward to make space between your thighs for your torso.
- Drive your hips forward as you stand to work your core muscles.
- Keep your knees over the top of your feet.

**Avoid**

- Leaning forward.
- Allowing your heels to come off the floor.

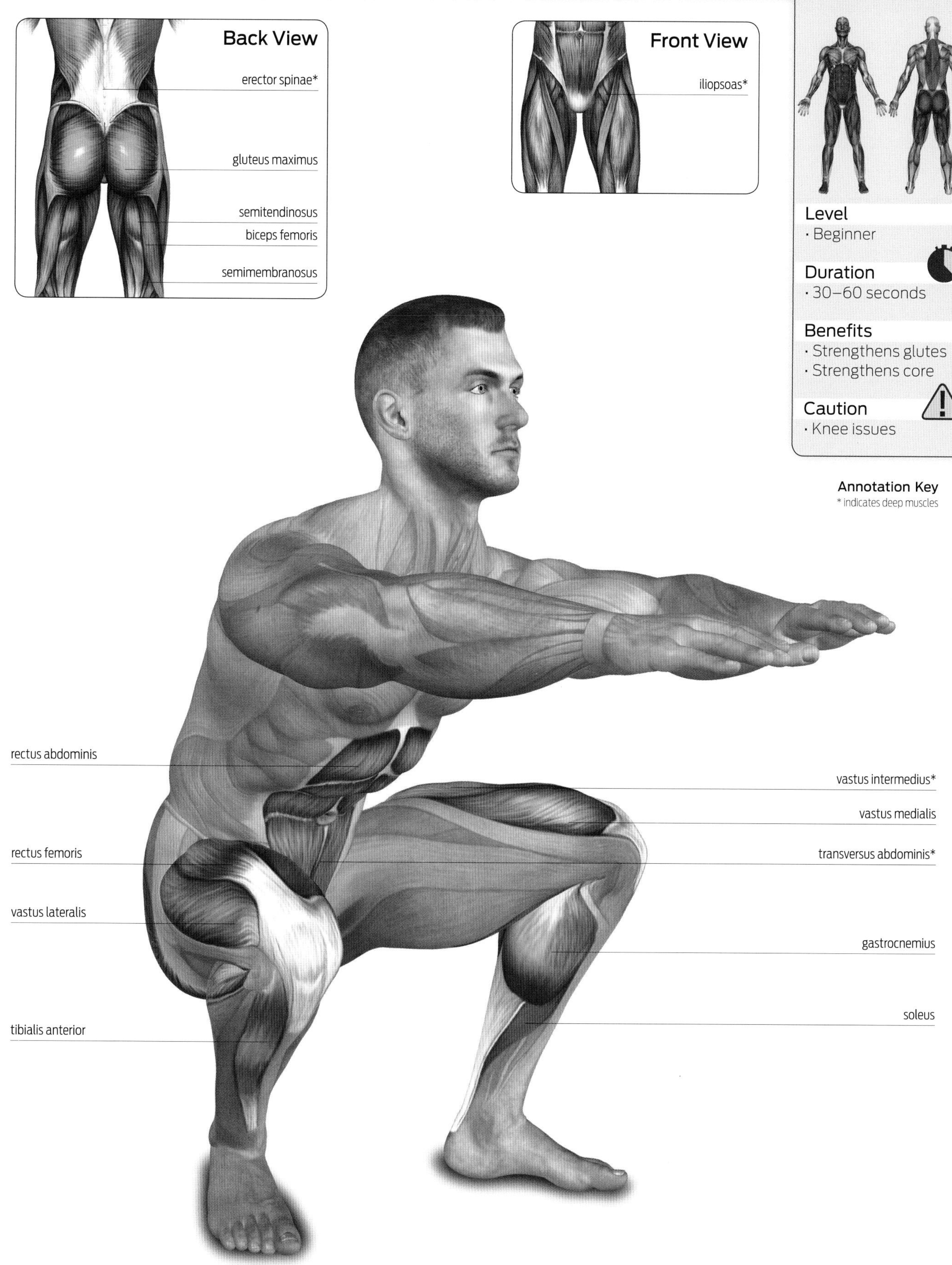


**Level**
· Beginner

**Duration**
· 30–60 seconds

**Benefits**
· Strengthens glutes
· Strengthens core

**Caution**
· Knee issues

**Annotation Key**
* indicates deep muscles

# Lunge

The Lunge is both a dynamic stretch and a hip, knee, and ankle stabilizer. It stretches your hip flexors, while strengthening your hamstrings, thighs, and glutes.

1 Stand with your left leg stepped out in front of your body. Keep a slight bend in your left knee.

2 Drop your right knee, touching it lightly on the floor.

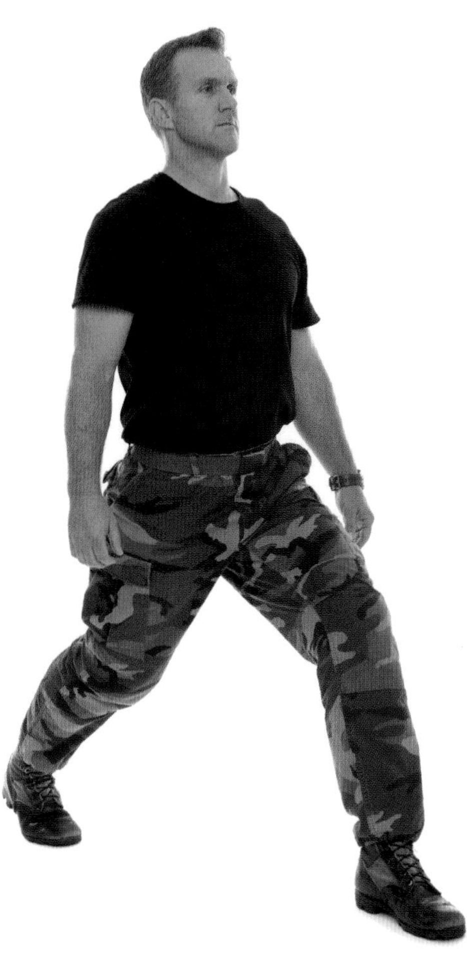

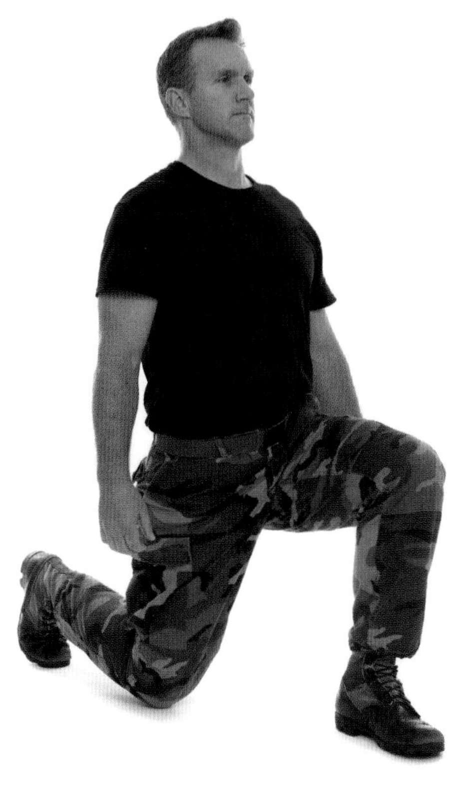

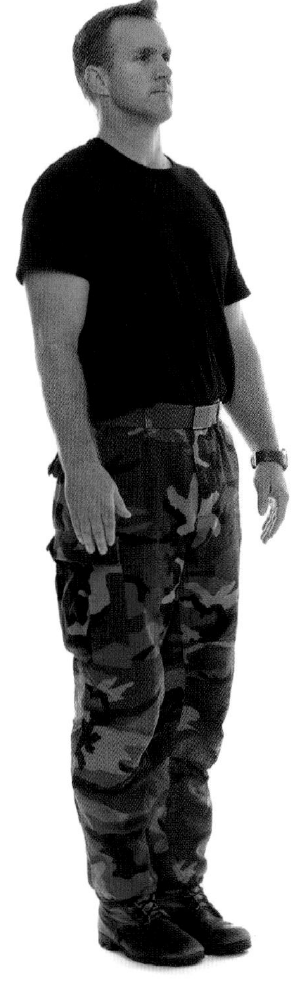

3 Stand back up, bringing your feet together. Switch legs, and repeat on the other side. Lunging once on each leg equals one repetition. Perform 10 reps.

**Correct form**
- As you drop your knee to the floor, make sure your front knee stays over the top of your foot.

**Avoid**
- Allowing your knee to bend forward of your toes; this will place stress on your knee.

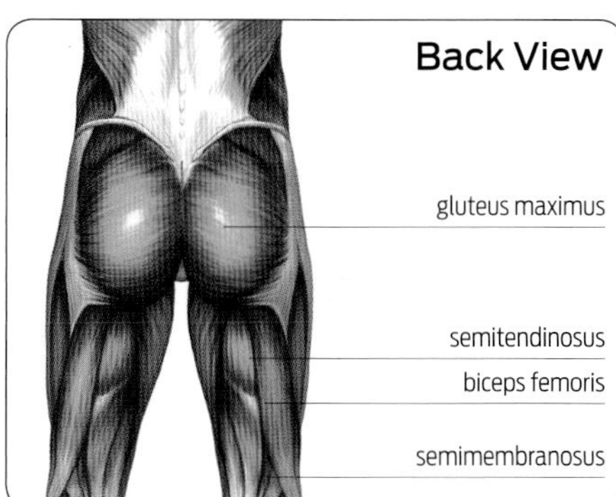

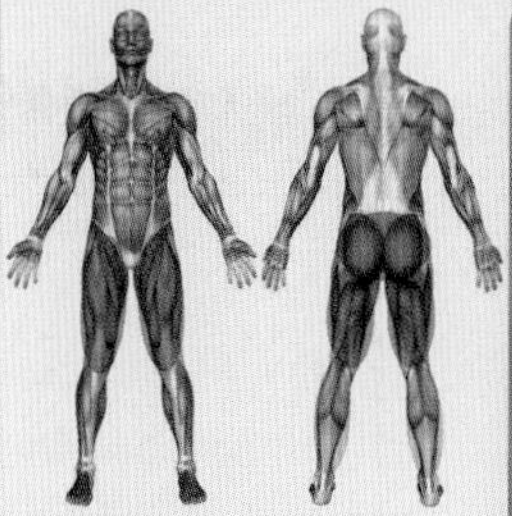

## Level
· Beginner

## Duration
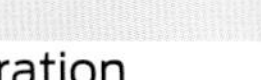
· 30–45 seconds

## Benefits
· Strengthens quadriceps
· Stabilizes hips

## Caution
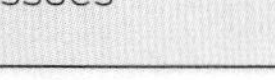
· Knee issues

**Annotation Key**
* indicates deep muscles

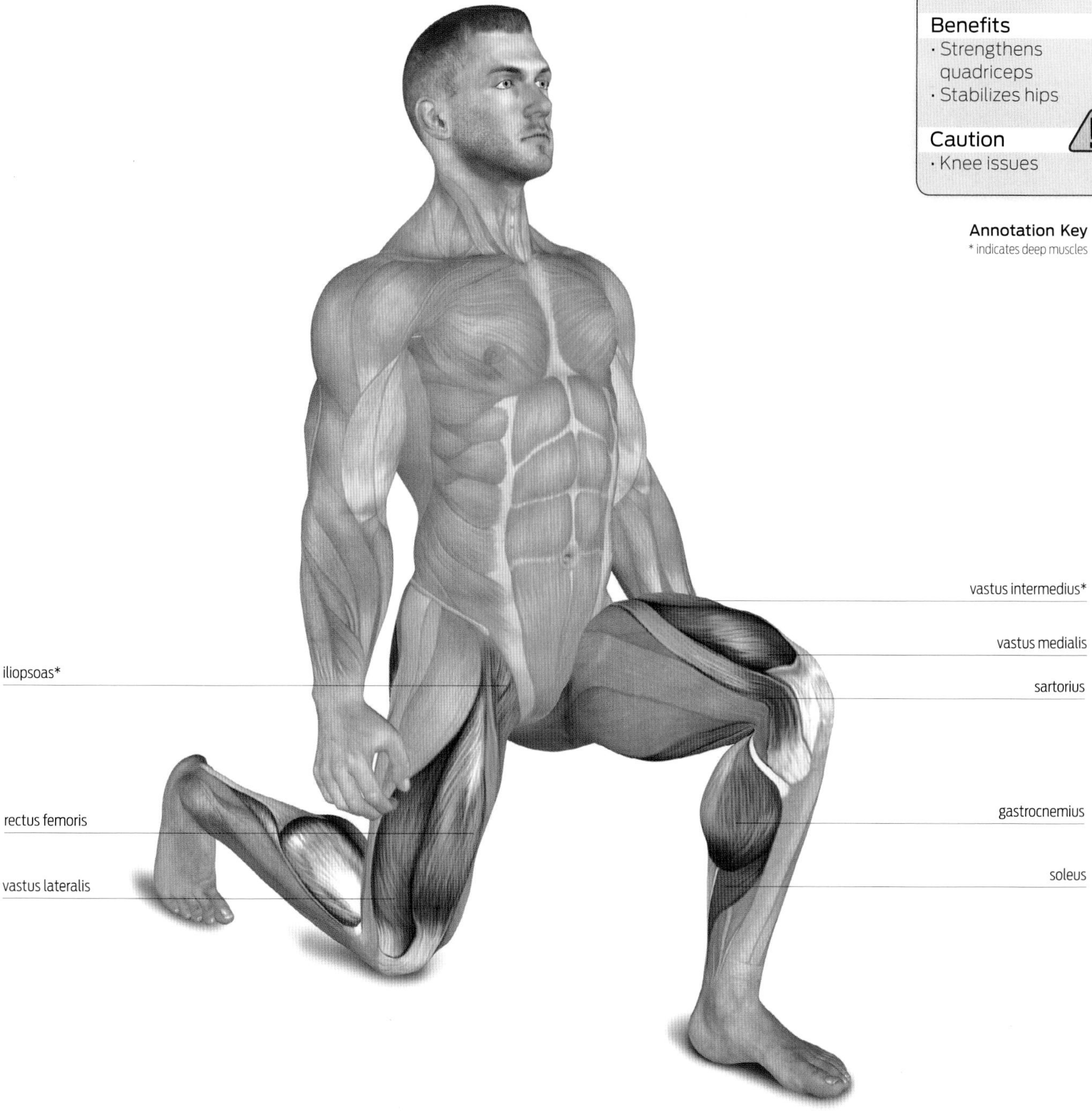

vastus intermedius*
vastus medialis
sartorius
iliopsoas*
rectus femoris
gastrocnemius
soleus
vastus lateralis

# Switch Lunge

The Switch Lunge takes the dynamic element of the Lunge a step further, calling for you to jump upward to switch legs. Like the Lunge, it will stabilize your hips, knees, and ankles, while stretching your hip flexors and strengthening your hamstrings, thighs, and glutes.

1 Stand with your left leg stepped out in front of your body. Keep a slight bend in your left knee.

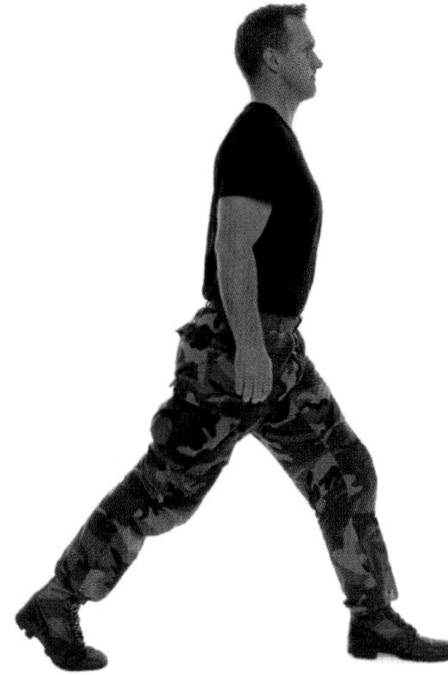

2 Drop your right knee, touching it lightly on the floor.

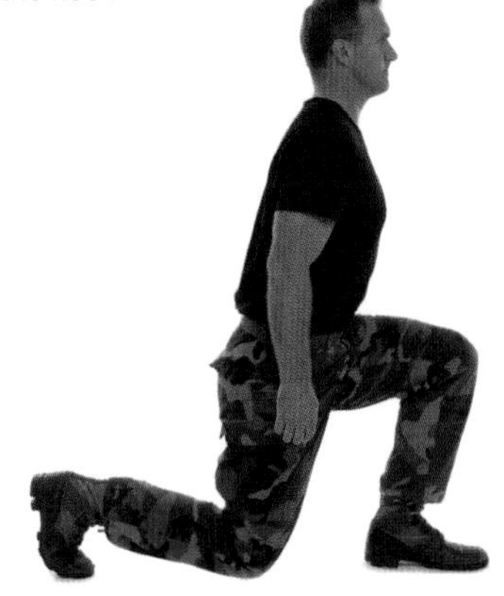

3 Jump up, switching your legs in the air.

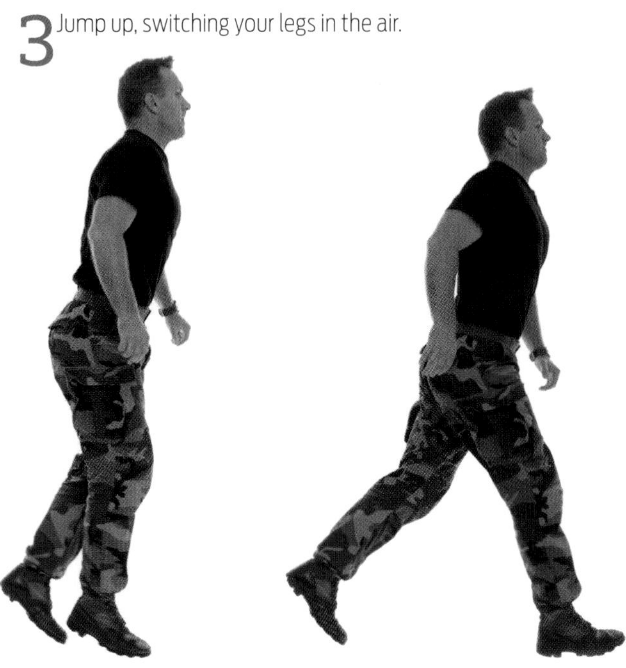

4 Land with your right leg forward and drop your left knee. Lunging and jumping once on each leg equals one repetition. Perform 10 reps.

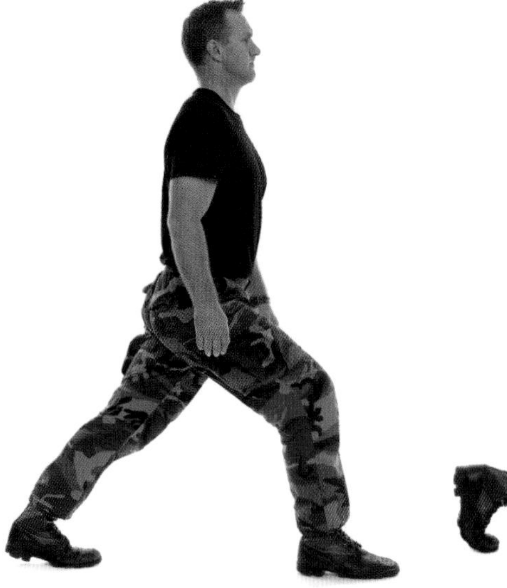

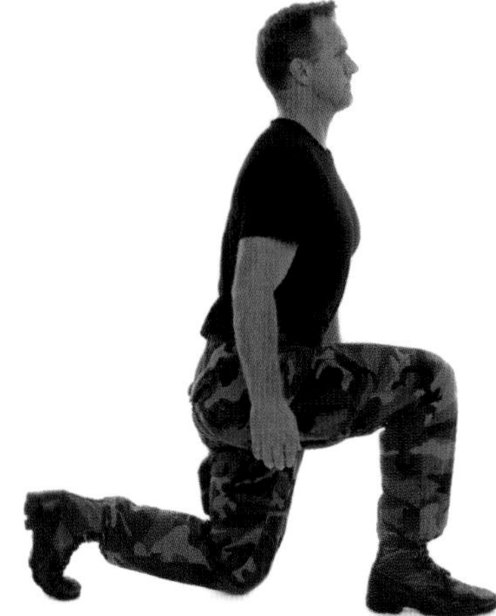

**Correct form**

- As you drop your knee to the floor, make sure your front knee stays over the top of your foot.

**Avoid**

- Allowing your knee to bend forward of your toes; this will place stress on your knee.

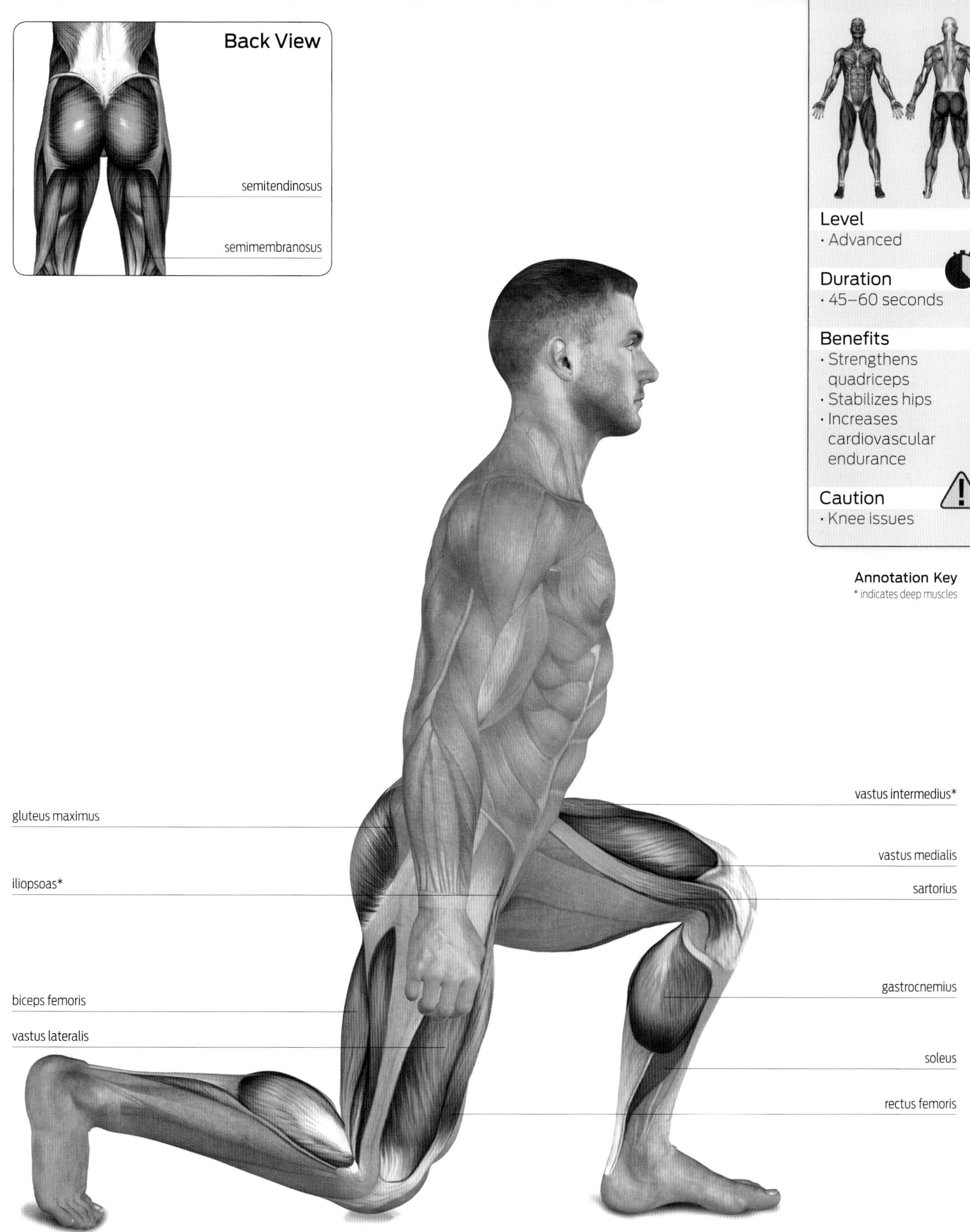


## Level
- Advanced

## Duration
- 45–60 seconds

## Benefits
- Strengthens quadriceps
- Stabilizes hips
- Increases cardiovascular endurance

## Caution
- Knee issues

**Annotation Key**
* indicates deep muscles

# Walking Lunge

Like the Lunge (pages 96–97), the Walking Lunge is a dynamic stretch that stabilizes your knees while building strength in your thighs. This exercise also works your glutes to firm and lift your butt.

1 Stand with your legs together and your arms at your sides.

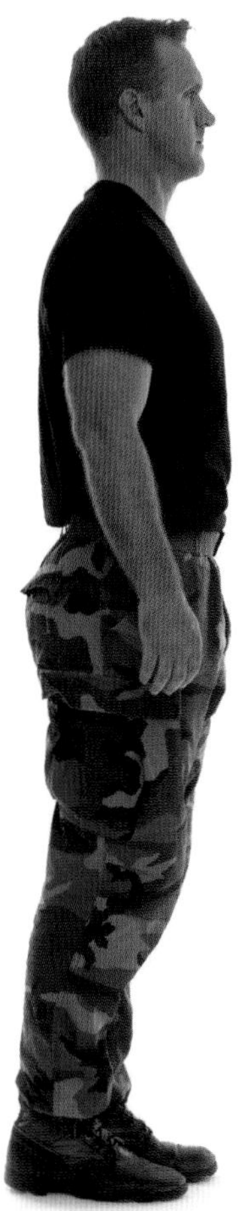

2 Step forward with your left leg.

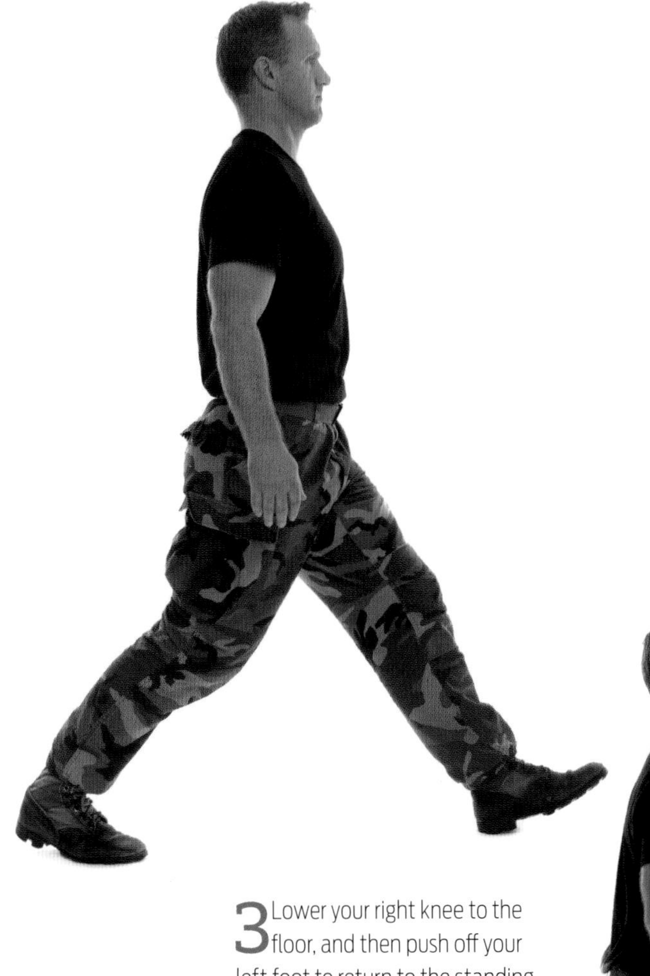

3 Lower your right knee to the floor, and then push off your left foot to return to the standing position. Repeat on the other side, for a total of 25 reps on each leg.

**Correct form**
- Keep your torso upright.
- Keep your forward knee over the top of the forward foot to prevent knee issues.

**Avoid**
- Leaning from side to side as you move forward.

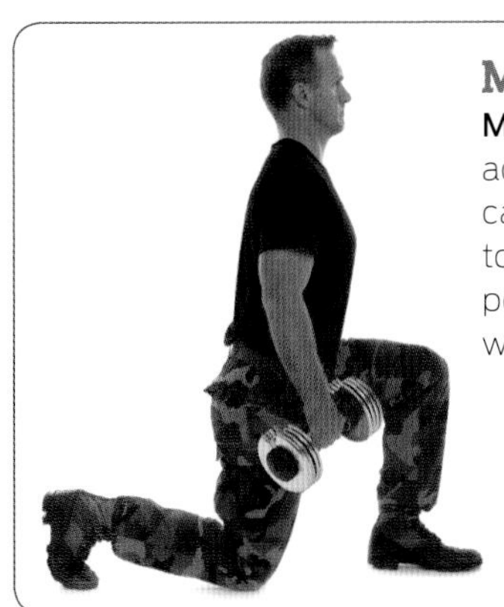

## Modification

**More difficult:** For an added challenge, you can add resistance to this exercise by performing it holding a weight in each hand.

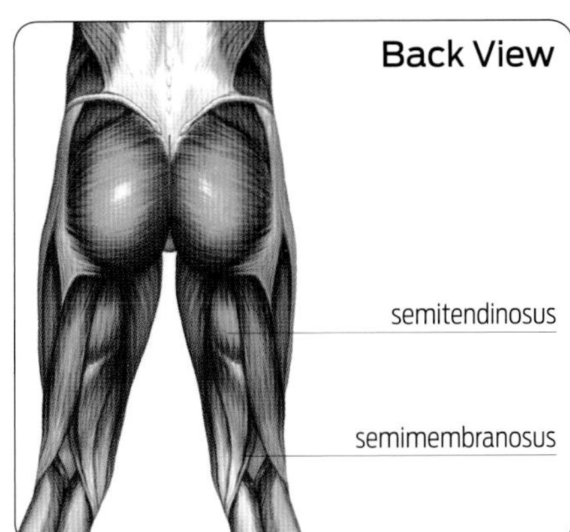


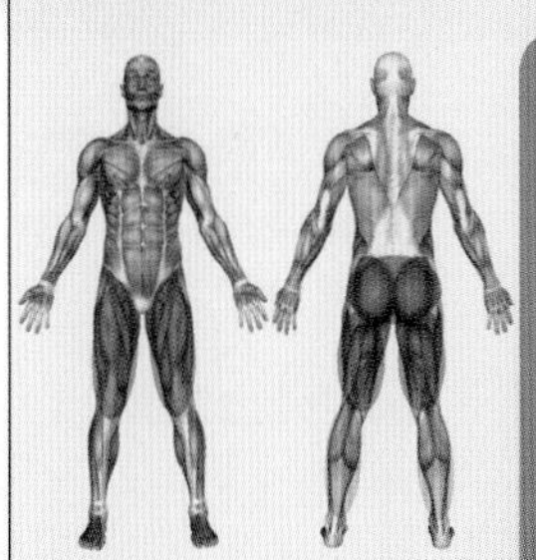

**Level**
- Intermediate

**Duration**

- 45–60 seconds

**Benefits**
- Strengthens quadriceps
- Stabilizes knee joint
- Strengthens core

**Caution**
- Knee issues

**Annotation Key**
* indicates deep muscles

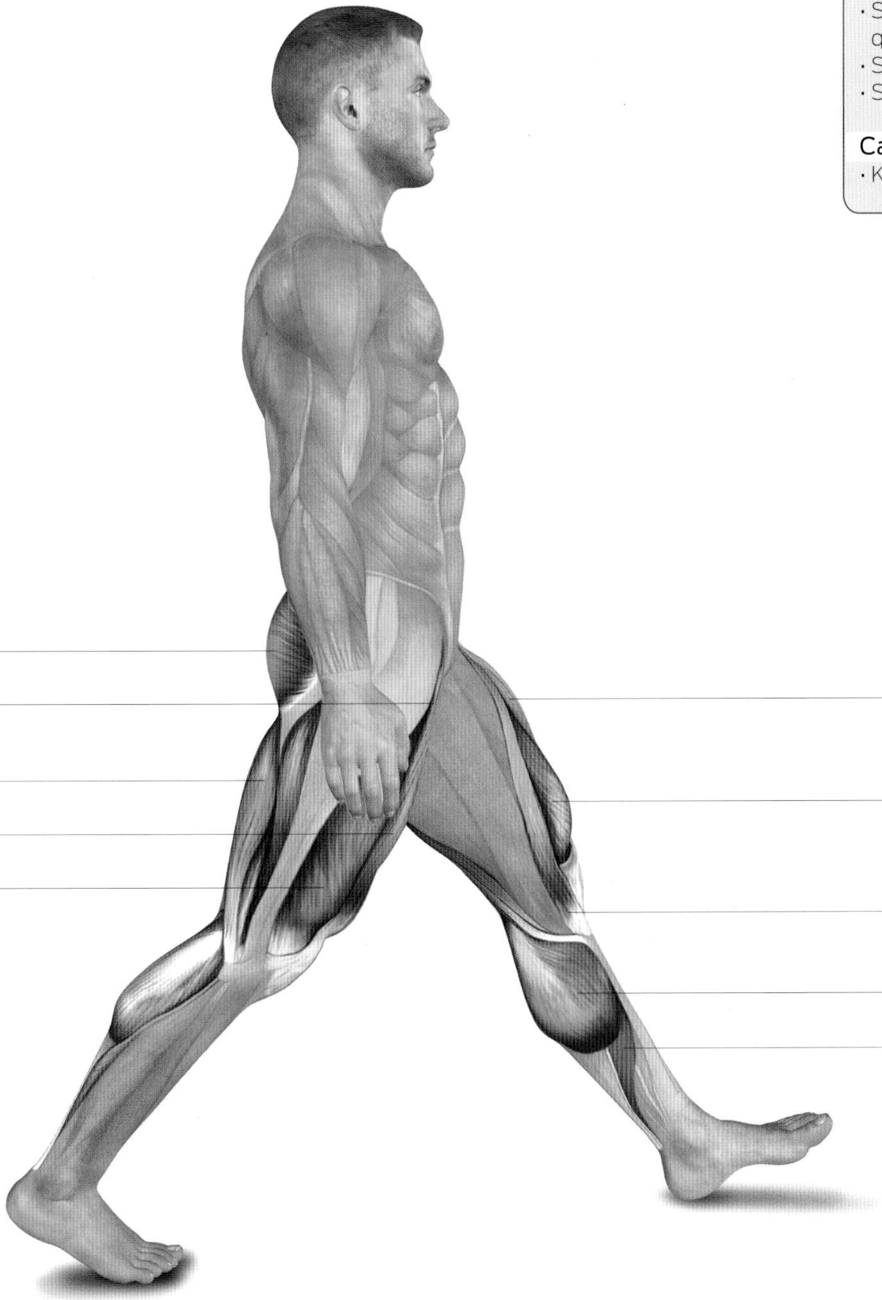

gluteus maximus
iliopsoas*
biceps femoris
rectus femoris
vastus lateralis
vastus intermedius*
vastus medialis
sartorius
gastrocnemius
soleus

# Lateral Lunge with Squat

The Lateral Lunge with Squat combines the benefits of two exercise mainstays: a sideways lunge and a squat. This isolation exercise targets the inner and outer thighs, which can help build strength and stability in the hip and lateral knee.

1 Stand tall with your feet together and your hands on your hips.

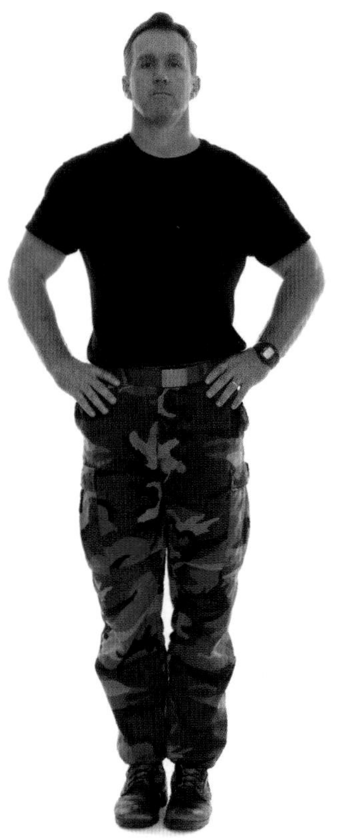

2 Contract your abdominals and glutes, and step out your right foot. Keeping your weight on your heels, bend your left knee and lower your hips as far as you can.

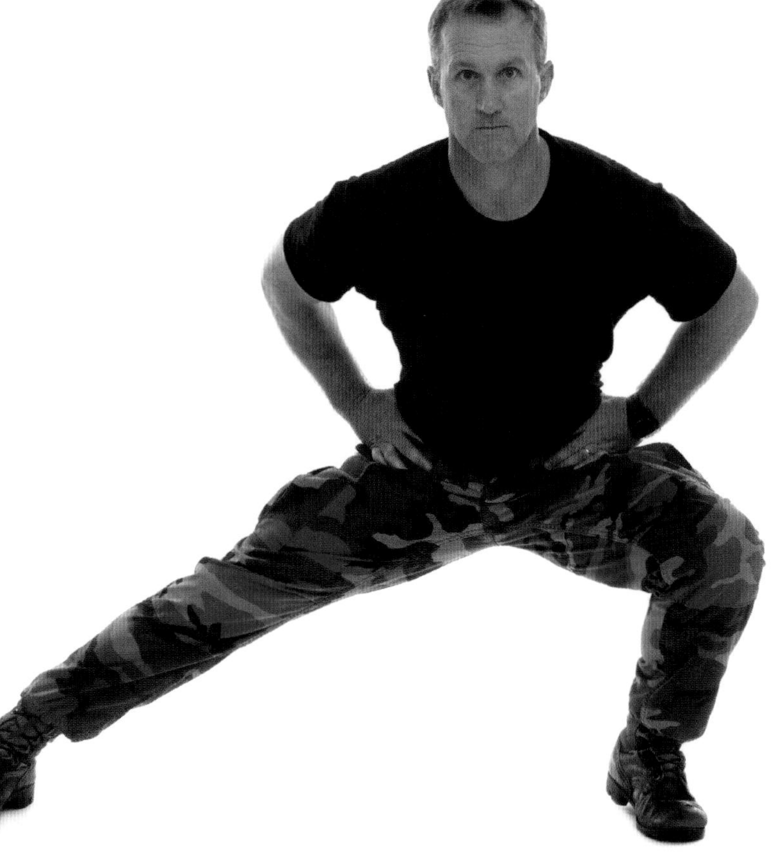

**Correct form**

- Keep your spine in neutral position as you bend your hips.
- Relax your shoulders and neck.
- Align your knee with the toe of your bent leg.
- Lower as far as you are able, but not beyond your thighs parallel to the floor.

**Avoid**

- Lifting your heels off the floor—squat only as deeply as you can while keeping your feet flat on the floor.
- Arching your back.

3 Push off the floor with your right foot, and return to the starting position. Repeat all steps with the left foot leading. Perform 20 reps on each leg.

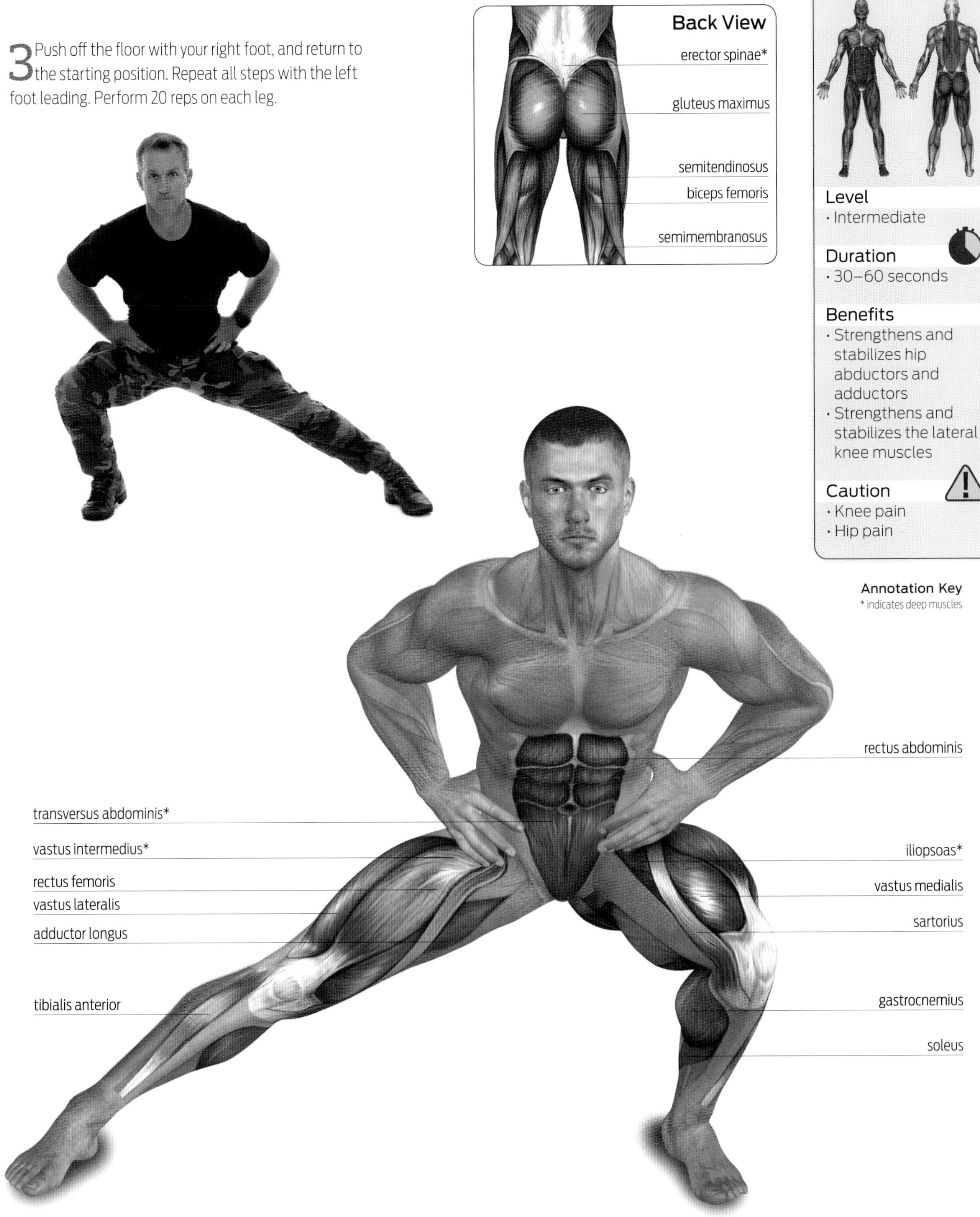


**Level**
- Intermediate

**Duration**
- 30–60 seconds

**Benefits**
- Strengthens and stabilizes hip abductors and adductors
- Strengthens and stabilizes the lateral knee muscles

**Caution**
- Knee pain
- Hip pain

**Annotation Key**
* indicates deep muscles

# Shoulder Flexing

Shoulder Flexing is a resistance exercise for the shoulders and upper back. This movement helps to build up strength when performed correctly. Shoulder flexion means moving your arms up and in front of you as you bend your shoulder joint. When performed correctly, the Shoulder Flexing exercise strengthens your shoulders while increasing their range of motion.

1 Stand with a dumbbell in each hand.

2 Lift both arms straight up in front of you to shoulder height.

3 Lower the weights slowly back to the starting position. Perform 25 reps.

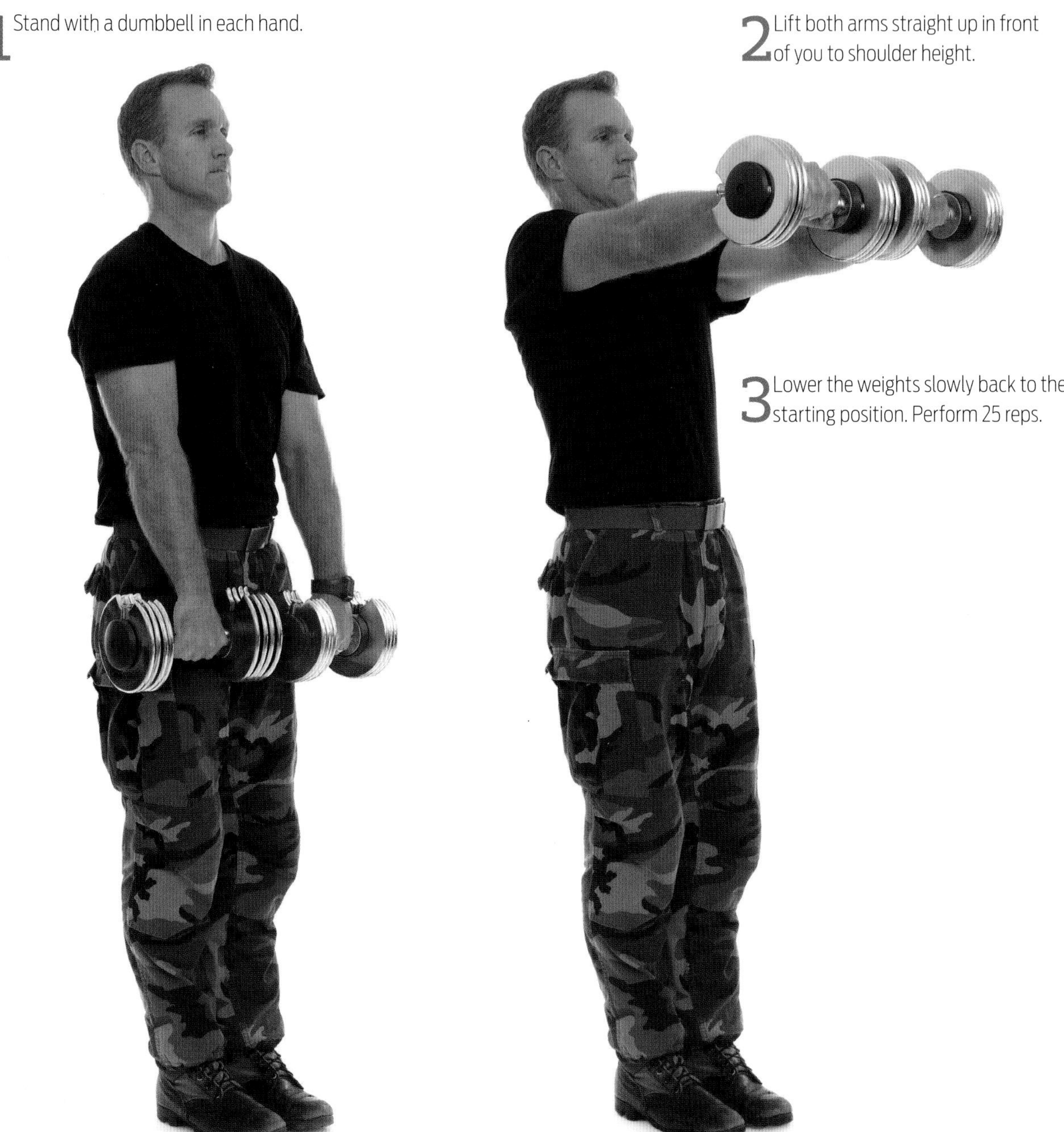

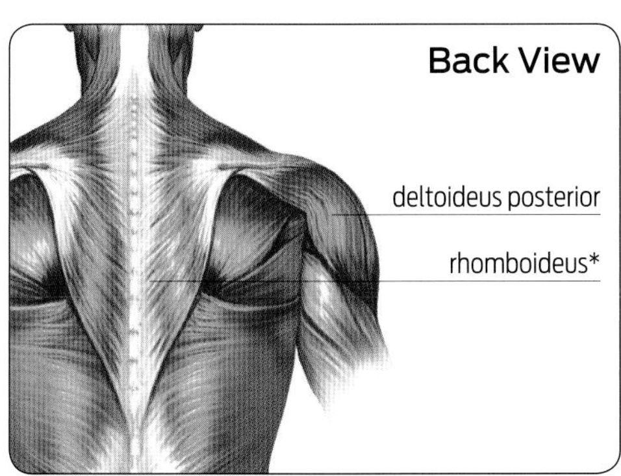


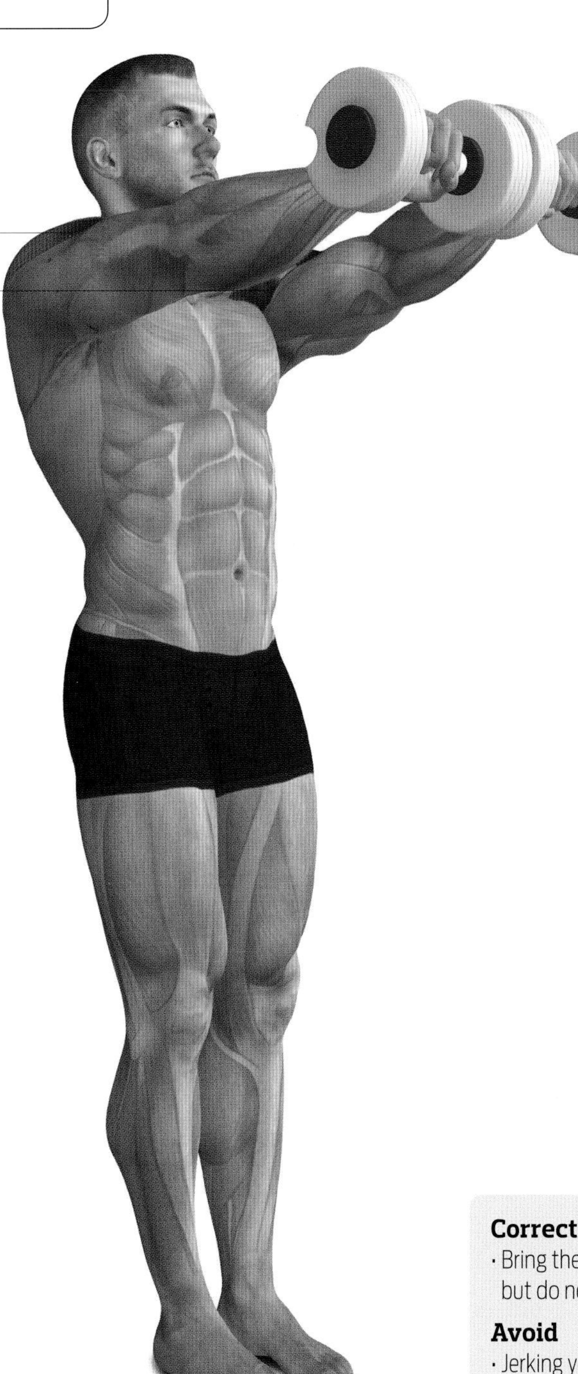


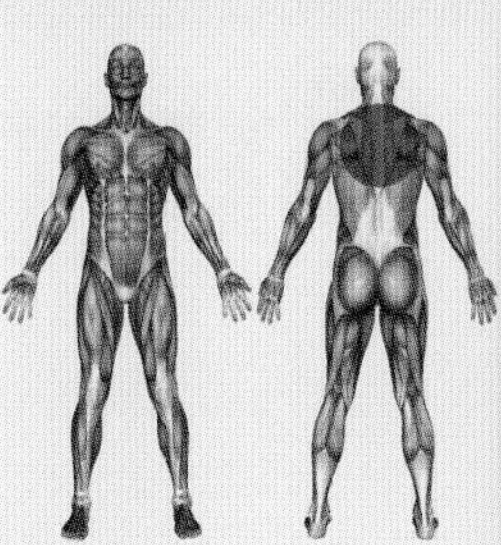

**Level**
- Beginner

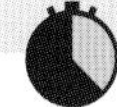

**Duration**
- 15–30 seconds

**Benefits**
- Stabilizes upper-back muscles
- Stabilizes shoulder muscles
- Increases Push-Up strength

**Caution**
- Lower-back issues

**Annotation Key**
* indicates deep muscles

**Correct form**
- Bring the weights down close to your sides, but do not rest the weight between reps.

**Avoid**
- Jerking your lower back to get the weights to shoulder height.

# Burpee

The Burpee, also known as the Squat Thrust, is a full-body strength-training exercise designed to benefit your cardiovascular system by using your entire muscle system. As with many military-style exercises, it can be performed to a four-count rhythm. It is a great exercise for military personnel, wrestlers and mixed martial arts fighters who rely on quickness, agility, strength and a strong cardio system.

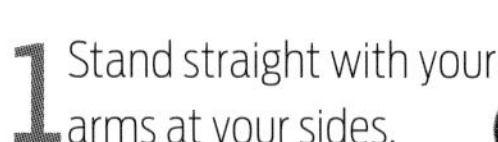

1 Stand straight with your arms at your sides.

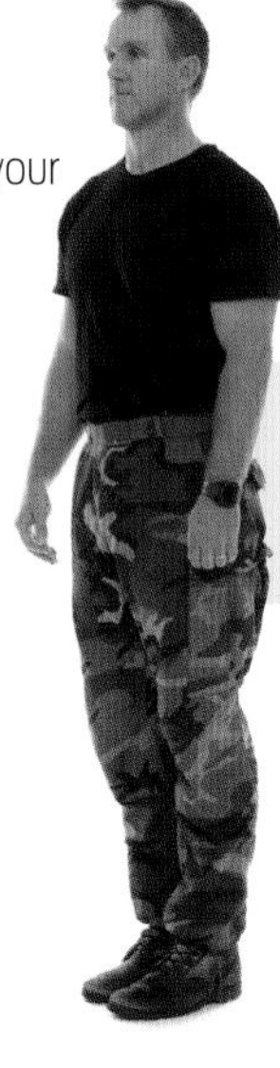

2 Drop into a squat position with your hands on the floor.

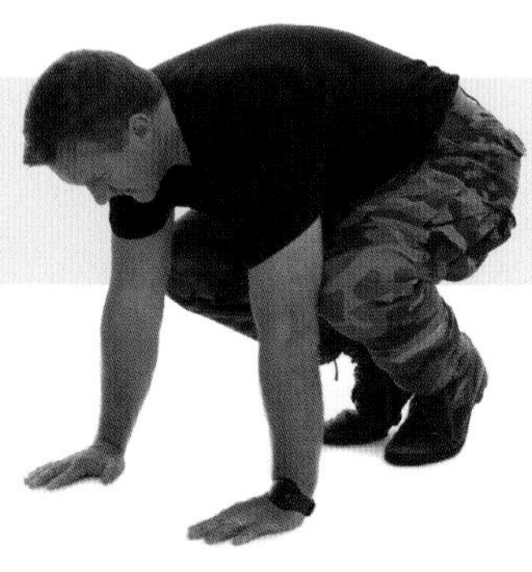

3 Kick your feet back as if you were assuming a Push-Up position while also dropping your chest to the floor.

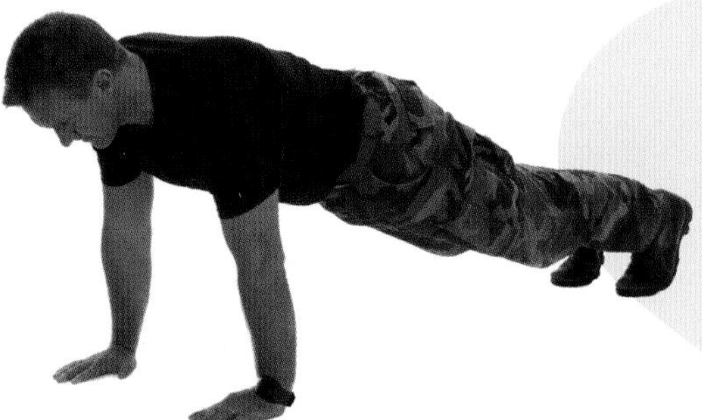

4 Perform a Push-Up.

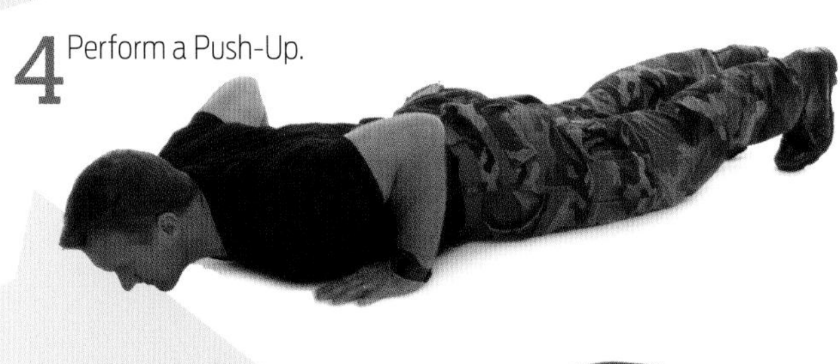

**Correct form**

- Make sure your chest touches the floor during step 3.
- Jump as high as you can as you rise from the squat.

**Avoid**

- Moving with floppy or jerky motions—your movement should be smooth and controlled.

5 Immediately return your feet to the squat position.

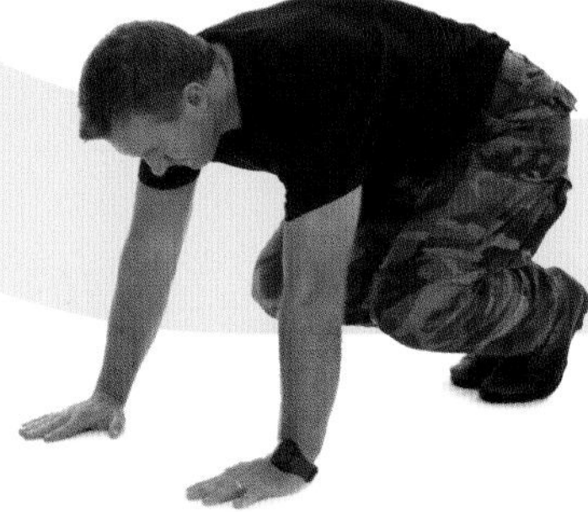

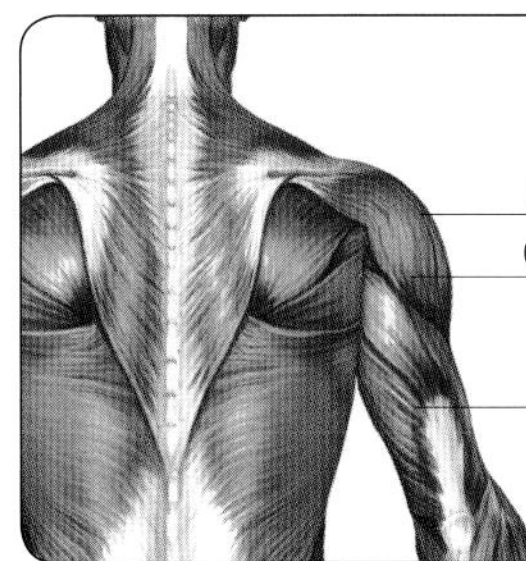


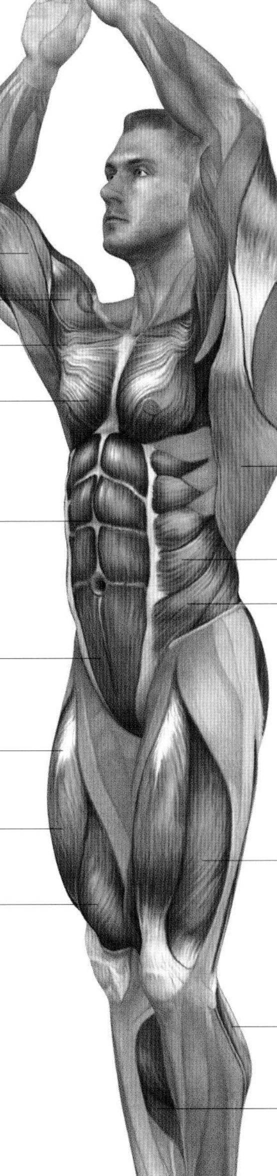


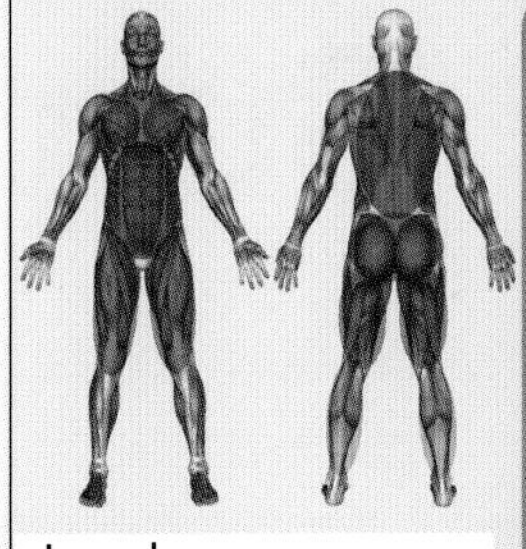

## Level
· Advanced

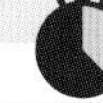

## Duration
· 60 seconds

## Benefits
· Increases cardiovascular endurance
· Increases agility and speed
· Strengthens entire body

## Caution
· Shortness of breath
· Shoulder issues
· Wrist issues
· Lower-back pain

**Annotation Key**
* indicates deep muscles

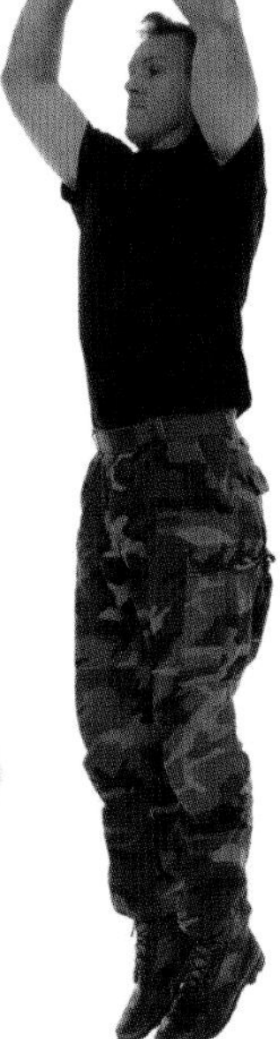

6 Jump back up to stand on your feet, and repeat the entire sequence. Perform as many reps as possible in 60 seconds.

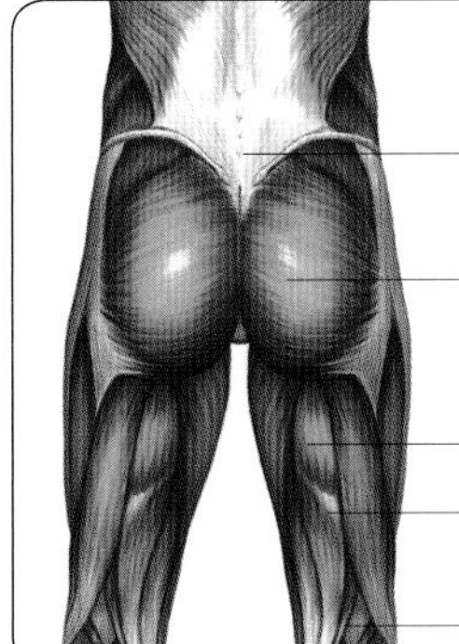

# Burpee with Pull-Up

As its names suggests, the Burpee with a Pull-Up adds another element to the traditional Burpee, making it even more of a strength-training challenge.

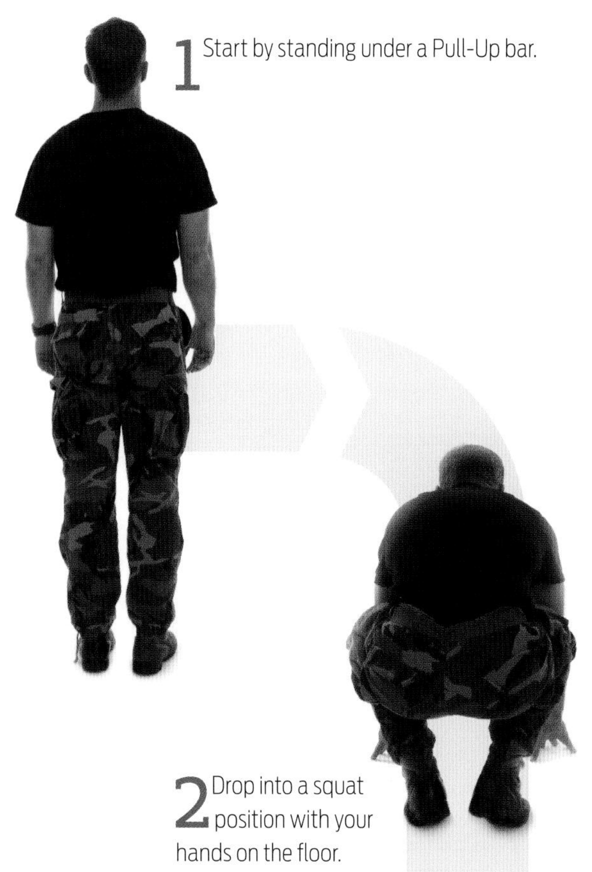

1 Start by standing under a Pull-Up bar.

2 Drop into a squat position with your hands on the floor.

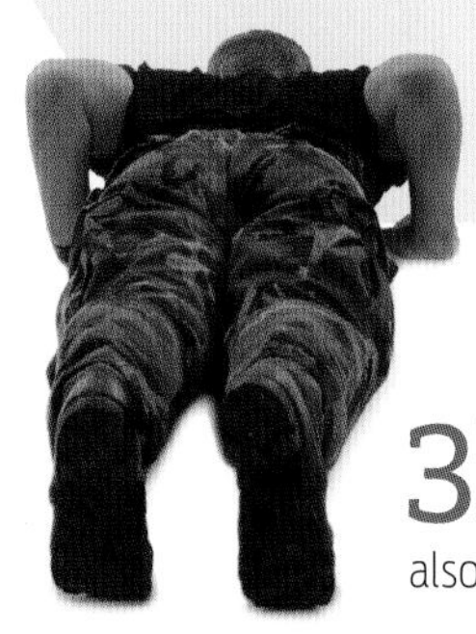

3 Kick your feet back as if you were assuming a Push-Up position while also dropping your chest to the floor.

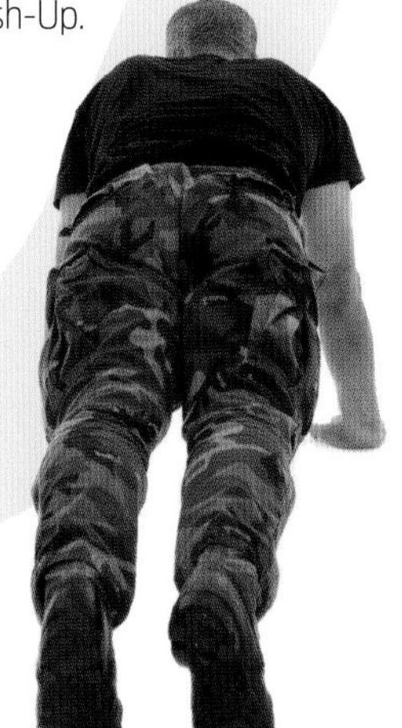

4 Perform a Push-Up.

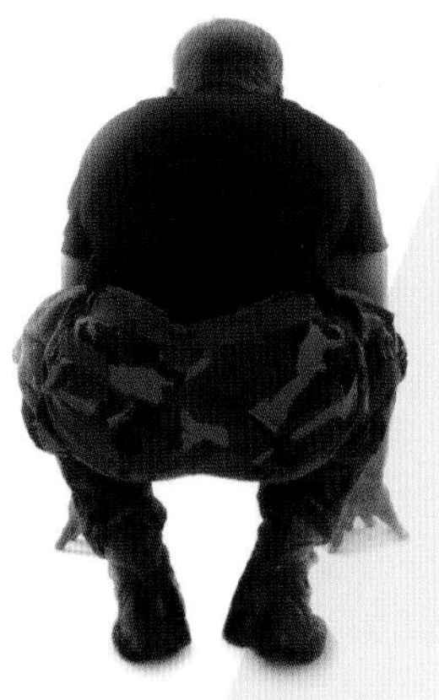

5 Immediately return your feet to the squat position.

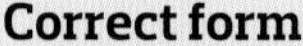

**Correct form**

- Make sure your chest touches the floor during step 3.
- Jump as high as you can as you rise from the squat.

**Avoid**

- Moving with floppy or jerky motions—your movement should be smooth and controlled.

**6** Jump back up to your feet and grab the Pull-Up bar.

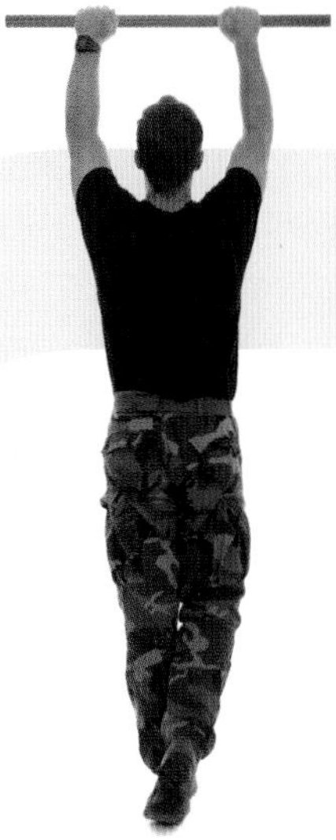

**7** Perform at least one Pull-Up, using the grip of your choice.

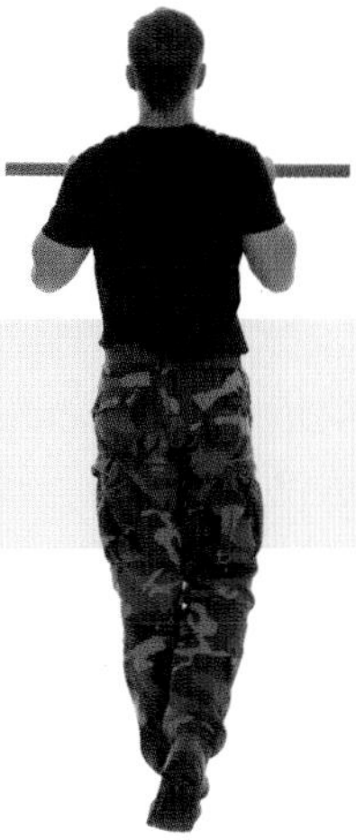

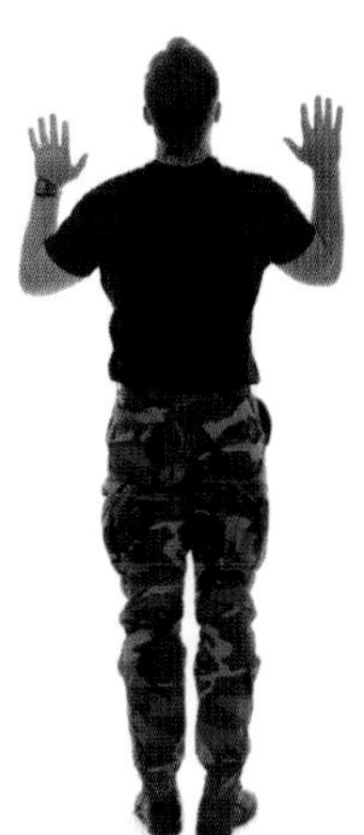

**8** Drop back to your feet, and repeat the entire sequence. Perform as many reps as possible in 60 seconds.

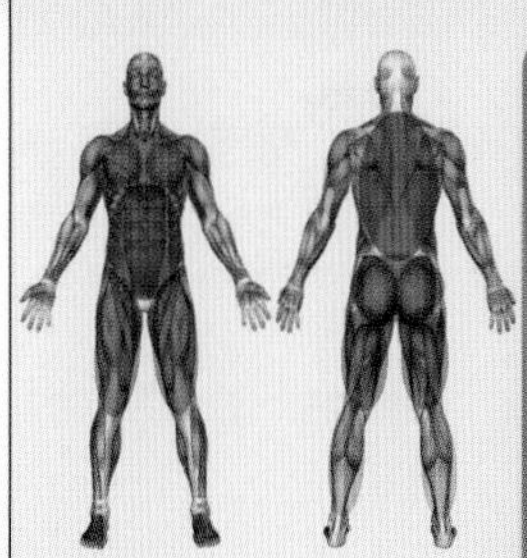

**Level**
- Advanced

**Duration**

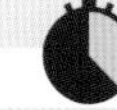

- 60 seconds

**Benefits**
- Increases cardiovascular endurance
- Increases agility and speed
- Strengthens entire body

**Caution**

- Shortness of breath
- Shoulder issues
- Wrist issues
- Lower-back pain

triceps brachii

rhomboideus*

latissimus dorsi

erector spinae*

gluteus maximus

semitendinosus

biceps femoris

semimembranosus

gastrocnemius

soleus

biceps brachii

deltoideus medialis

deltoideus posterior

**Annotation Key**
* indicates deep muscles

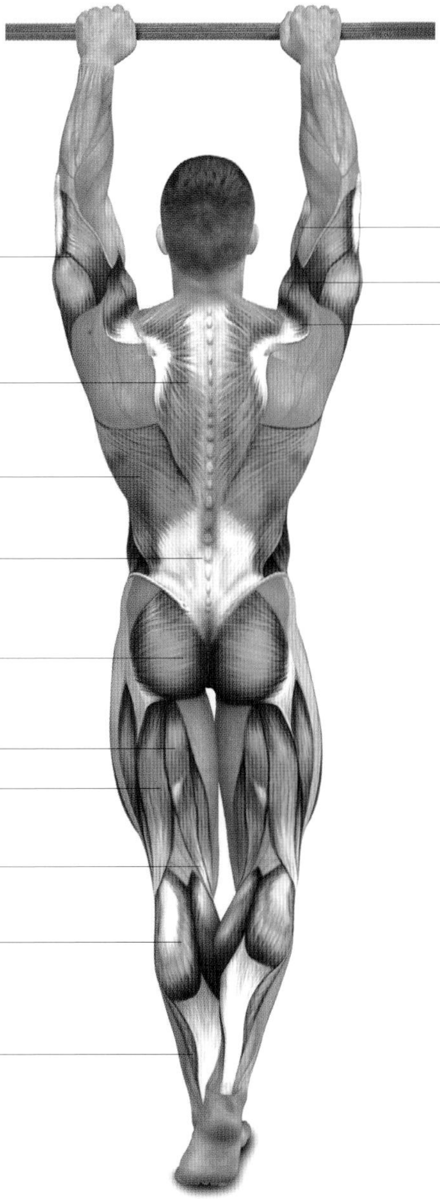

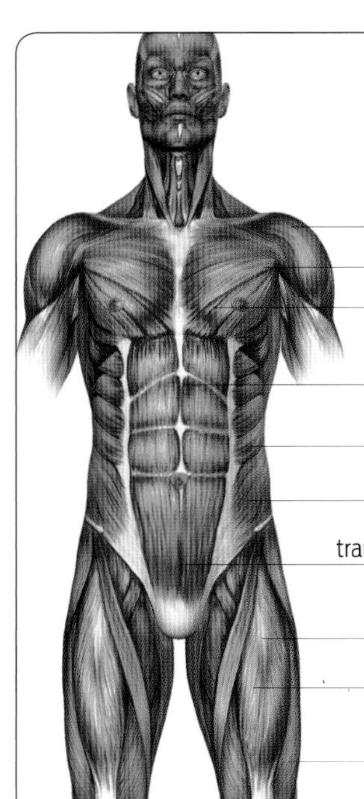

# Speed Skater

The Speed Skater exercise targets your iliotibial bands, hip adductors, and hip abductors, which all work to keep your knees and hips stable. If you include running in your overall fitness program, regularly performing this exercise can help avoid knee injury. Running is a staple component of special forces training, with candidates required to run long distances on various terrain such as unstable sand and dirt, which can place stress on the knees.

1 Stand in a half-squat position, and place your left leg slightly behind your right.

2 Jump to your left as far as possible while swinging your arms toward the left. Land in a half-squat position with your right leg slightly behind your left.

3 Immediately jump back toward the right as far as possible, as if you were skating in long strides. Switching back and forth equals one repetition. Perform 10 reps.

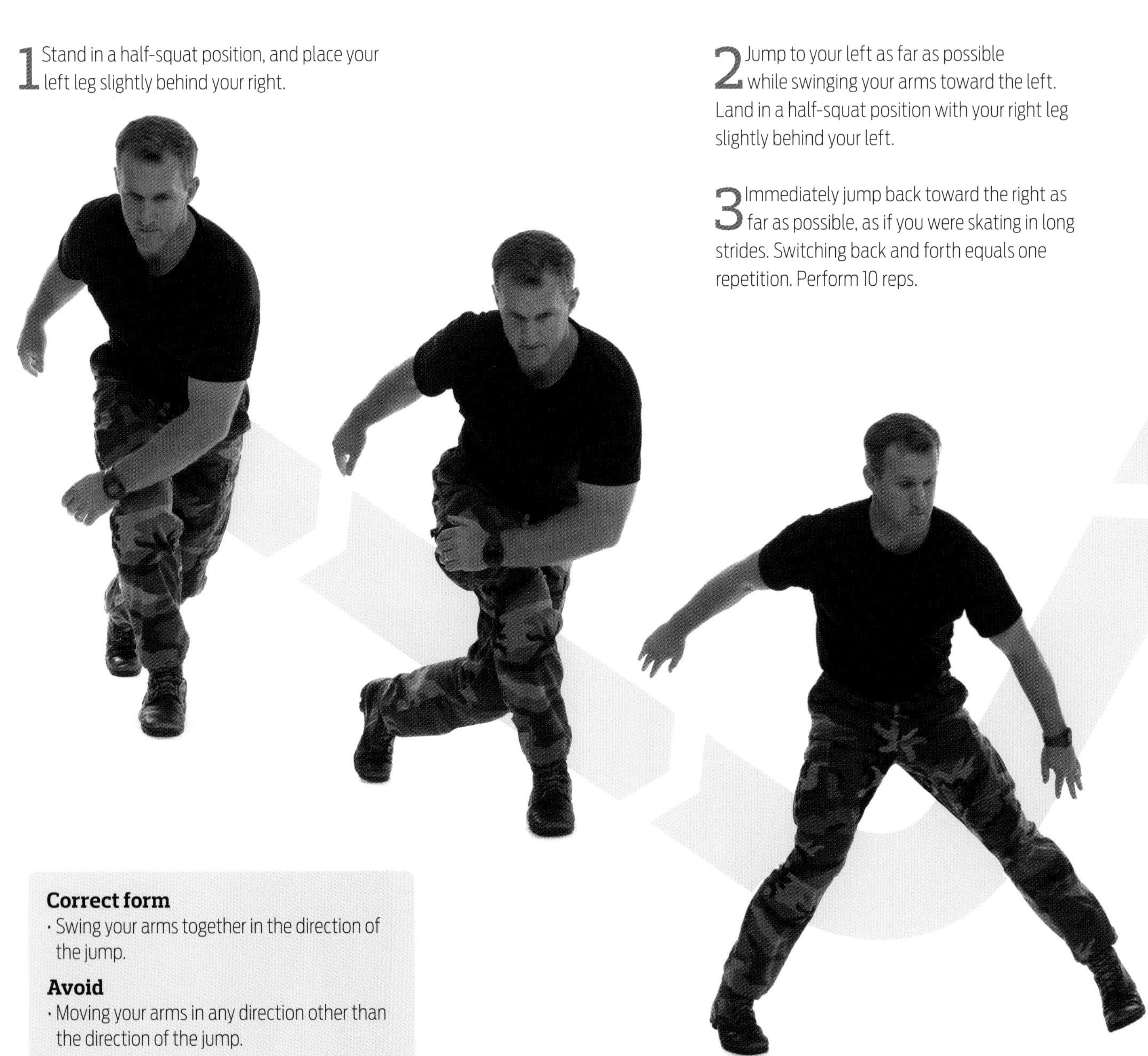

**Correct form**

- Swing your arms together in the direction of the jump.

**Avoid**

- Moving your arms in any direction other than the direction of the jump.

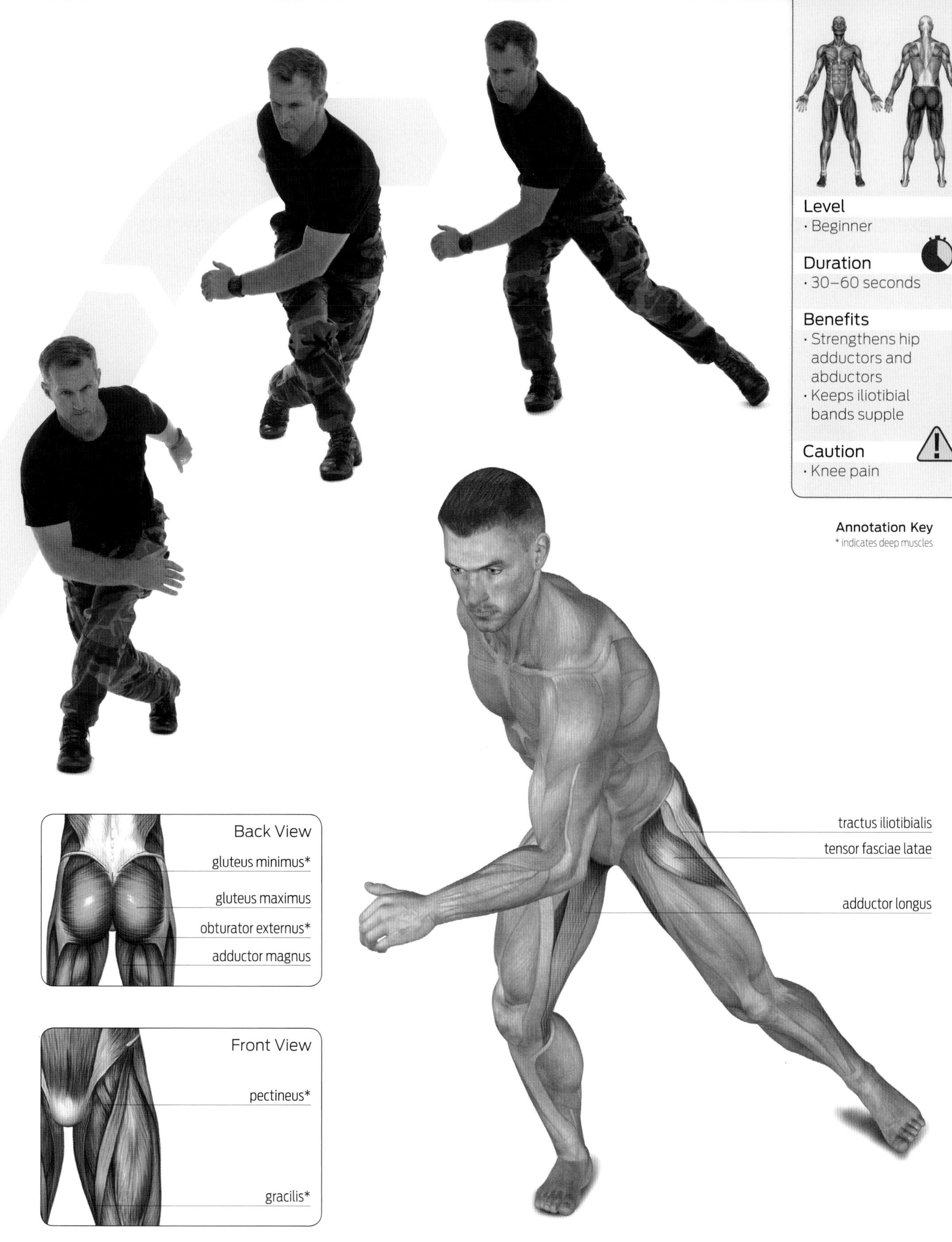


Level
· Beginner

Duration
· 30–60 seconds

Benefits
· Strengthens hip adductors and abductors
· Keeps iliotibial bands supple

Caution
· Knee pain

Annotation Key
* indicates deep muscles

# Straight-Leg Skater

A variation of the Speed Skater (pages 110–111), the Straight-Leg Skater targets your inner and outer thighs, including your hip adductor and abductor muscles and iliotibial bands. Like the Speed Skater, it is a great exercise for runners, counterbalancing the effects of repetitive flexion and extension and alleviating the resulting strength imbalance between the inner and outer thigh muscles and the quadriceps and hamstrings.

1 Stand straight, and place your left leg slightly behind your right.

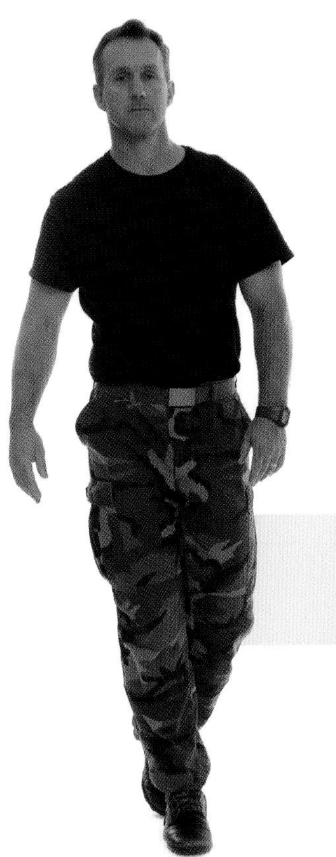

2 Keeping your legs and back straight, jump to your left as far as possible while swinging your arms toward the left.

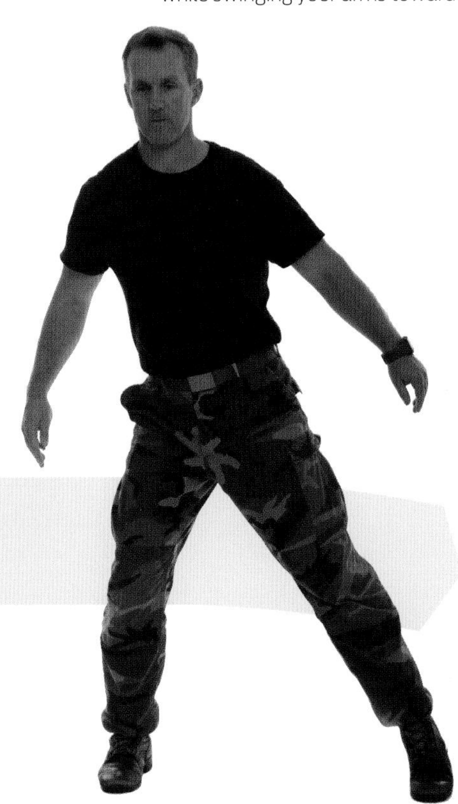

3 Land in a standing position with your right leg slightly behind your left.

**Correct form**
- Keep your torso upright.

**Avoid**
- Leaning forward as you move from side to side.

4 Continue jumping side-to-side, crossing one leg behind the other. Switching back and forth equals one repetition. Perform 25 reps.

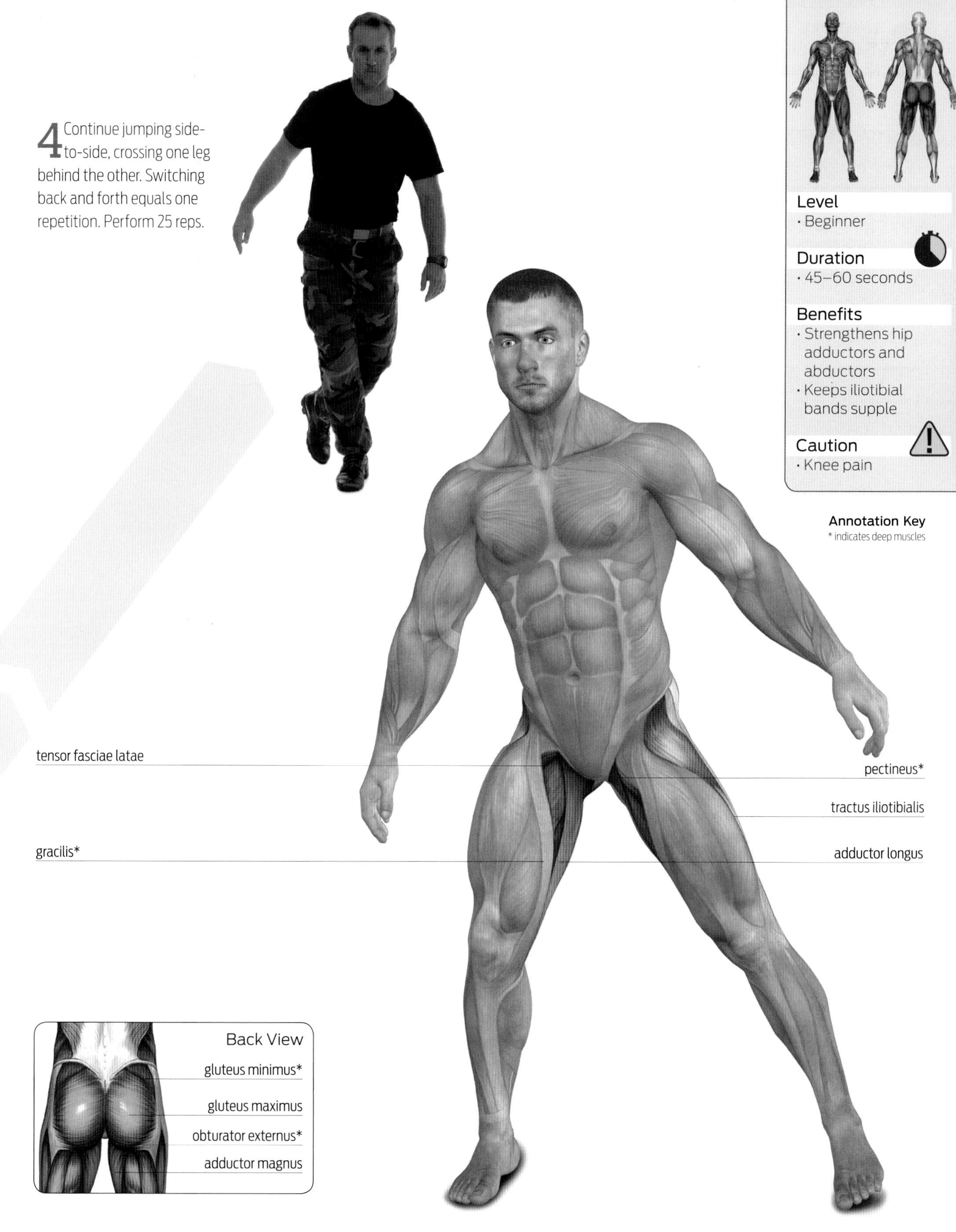


**Level**
- Beginner

**Duration**
- 45–60 seconds

**Benefits**
- Strengthens hip adductors and abductors
- Keeps iliotibial bands supple

**Caution**
- Knee pain

**Annotation Key**
* indicates deep muscles

# DFRB

"DFRB" stands for Drop, Face, Recover, and Back. During this agility exercise you will assume these four positions in rapid succession. "Drop" means to get into the push-up position. "Face" means to lower your body until your chest touches the floor. "Recover" means to jump both feet to your chest and stand up. "Back" means to flip onto your back. Begin by performing the moves in DFRB order, as outlined below, but as you progress, you can repeat the moves in any order—just remember that one repetition equals one movement in each position.

1 Begin in the standing position.

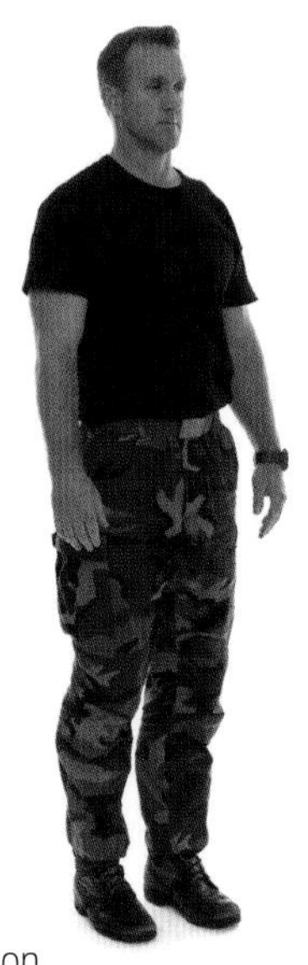

2 Drop forward into a Push-Up Position.

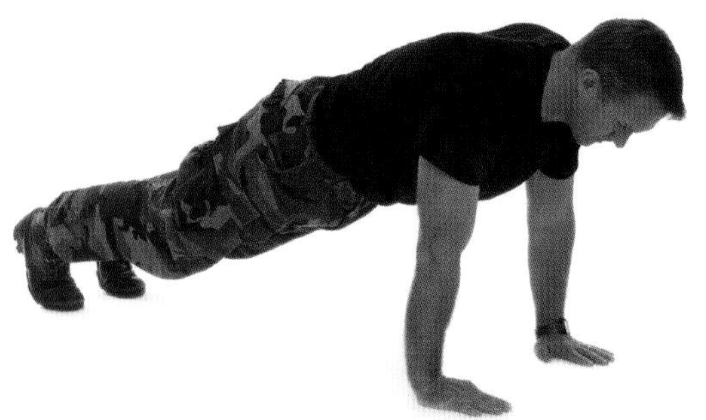

3 Lower your chest to the floor to assume the Face Position.

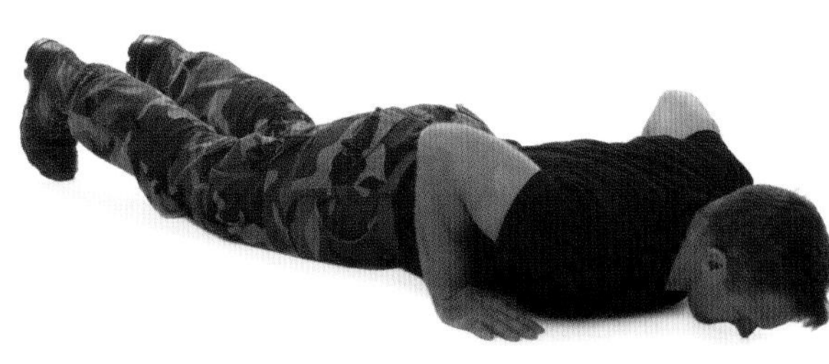

4 Rapidly jump both feet forward to your chest, so that you are in a full squat position, and then quickly stand up. This is the Recover Position.

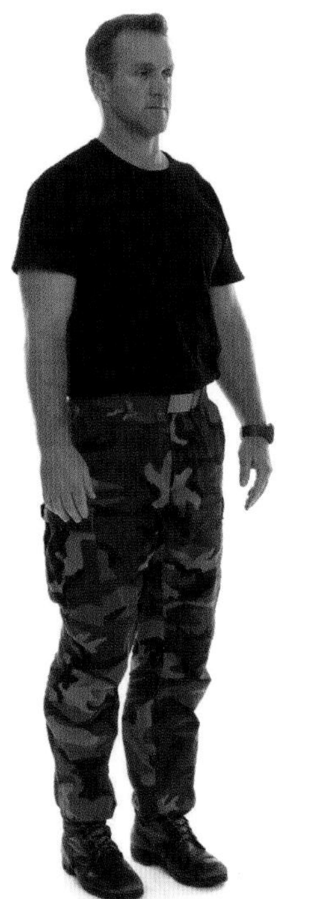

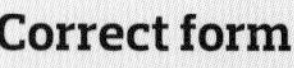

**Correct form**

- If you are working with someone, your partner can call the commands for you.

**Avoid**

- Moving slowly: an agility exercise requires quick movement into each position.

5 To assume the Back position, quickly drop your body to the floor and lie back, with your head landing where your feet were in the Face Position.

6 Jump to your feet, and repeat the sequence in any order. Performing all four positions equals one repetition. Perform 10 reps.

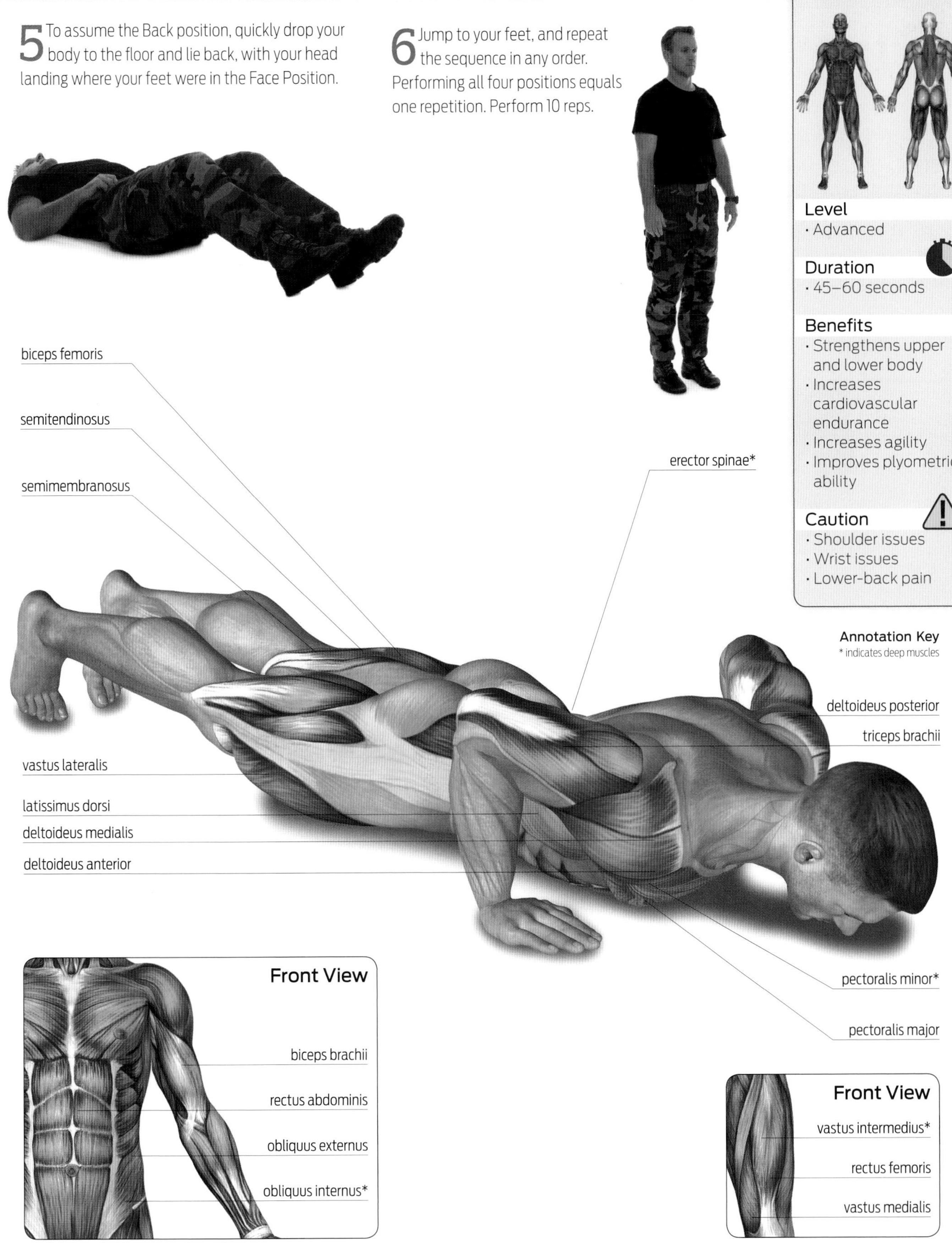


**Level**
- Advanced

**Duration**
- 45–60 seconds

**Benefits**
- Strengthens upper and lower body
- Increases cardiovascular endurance
- Increases agility
- Improves plyometric ability

**Caution**
- Shoulder issues
- Wrist issues
- Lower-back pain

**Annotation Key**
* indicates deep muscles

# Plank

The Plank is an isometric exercise, designed to work your entire core. SEALs perform this core-stabilizing exercise for a good reason: it is a reliable way to build endurance in the abdominals and back, as well as in the stabilizer muscles.

1 Lie on your stomach on the floor, balancing your feet on your toes.

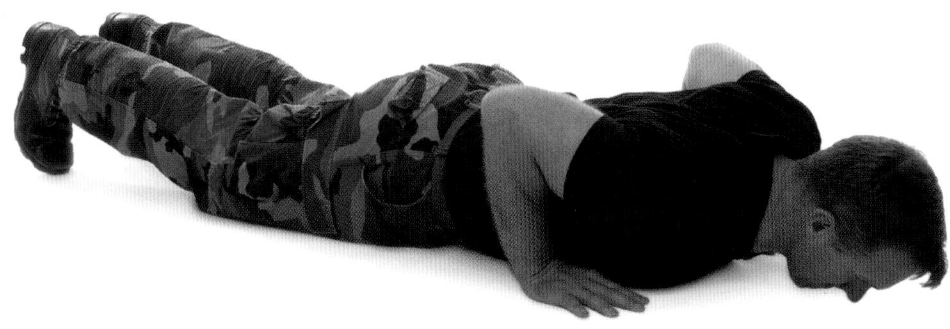

2 Bend your elbows and place your forearms on the floor with your palms toward each other, and make your hands into fists. Contract your glutes and legs and lift your hips and thighs off the floor.

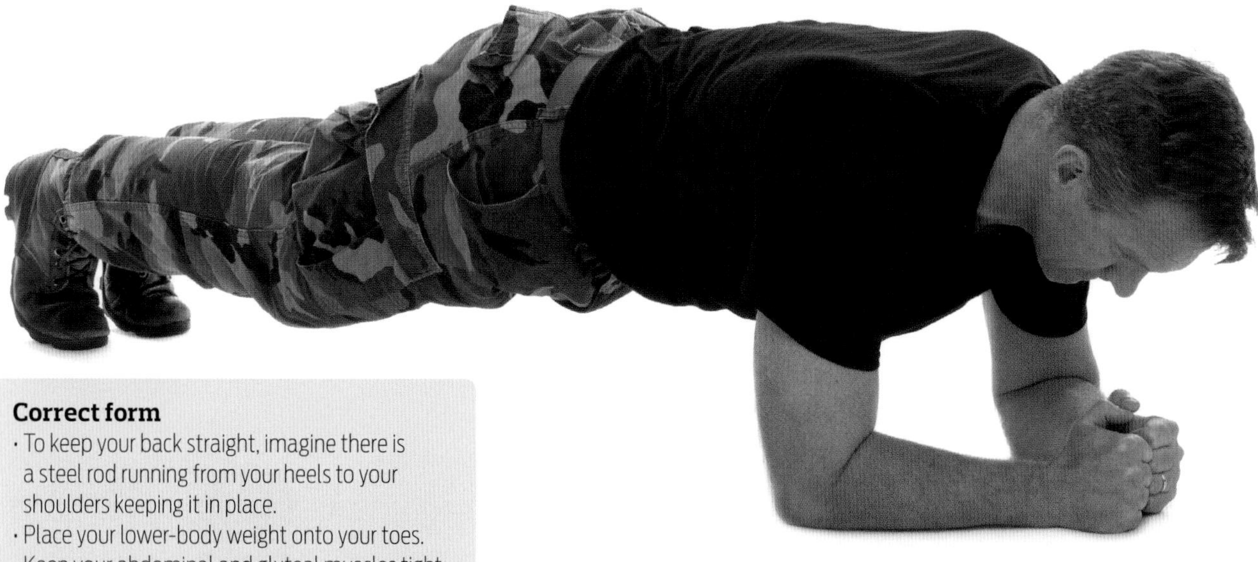

**Correct form**

- To keep your back straight, imagine there is a steel rod running from your heels to your shoulders keeping it in place.
- Place your lower-body weight onto your toes.
- Keep your abdominal and gluteal muscles tight.

**Avoid**

- Bridging too high, which can take stress off working muscles.

3 Tighten your abdominals, look down at the floor, and keep your back straight. Remain suspended in Plank for 60 seconds.

Back View
subscapularis*
supraspinatus*
infraspinatus*
teres minor

Back View
erector spinae*
semitendinosus
semimembranosus

Front View
deltoideus anterior
pectoralis major
rectus abdominis
trnasversus abdominis*
soleus
vastus medialis
tibialis anterior

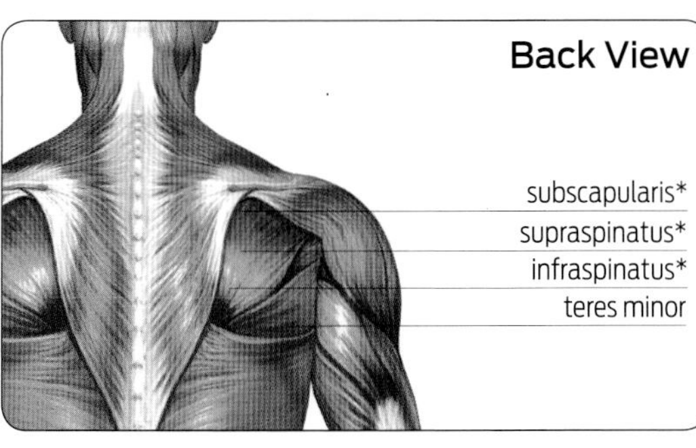

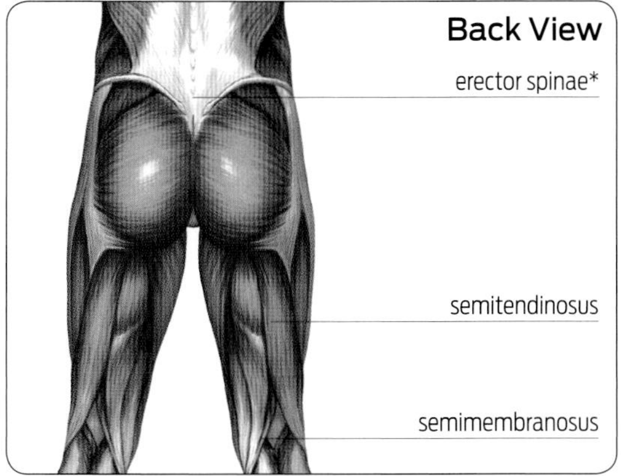

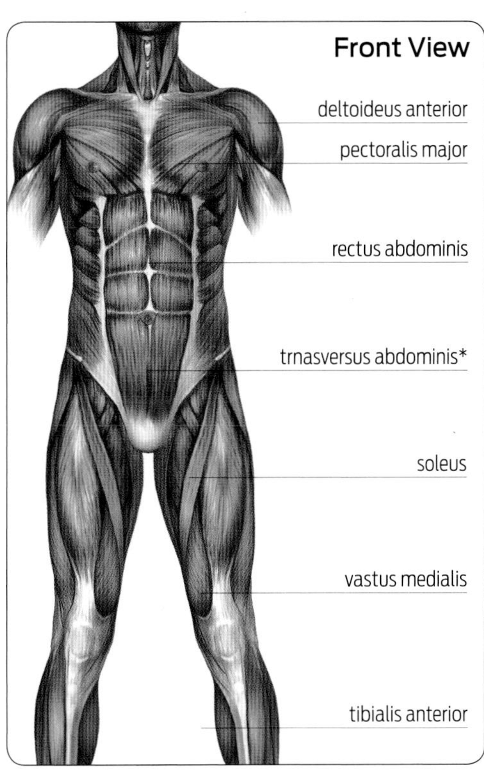

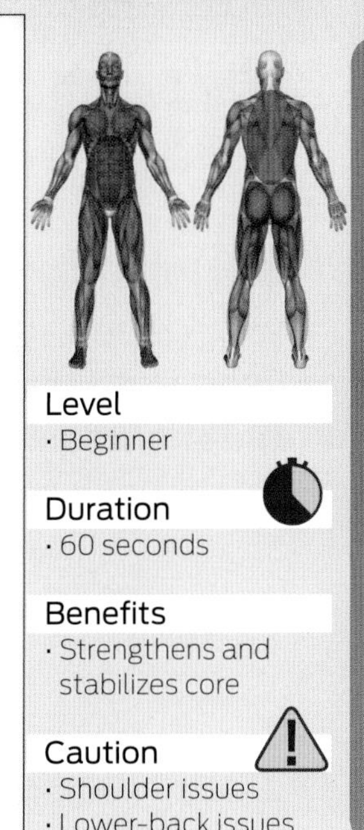

**Level**
- Beginner

**Duration**
- 60 seconds

**Benefits**
- Strengthens and stabilizes core

**Caution**
- Shoulder issues
- Lower-back issues

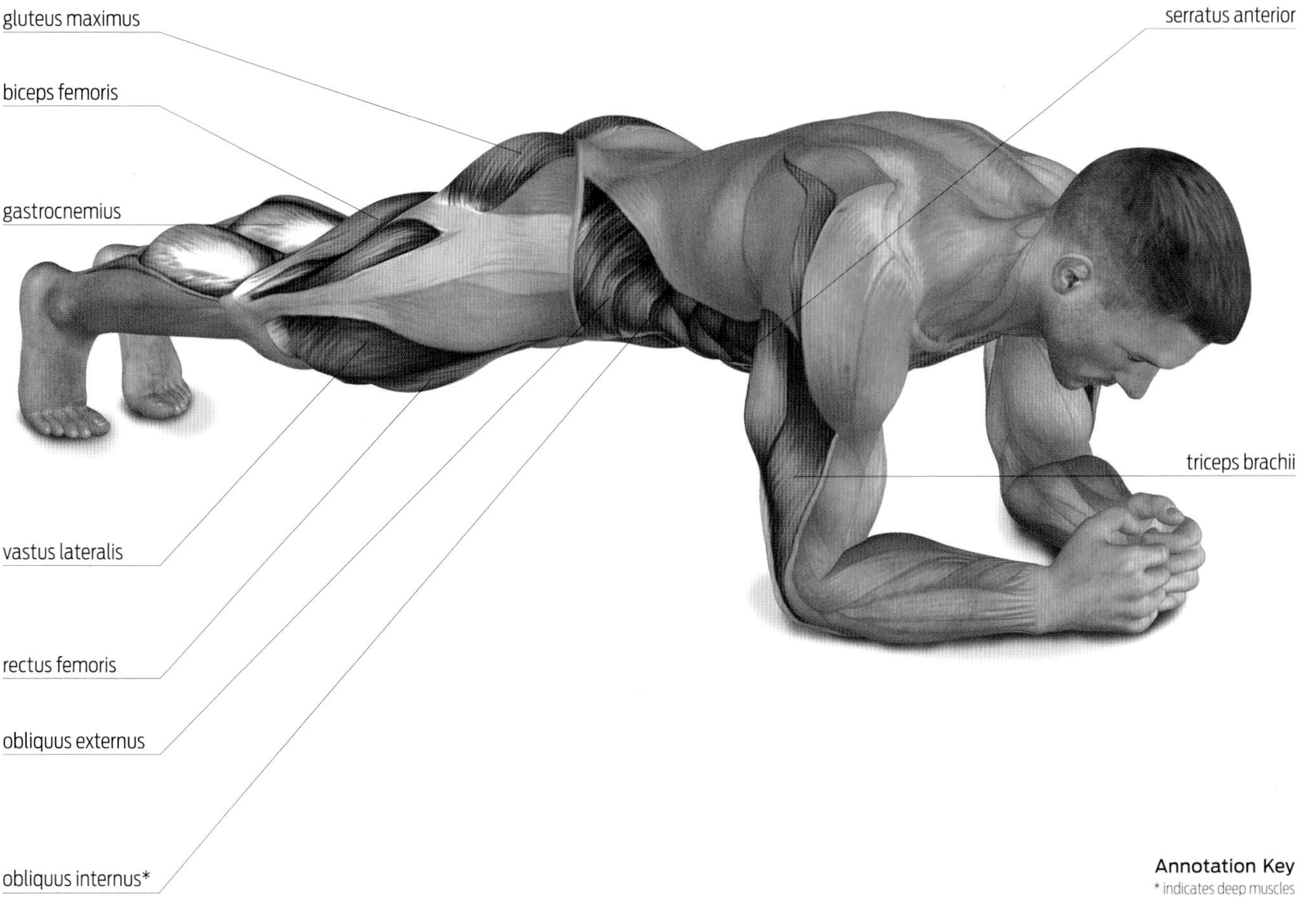

gluteus maximus
biceps femoris
gastrocnemius
vastus lateralis
rectus femoris
obliquus externus
obliquus internus*
serratus anterior
triceps brachii

**Annotation Key**
* indicates deep muscles

# High Plank

The High Plank is an amazing upper-body stabilizing exercise that teaches you to keep your body firm and steady. It calls for you to hold your body in Drop Position, which serves to increase Push-Up strength while stabilizing the shoulders and upper back. Increased stability of the shoulders and upper back can help prevent injuries.

1 With your hands shoulder-width apart, place your palms on the floor, keeping your feet together and back straight. Push your body up until your arms are straight.

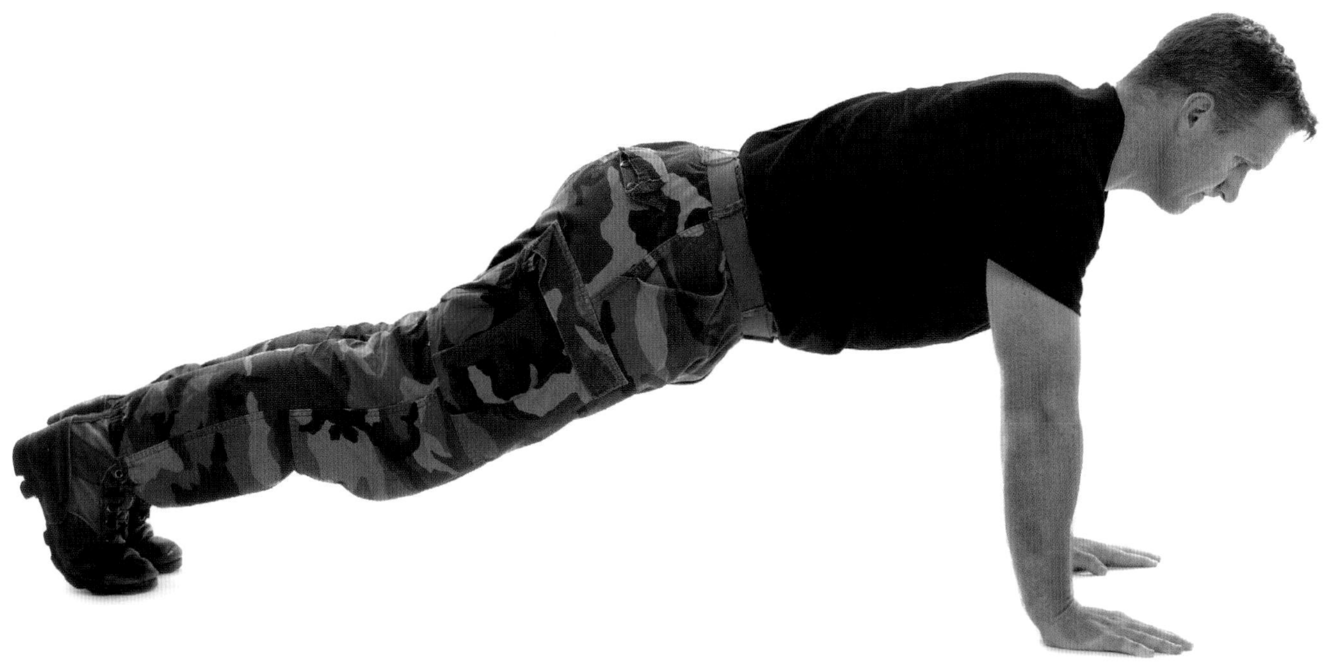

2 Remain suspended in High Plank for 60 seconds.

**Correct form**

- Keep your back straight.
- Place your lower-body weight onto your toes.
- Keep your abdominal and gluteal muscles tight.

**Avoid**

- Dropping your chin to your chest—keep your head up.
- Pushing your hips into the air.

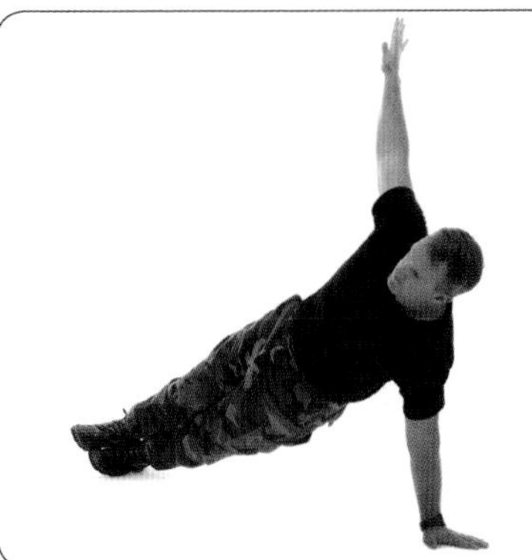

## Modification

**More diffcult:** T-Stabilization will further improve your balance and stability. From High Plank, shift your weight onto the outside of your left foot and onto your left arm. Roll to the side, guiding with your hips and bringing your right shoulder back. Stack your right foot on top of the left, squeezing both legs together. Bring your right arm up toward the ceiling, and elongate your body, making a straight line from your head to your heels. Hold for 15 to 30 seconds. Release, and then repeat on the other side.

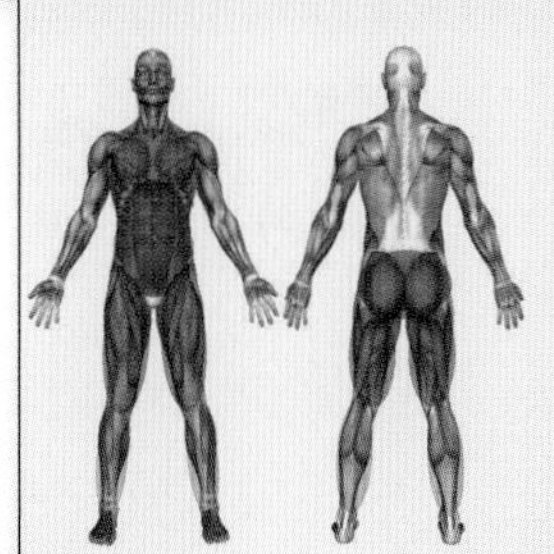

**Level**
- Beginner

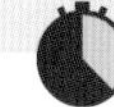

**Duration**
- 60 seconds

**Benefits**
- Strengthens and stabilizes core

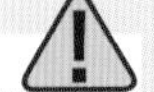

**Caution**
- Shoulder issues
- Lower-back issues
- Wrist issues

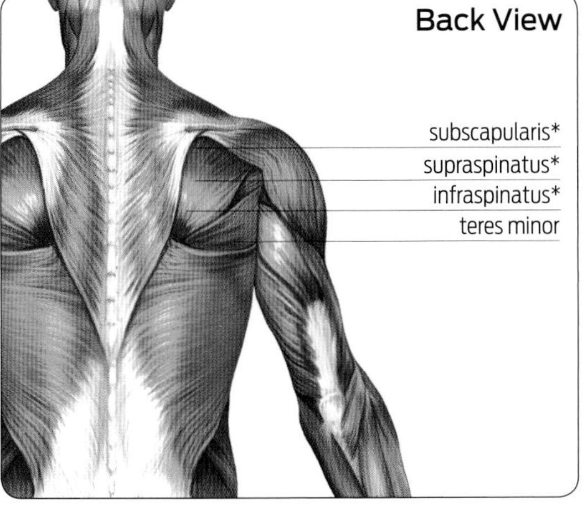


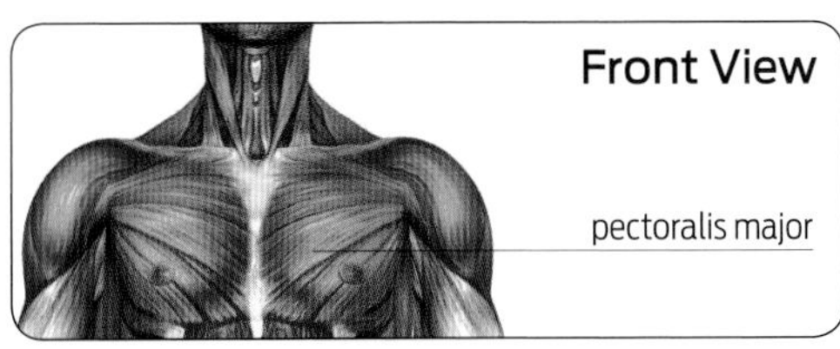


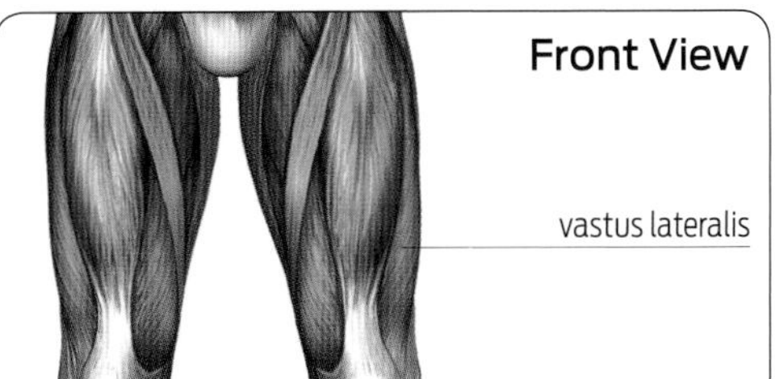


**Annotation Key**
* indicates deep muscles

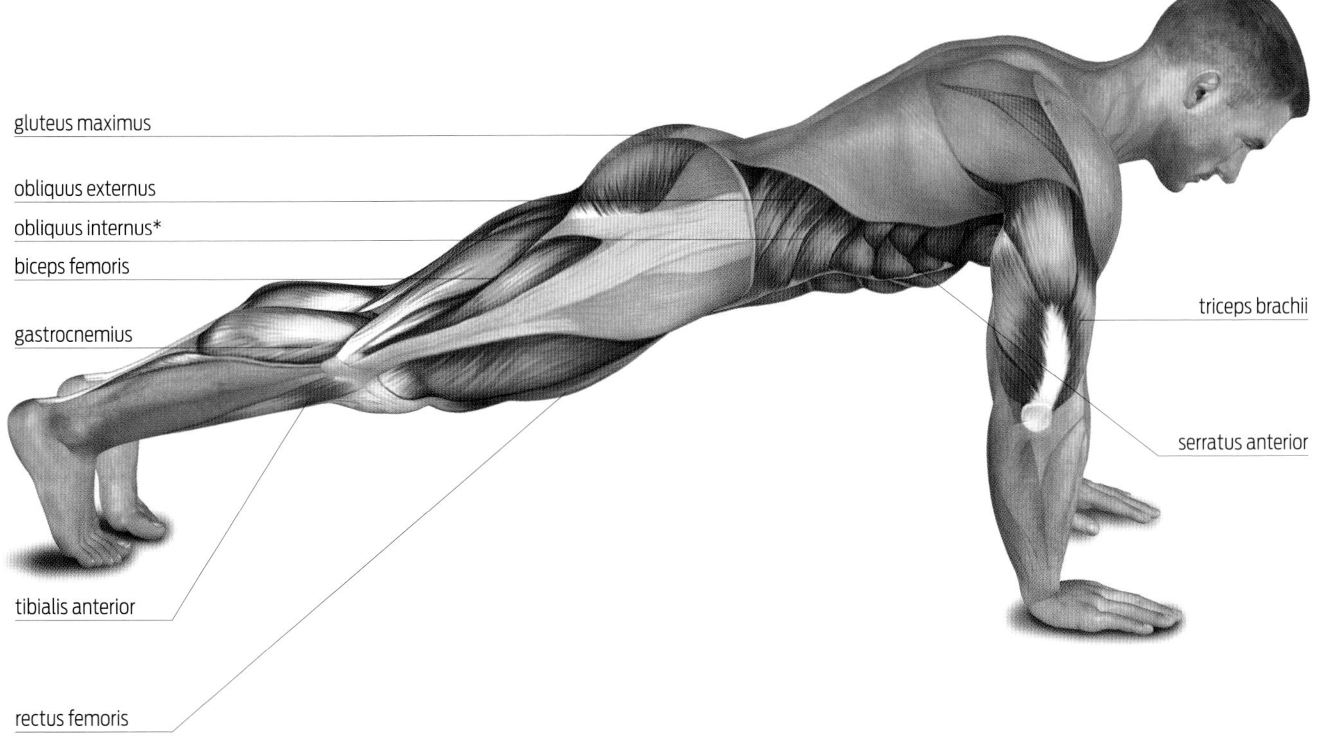

# Side Plank

Side Plank stabilizes your spine, and it is also an effective shoulder, abdominal, and lower-back strengthener. Like other versions of Plank, it increases both strength and stability, which helps prevent injuries.

1 Lie on your left side with your legs straight and parallel to each other. Keep your feet flexed.

2 Bend your left arm to form a 90-degree angle with the knuckles of your hand facing forward. Place your right hand on your waist.

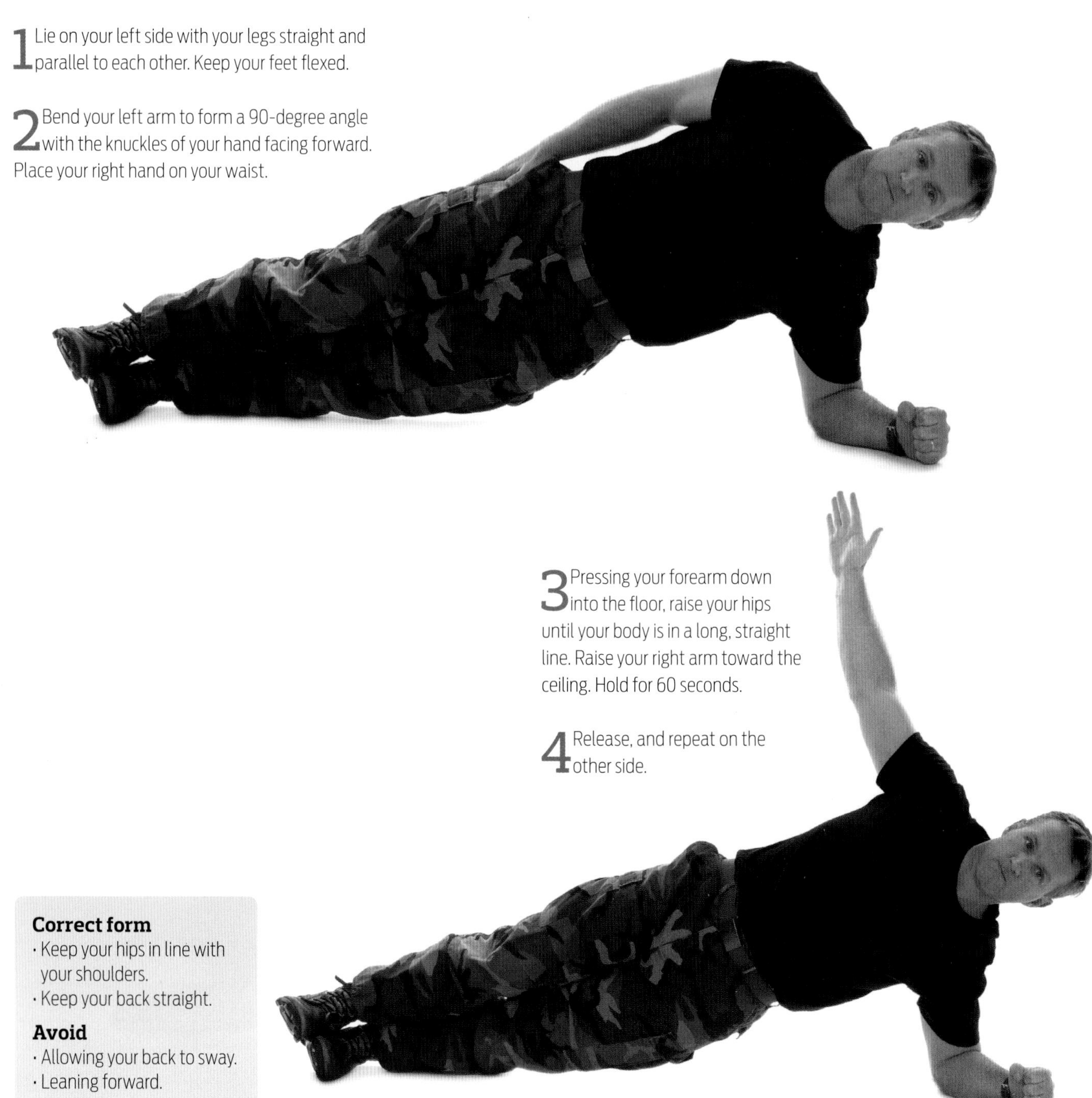

3 Pressing your forearm down into the floor, raise your hips until your body is in a long, straight line. Raise your right arm toward the ceiling. Hold for 60 seconds.

4 Release, and repeat on the other side.

**Correct form**
- Keep your hips in line with your shoulders.
- Keep your back straight.

**Avoid**
- Allowing your back to sway.
- Leaning forward.

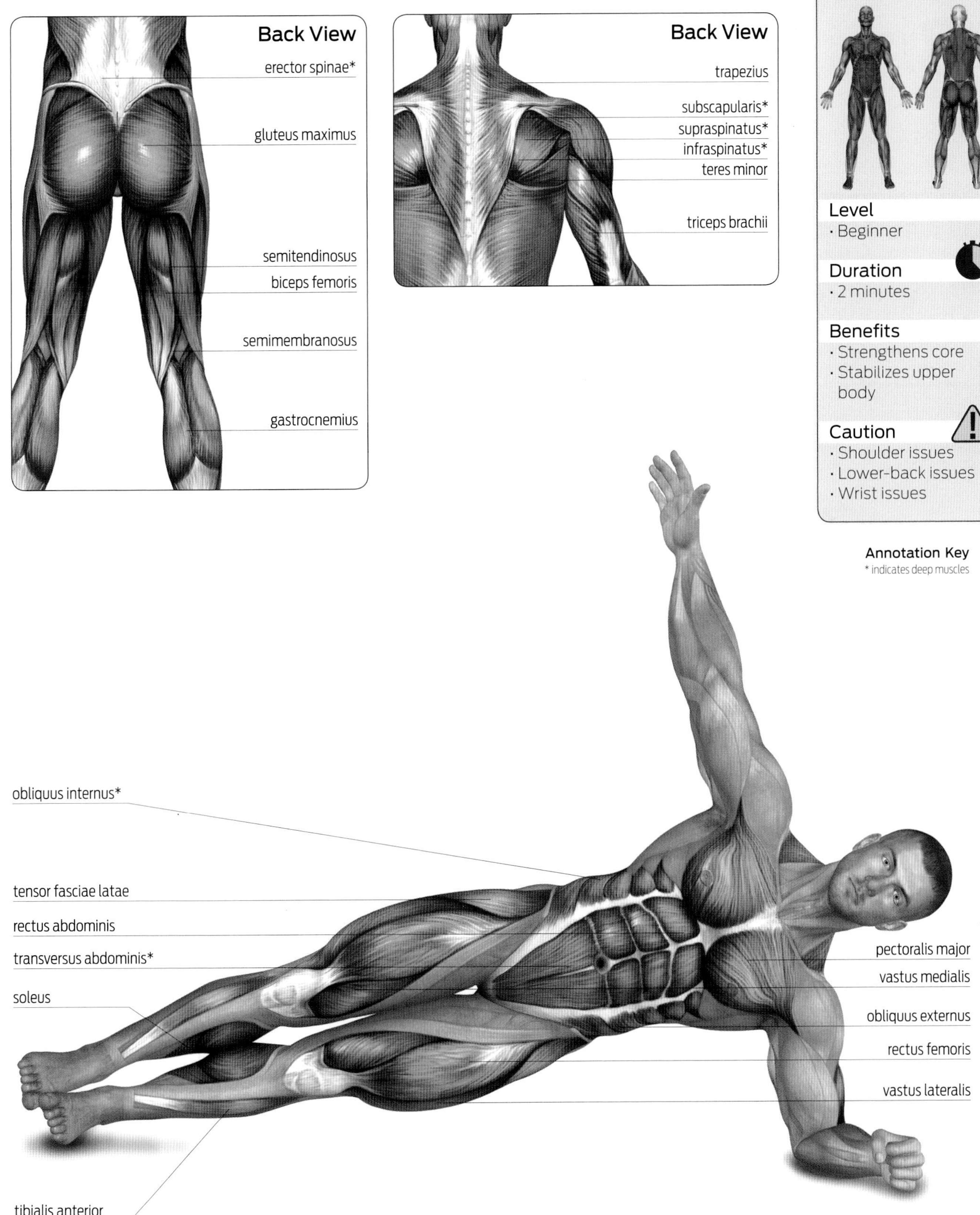


**Level**
- Beginner

**Duration**
- 2 minutes

**Benefits**
- Strengthens core
- Stabilizes upper body

**Caution**
- Shoulder issues
- Lower-back issues
- Wrist issues

**Annotation Key**
* indicates deep muscles

# Bird Dog

Bird Dog, so named because it resembles a pointing bird dog, is a lower-back stabilization exercise, as well as a shoulder and upper-back stabilizer. The Bird Dog may look like a simple exercise, but it really challenges your sense of balance and coordination. It is an isometric exercise, meaning you contract and hold a muscle in a static position. Isometric exercises also contract the ligament associated with a muscle. This can have the added benefit of stabilizing the joint associated with the movement.

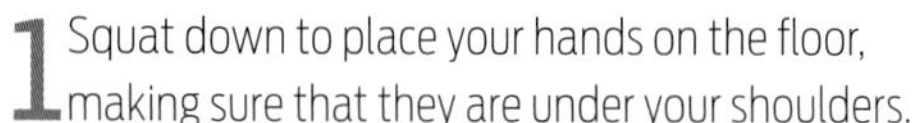

1 Squat down to place your hands on the floor, making sure that they are under your shoulders.

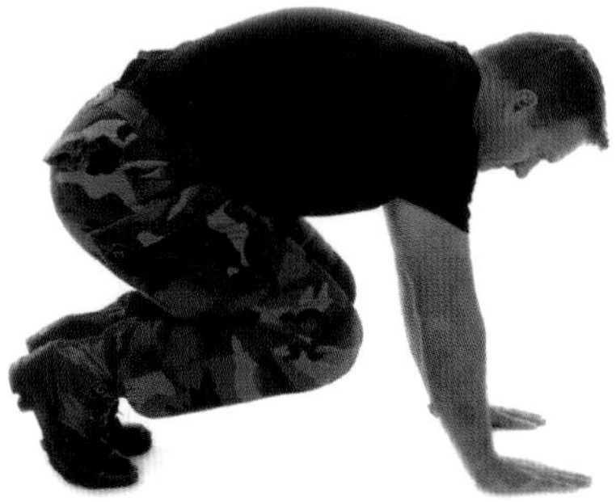

2 Extend your legs to assume the Drop Position.

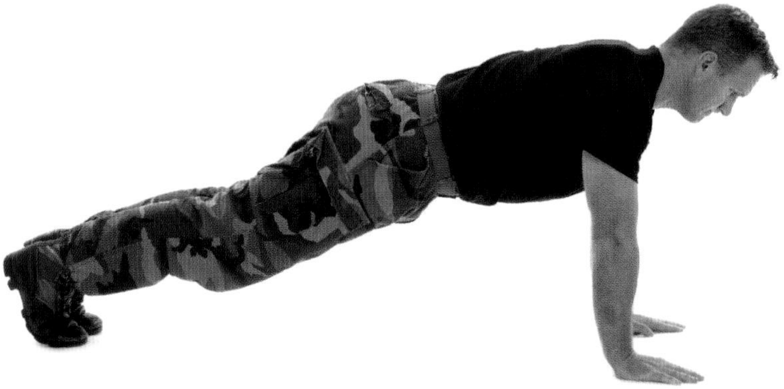

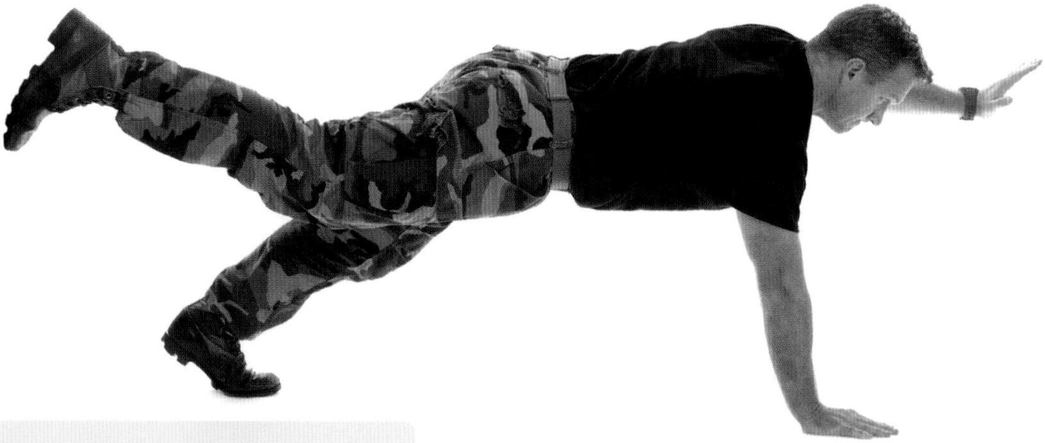

**Correct form**

- Be sure to raise both the extended arm and leg high enough so that they are parallel with the floor.
- Engage your abs by drawing your navel toward your spine.
- Practice makes perfect—it will take you a few tries to get your balance.

**Avoid**

- Allowing your lower back to sag.

3 Extend your left arm parallel to the floor, while lifting your right leg and extending it behind you.

4 Hold for 30 seconds, return to Drop Position, and then repeat on the other side.

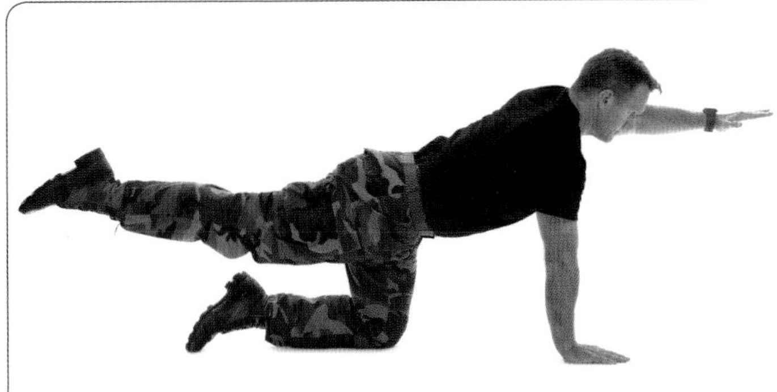

## Modification

**Easier:** Start on your hands and knees, making sure that your hands are under your shoulders and your knees are under your hips. Extend one arm parallel to the floor, while lifting your opposite leg and extending it behind you. Hold for 30 seconds, and then repeat on the other side.

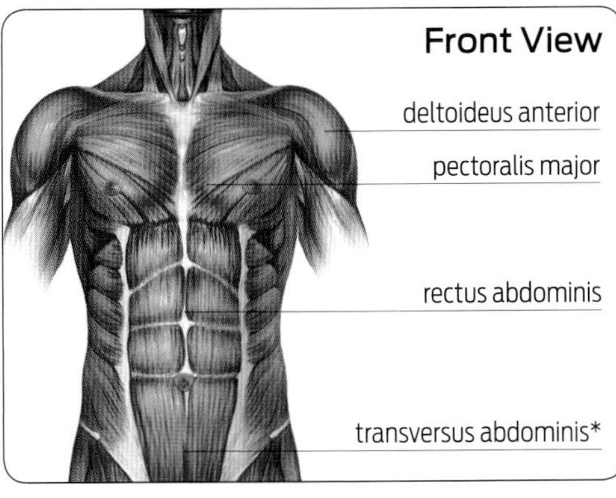


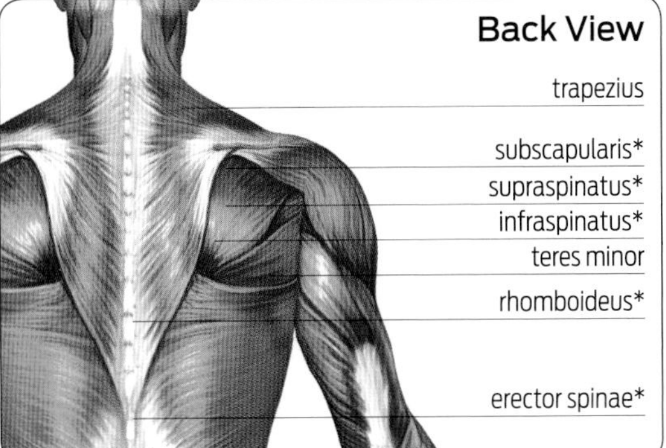


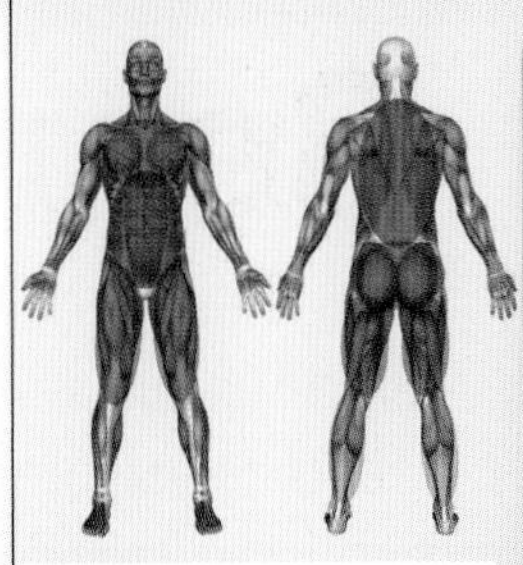

**Level**
· Advanced

**Duration** 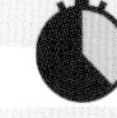
· 60 seconds

**Benefits**
· Stabilizes lower back
· Stabilizes shoulders and upper back
· Improves balance and coordination

**Caution** 
· Shoulder issues
· Wrist injury
· Lower-back injury

**Annotation Key**
* indicates deep muscles

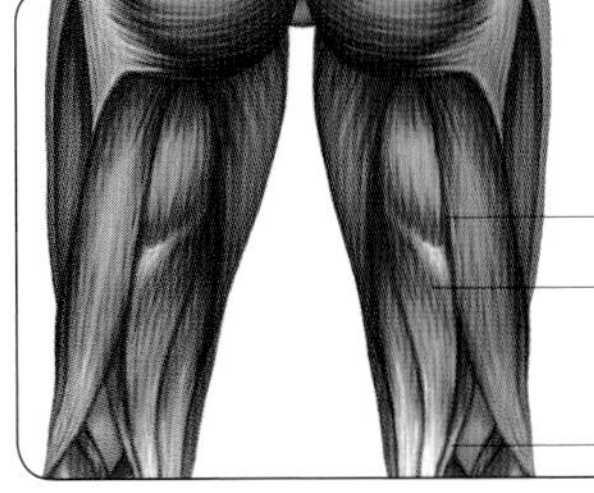


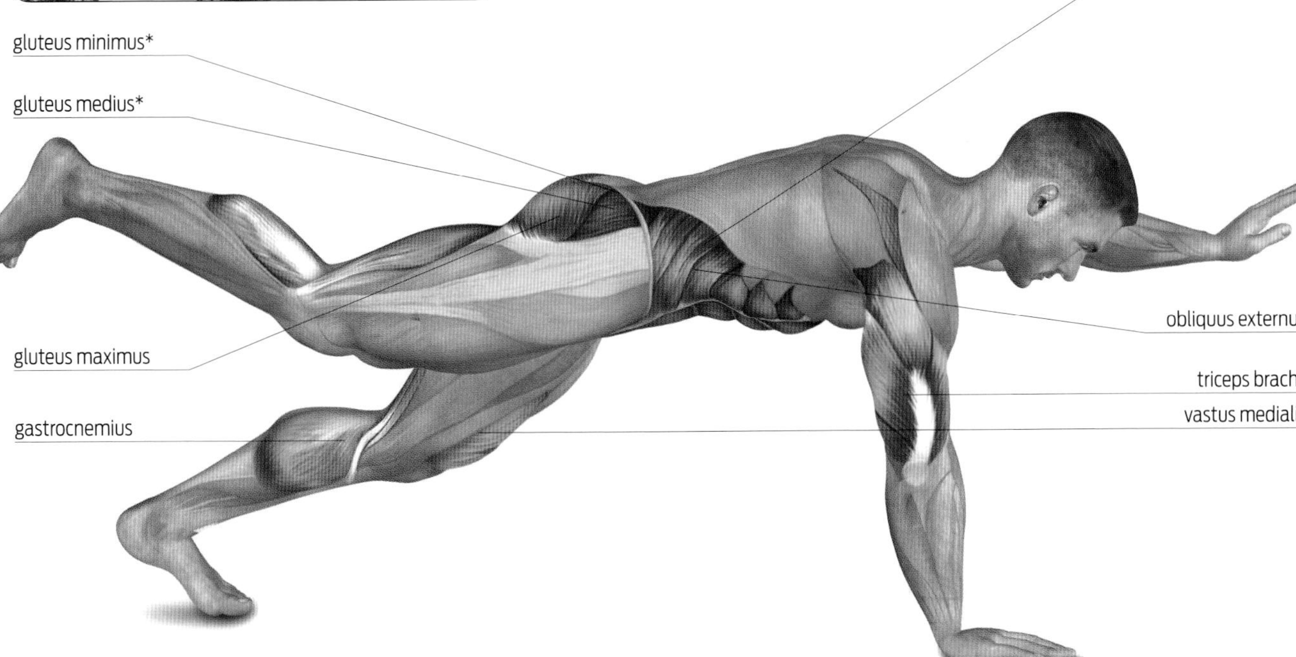

# Bear Crawl

Bear Crawl is a tough exercise, but it is great for increasing agility, cardiovascular health, and upper-body strength. This anaerobic exercise is a staple for special forces operatives, both in training and in the field. Anaerobic exercise triggers lactic acid formation, which promotes strength, speed, and power.

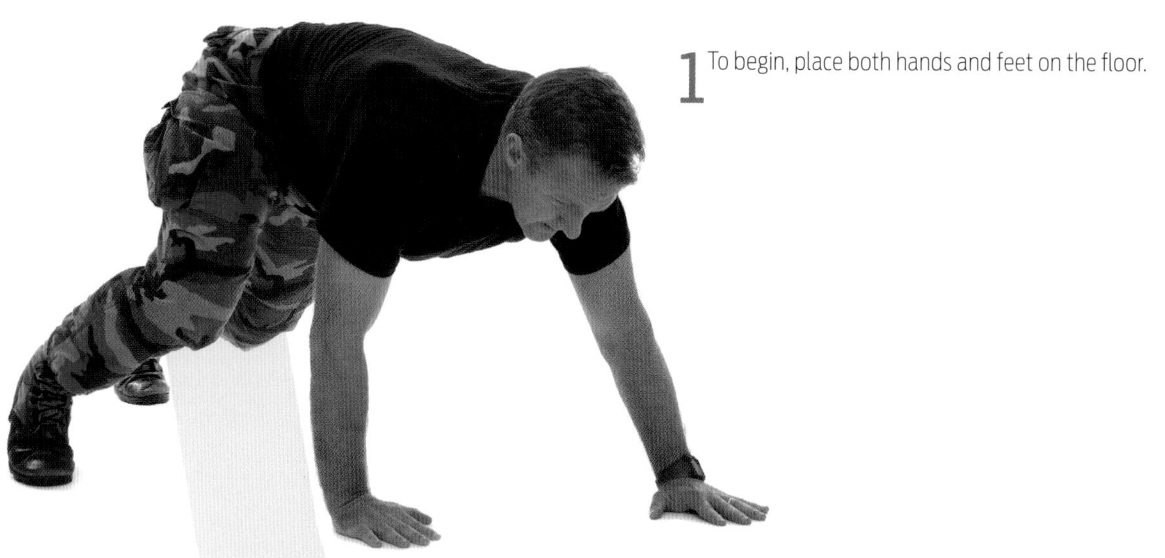

1 To begin, place both hands and feet on the floor.

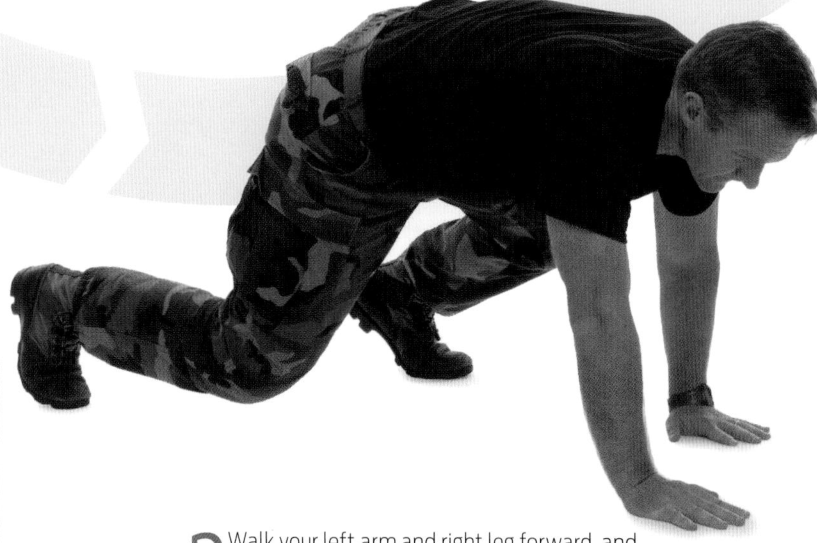

2 Walk your left arm and right leg forward, and then your right arm and left leg.

**Correct form**

- Move as steadily and as smoothly as possible.

**Avoid**

- Placing all of your weight on your arms and shoulders, which can stress your rotator cuffs.
- Touching your knees to the floor.

3 Keep moving forward and backward in this position, keeping your weight evenly distributed between your arms and legs. Perform for 60 seconds.

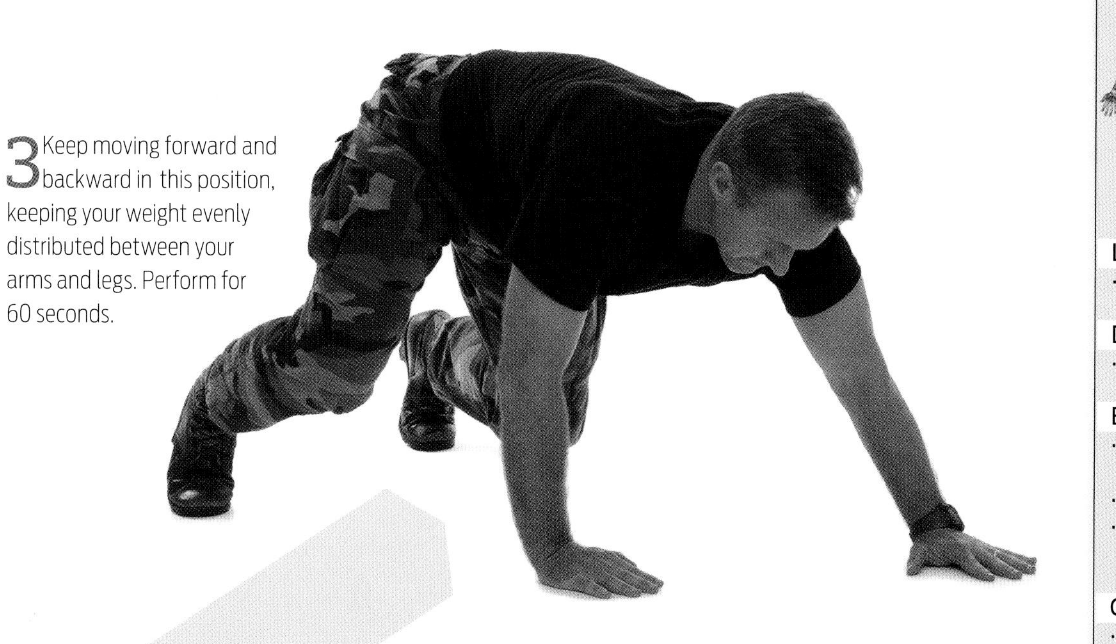

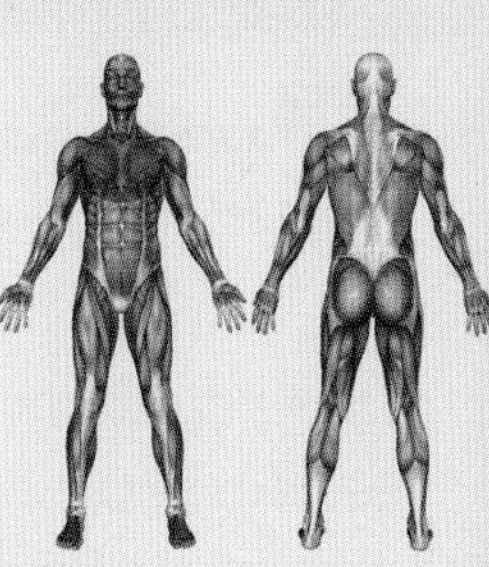

**Level**
- Intermediate

**Duration** 
- 60 seconds

**Benefits**
- Strengthens upper body
- Increases agility
- Improves coordination

**Caution**
- Shoulder issues
- Wrist injury
- Lower-back injury

**Annotation Key**
* indicates deep muscles

deltoideus anterior
pectoralis minor*
triceps brachii
biceps brachii
pectoralis majo

# Crab Crawl

Like its opposite, the Bear Crawl (pages 124–125), the Crab Crawl is an anaerobic exercise that triggers lactic acid formation, promoting strength, speed, and power while giving you a cardio workout. The Crab Crawl is a challenge to execute properly, demanding agility and coordination.

1 Begin with both hands and feet on the floor. Lift your body slightly so that your butt is just above the floor.

3 Walk your left foot forward. Continue moving forward, taking several steps with each leg.

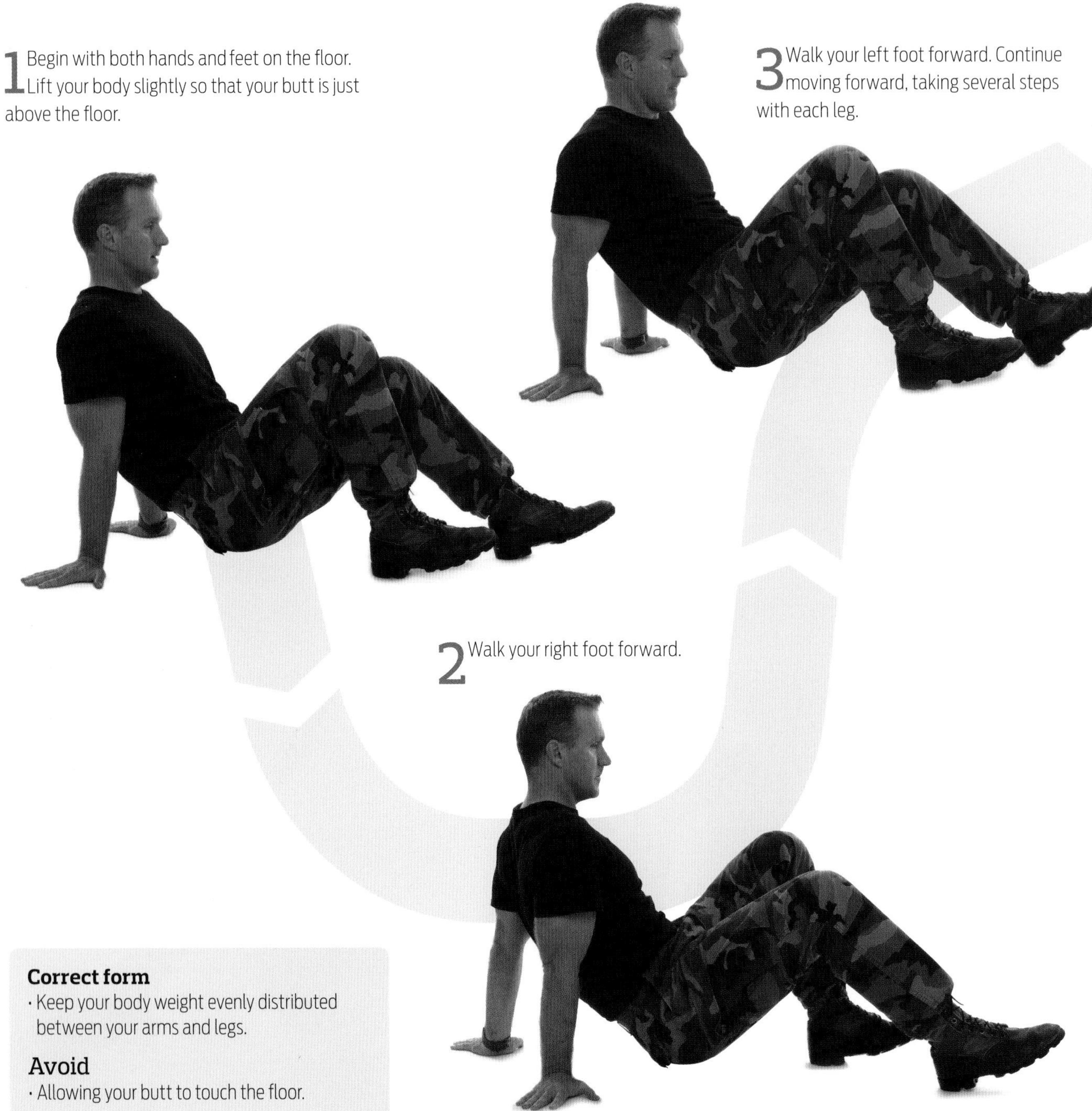

2 Walk your right foot forward.

**Correct form**
- Keep your body weight evenly distributed between your arms and legs.

**Avoid**
- Allowing your butt to touch the floor.

**4** Next, walk each leg back. Alternate moving backward and forward for 60 seconds.

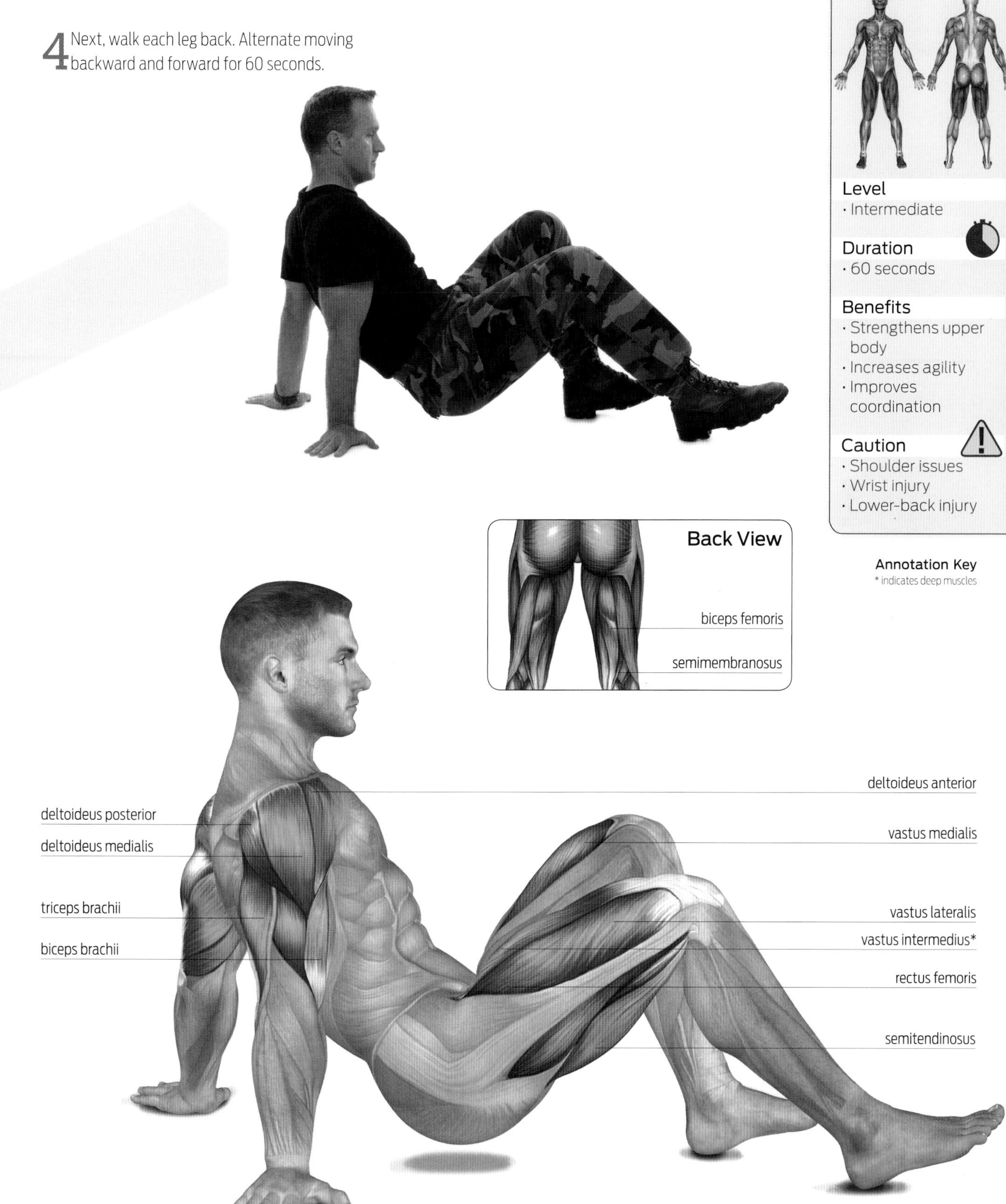


**Level**
- Intermediate

**Duration**
- 60 seconds

**Benefits**
- Strengthens upper body
- Increases agility
- Improves coordination

**Caution**
- Shoulder issues
- Wrist injury
- Lower-back injury

**Annotation Key**
* indicates deep muscles

# Alligator Crawl

The Alligator Crawl works your chest, shoulders, back, and arms. It calls for you to imitate an alligator stalking its prey, holding your body in a hover position similar to a half push-up while steadily moving forward. You can also reverse your movements to slither backward as if in retreat.

1 Start in the Drop Position, with your hands shoulder-width apart, your palms on the floor, your feet together, and your back straight. Lower down into a half push-up position, keeping your back straight.

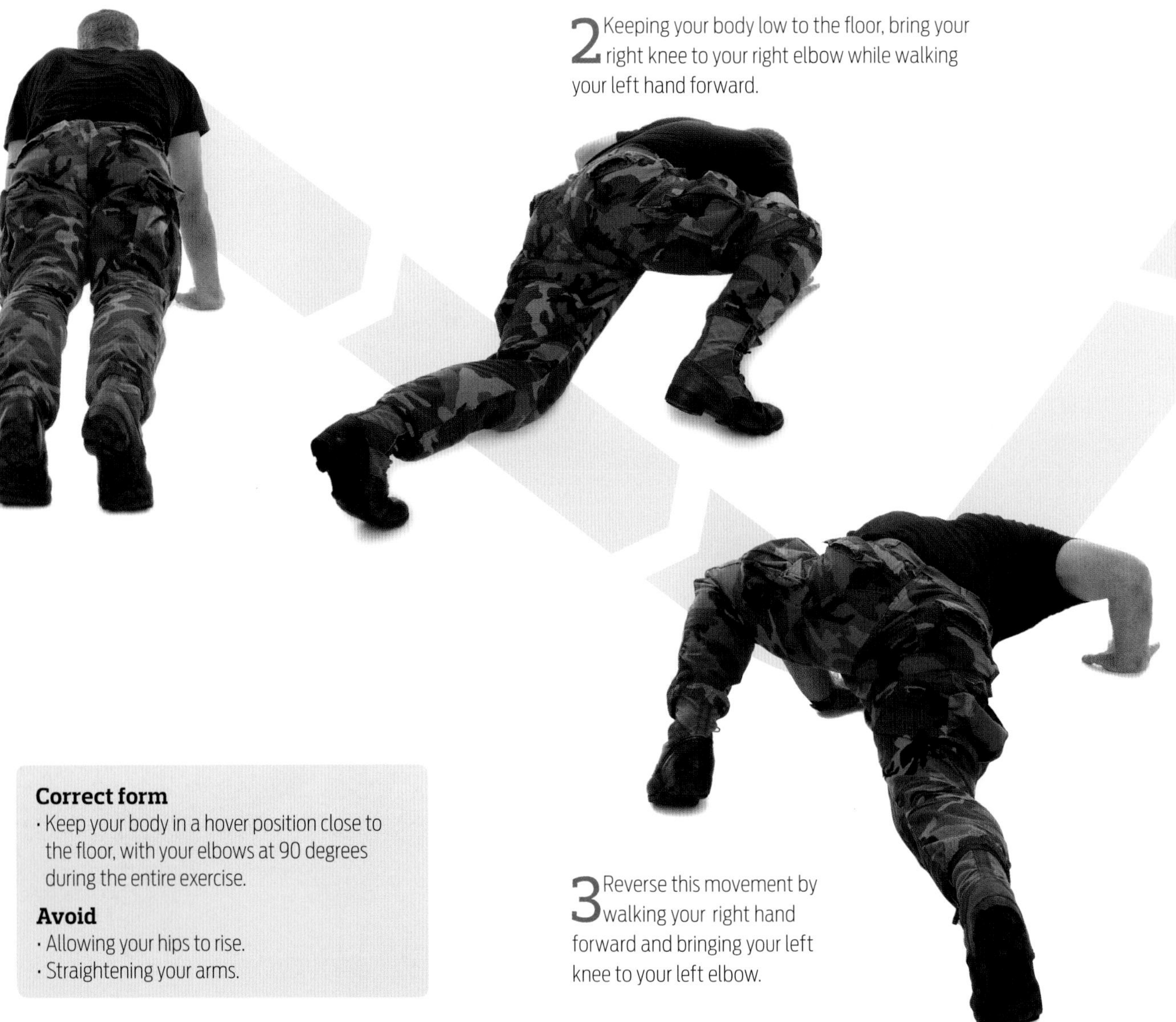

2 Keeping your body low to the floor, bring your right knee to your right elbow while walking your left hand forward.

3 Reverse this movement by walking your right hand forward and bringing your left knee to your left elbow.

**Correct form**

- Keep your body in a hover position close to the floor, with your elbows at 90 degrees during the entire exercise.

**Avoid**

- Allowing your hips to rise.
- Straightening your arms.

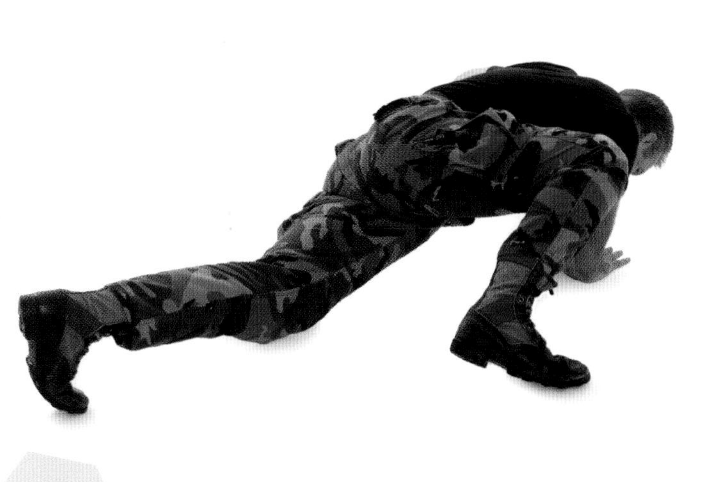

4 Continue moving forward, reversing your hand and knee positions. Perform for 60 seconds.

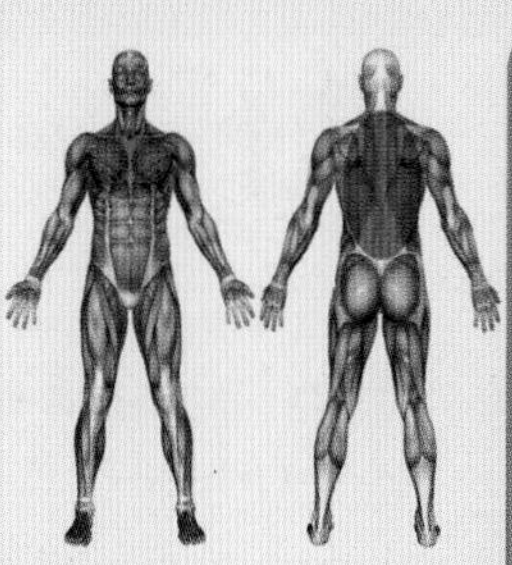

**Level**
- Intermediate

**Duration**
- 60 seconds

**Benefits**
- Strengthens upper body
- Increases agility
- Improves coordination

**Caution**
- Shoulder issues
- Wrist injury
- Lower-back injury

**Annotation Key**
* indicates deep muscles

latissimus dorsi

triceps brachii

biceps brachii

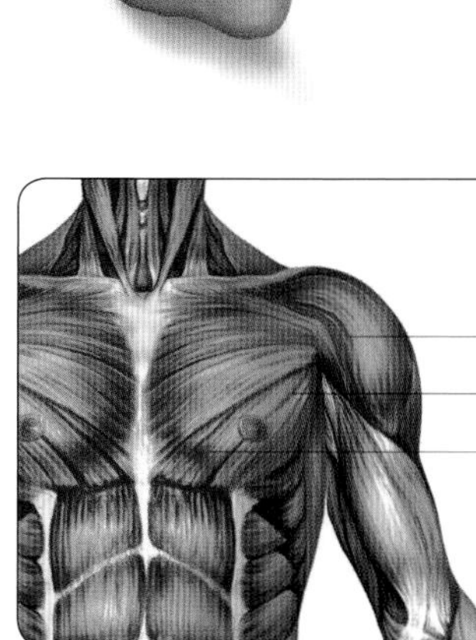

# Star Jump

The Star Jump exercise helps develop leg strength and cardiovascular endurance. It is a very tough movement to perform—you must be able to jump high enough to simultaneously extend your legs and arms outward. Special forces candidates must often perform so many repetitions that they throw up. You don't need to go to this extreme, but challenge yourself to perform as many as you safely can in quick succession.

1 Stand with your feet together.

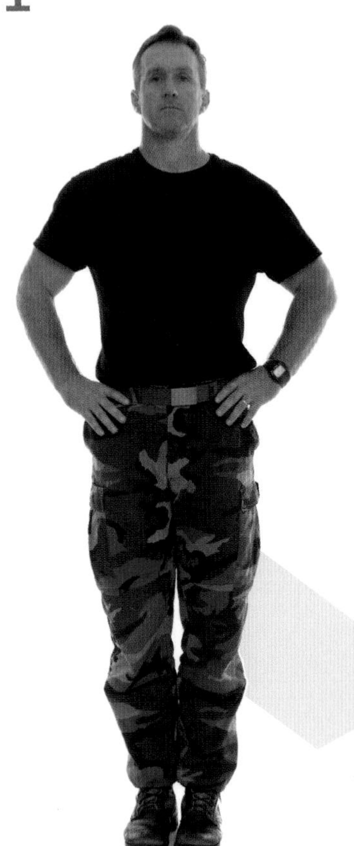

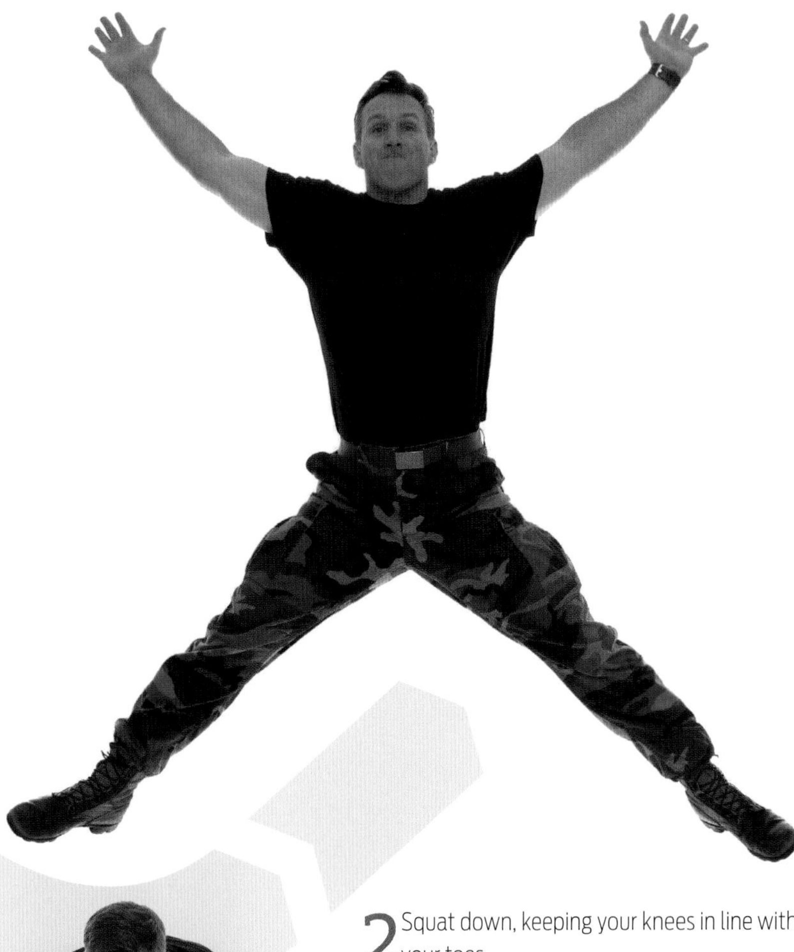

2 Squat down, keeping your knees in line with your toes.

3 In one explosive movement, jump as high as possible while spreading your arms and legs as wide as you can. Your body will make a star shape in the fully extended point of the jump.

4 Bend your knees slightly as you land in the standing position. Sink back to a squat, and repeat. Each jump equals one repetition. Perform 10 reps.

**Correct form**

- Perform these on a soft surface such as an exercise mat or padded carpeting to reduce the impact of your landing.
- Flare out your legs as far as possible.

**Avoid**

- Twisting in the jump—landing in an awkward position could cause a torque injury.

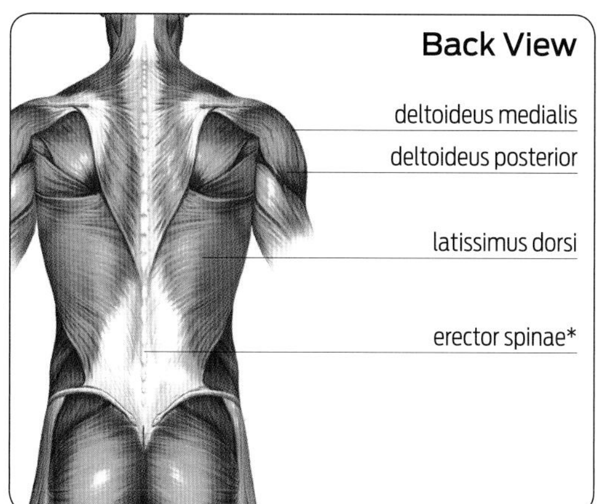


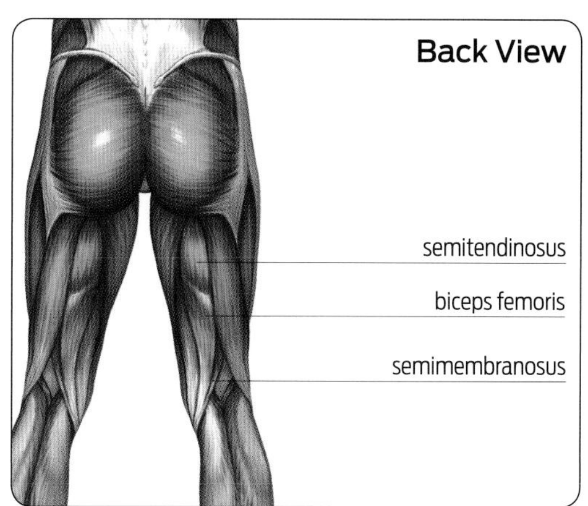

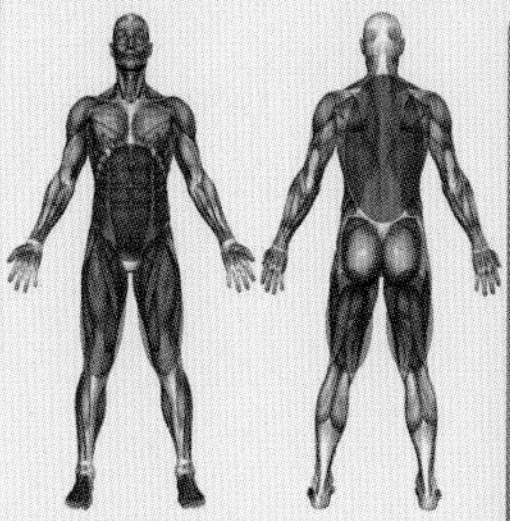

**Level**
- Advanced

**Duration**
- 30–45 seconds

**Benefits**
- Strengthens upper and lower body
- Increases agility
- Improves coordination
- Increases cardiovascular endurance

**Caution**
- Ankle issues

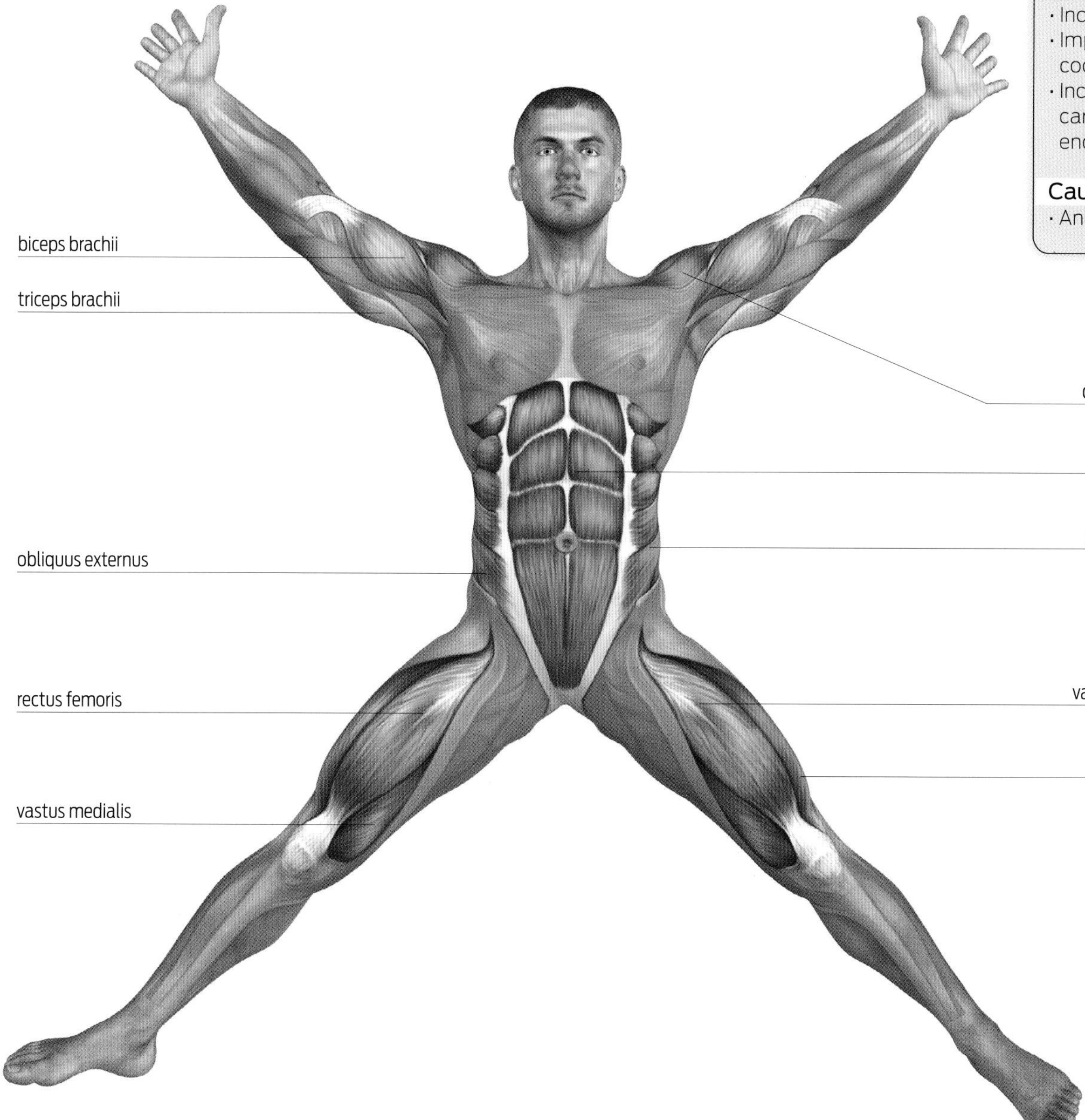

**Annotation Key**
* indicates deep muscles

biceps brachii
triceps brachii
deltoideus anterior
rectus abdominis
obliquus internus*
obliquus externus
rectus femoris
vastus intermedius*
vastus lateralis
vastus medialis

# Shoulder Crusher

The Shoulder Crusher exercise is much like the DFRB (pages 114–115), in which you perform a series of positions in rapid succession. Each of the 8 counts can be called as a command in any sequence, or you can perform the counts in the order listed below. As its name implies, this is a tough exercise that gives your shoulders a thorough workout.

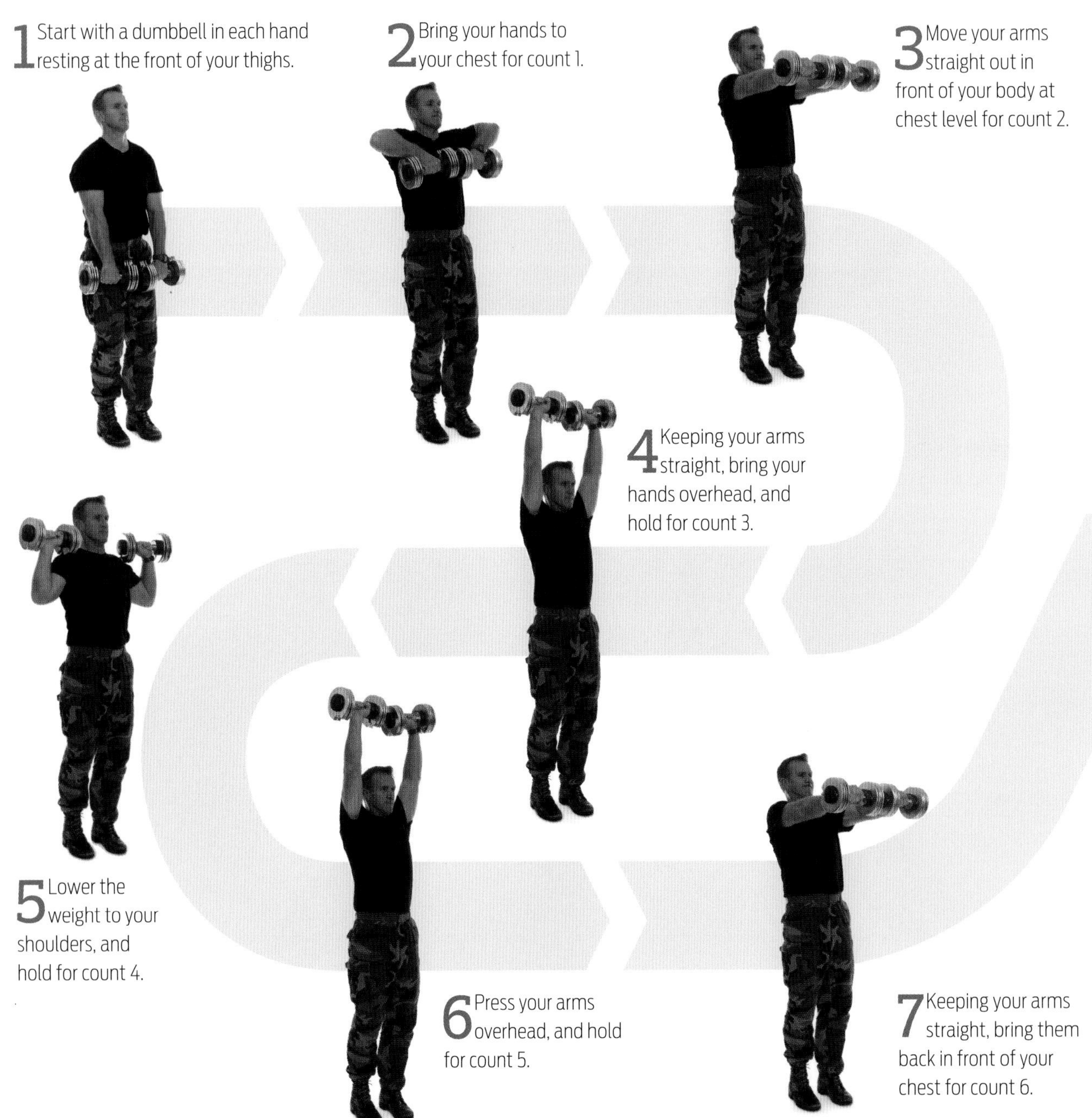

1 Start with a dumbbell in each hand resting at the front of your thighs.

2 Bring your hands to your chest for count 1.

3 Move your arms straight out in front of your body at chest level for count 2.

4 Keeping your arms straight, bring your hands overhead, and hold for count 3.

5 Lower the weight to your shoulders, and hold for count 4.

6 Press your arms overhead, and hold for count 5.

7 Keeping your arms straight, bring them back in front of your chest for count 6.

8 Pull your hands into the chest for count 7.

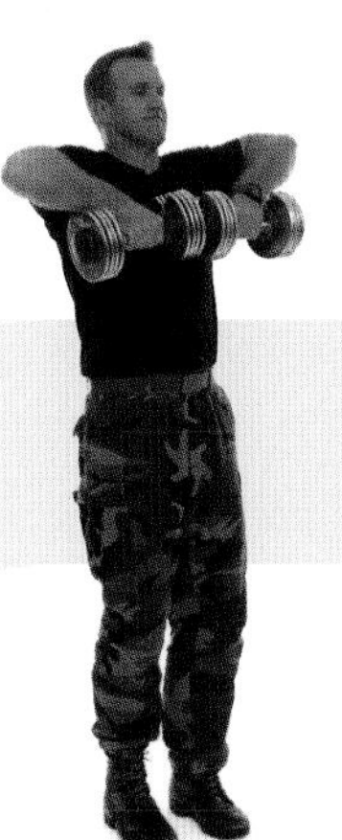

9 Drop your arms to the front of each thigh for count 8. Each time your hands hit your thighs equals one repetition. Perform 10 reps.

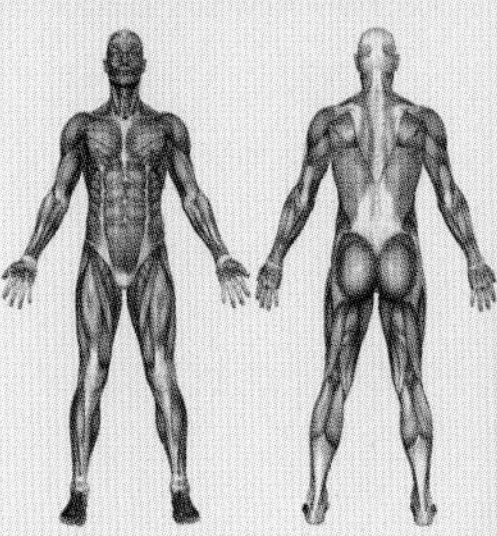

**Level**
· Advanced

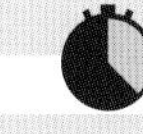

**Duration**
· 1–2 minutes

**Benefits**
· Strengthens shoulders

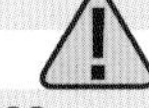

**Caution**
· Shoulder issues
· Lower-back pain
· Wrist issues

deltoideus medialis

deltoideus posterior

deltoideus anterior

**Annotation Key**
* indicates deep muscles

**Correct form**
· Keep your arms straight.
· When bringing the dumbbells overhead, make sure that your hands are directly overhead and not in front of your center of gravity.

**Avoid**
· Using a weight too heavy for your strength level.

# 4-Count Overhead

As part of their stamina/endurance training, special forces students and teams work together under a log to perform a variety of exercises, including overhead presses. Instructors call the steps so that teams move in concert. The 4-Count Overhead simulates this kind of training while it works the muscles of your shoulders. Perform the steps to a steady 4-count beat.

1 With both hands, grasp a dumbbell of any weight you can press overhead, and bring it to your right shoulder. This is your starting position.

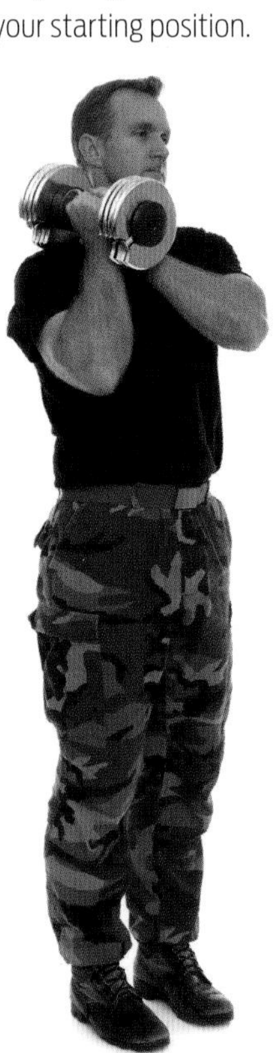

2 Press the weight overhead with your arms straight for count 1.

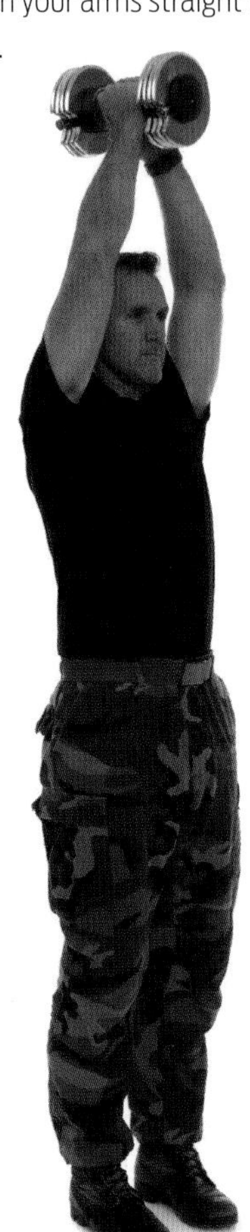

3 Lower the weight to your left shoulder for count 2.

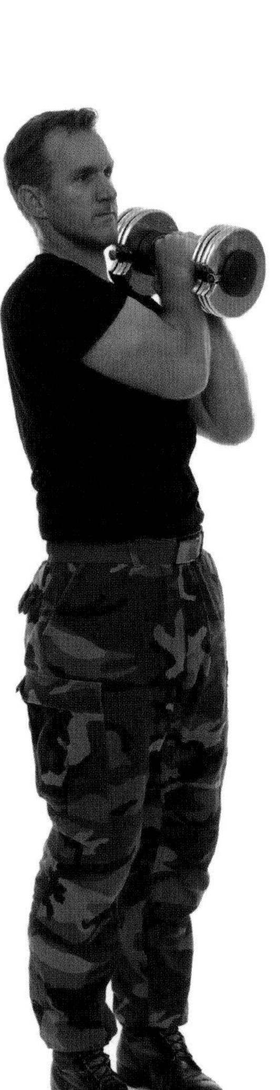

4 Press the weight overhead with your arms straight for 3.

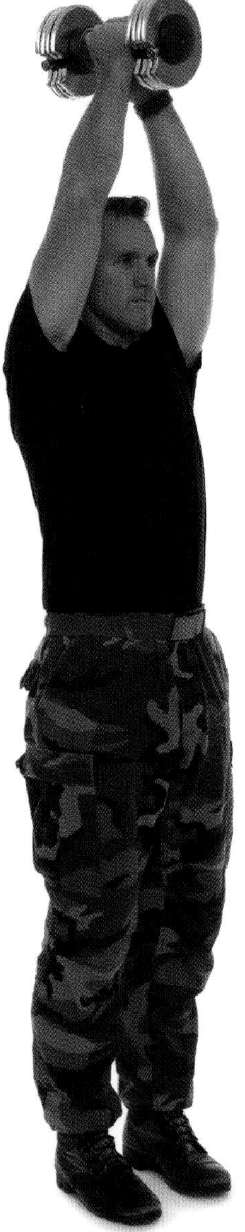

**Correct form**

- Move the weight around your head, and not your head around the weight.
- Keep your glutes and abdominals tight.

**Avoid**

- Arching your lower back.

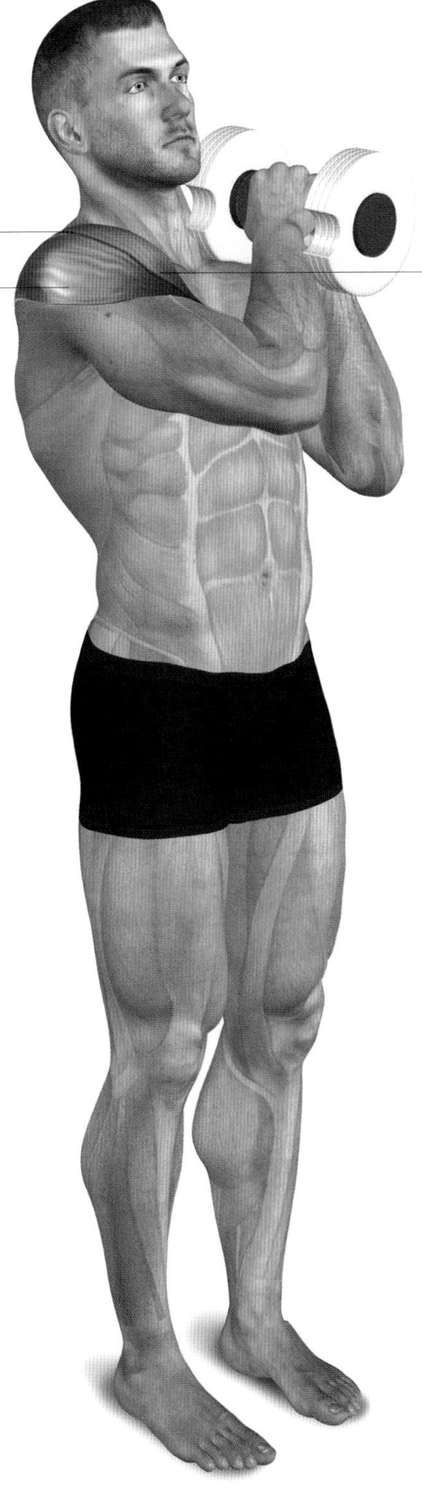


5 Lower the weight to your right shoulder for count 4. Each time the weight touches your right shoulder equals one repetition. Perform 10 reps.

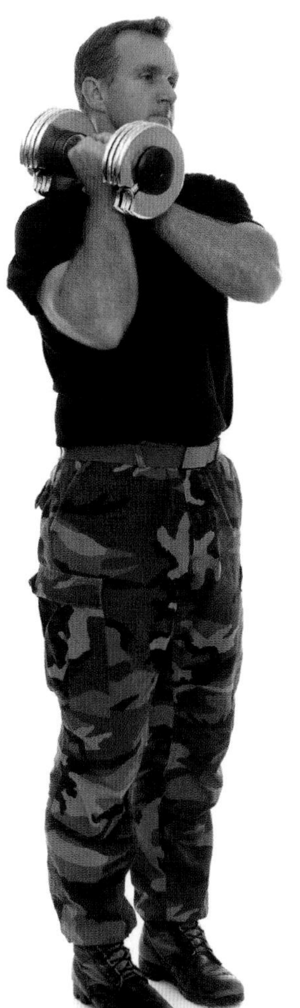

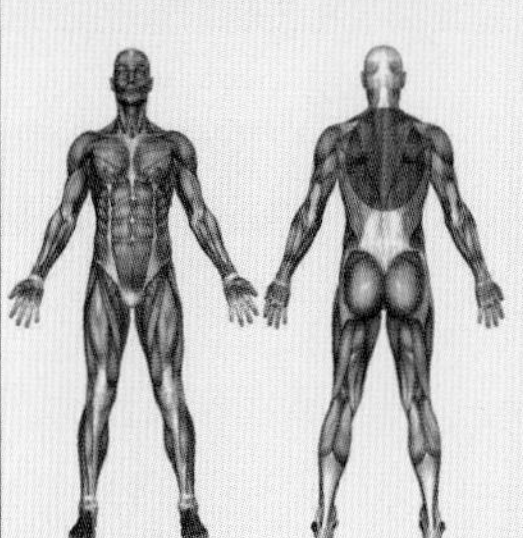

**Level**
- Advanced

**Duration**

- 30–45 seconds

**Benefits**
- Strengthens shoulders

**Caution**
- Shoulder issues
- Lower-back pain
- Wrist issues

**Annotation Key**
* indicates deep muscles

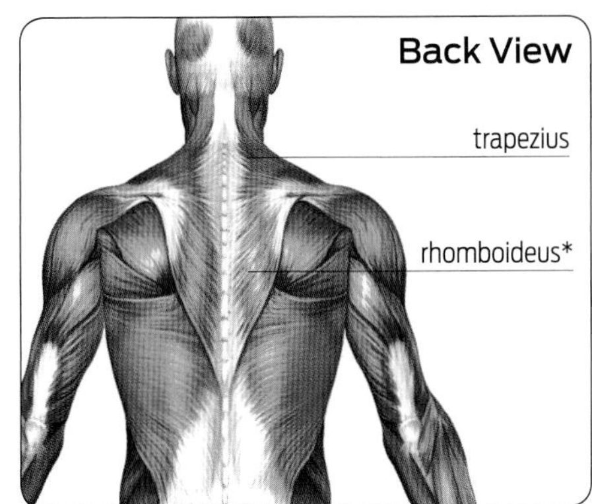

# Arm Hauler

The Arm Hauler exercise is primarily for stabilizing and building the strength of the upper back and rear shoulders. It is also a effective exercise for the prevention of shoulder injuries.

1 Lie flat on your stomach on the floor, and spread your arms wide, keeping them level with your shoulders.

2 Lift your head, keeping your chin up while arching your lower back. Bring your arms off the floor and reach as far behind you as possible.

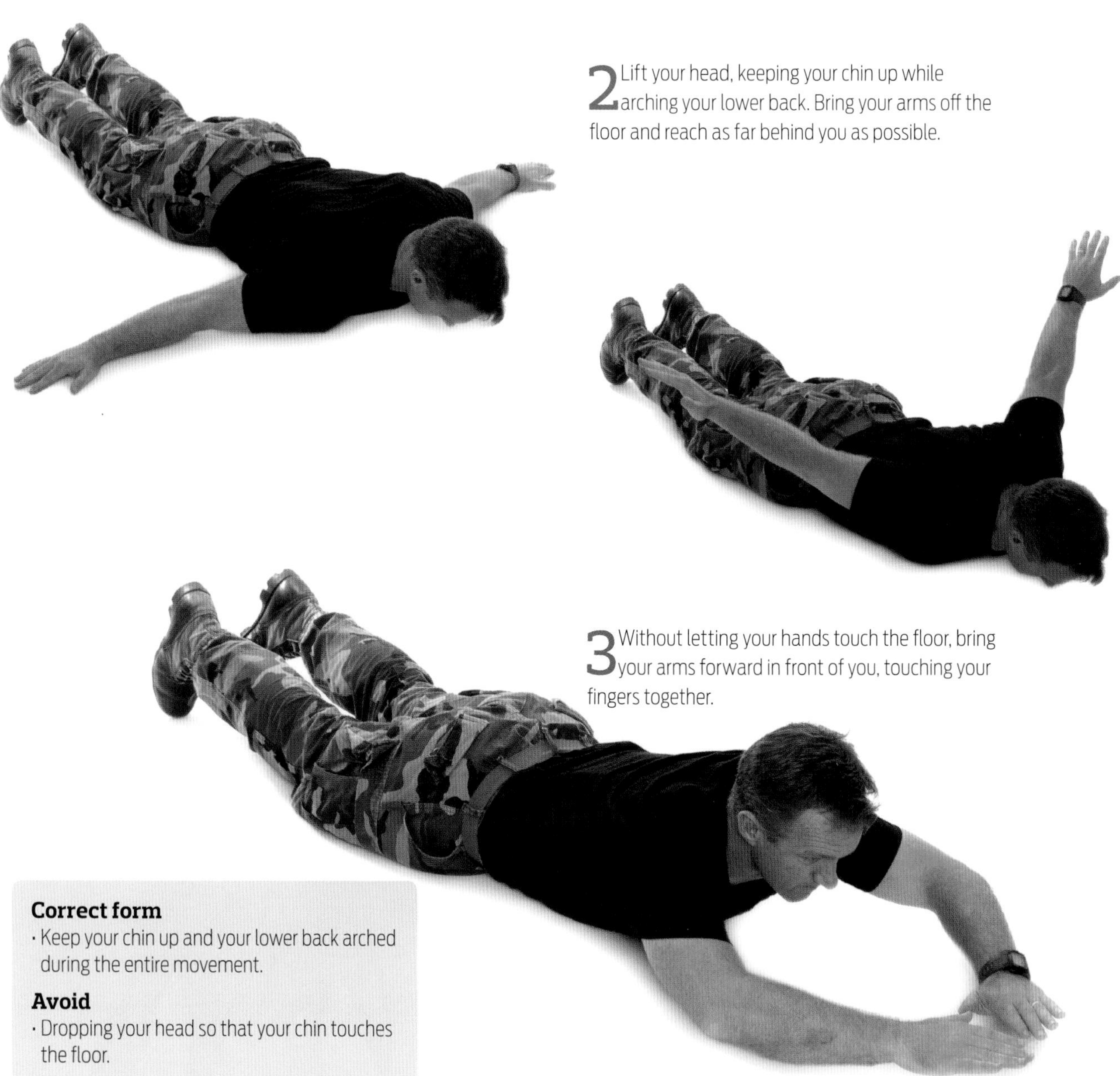

3 Without letting your hands touch the floor, bring your arms forward in front of you, touching your fingers together.

**Correct form**

- Keep your chin up and your lower back arched during the entire movement.

**Avoid**

- Dropping your head so that your chin touches the floor.

**4** Finish the move by bringing your hands back to the starting position. Perform 10 reps.

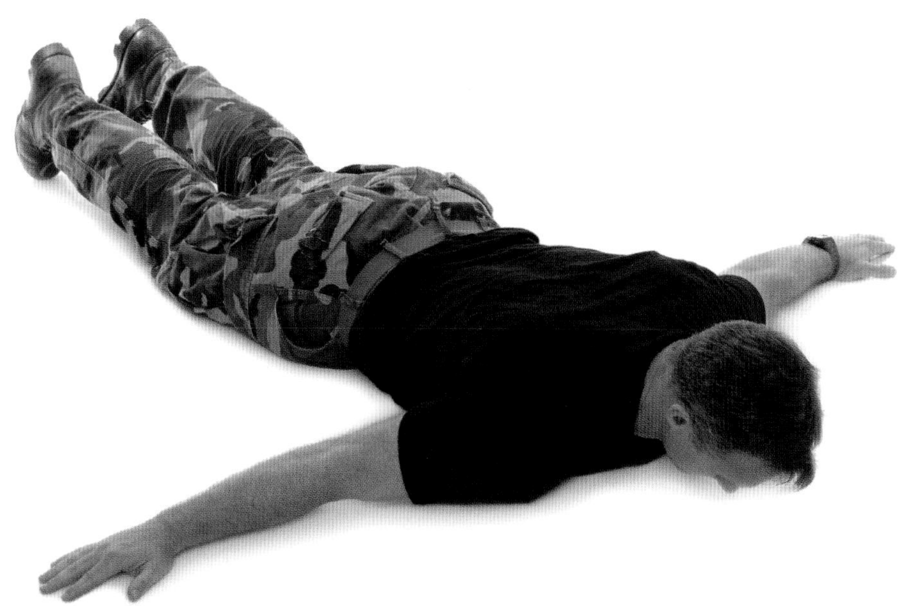

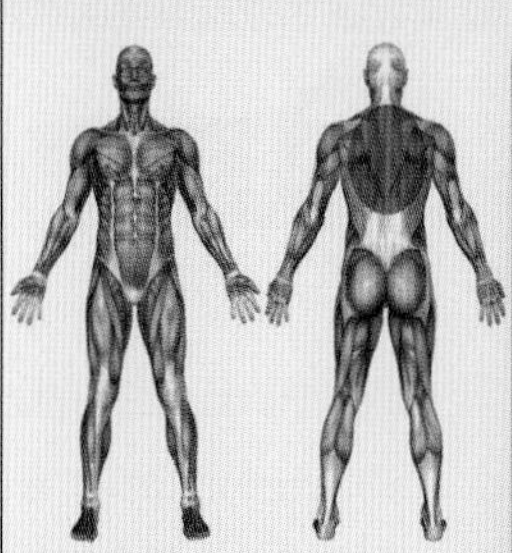

**Level**
- Intermediate

**Duration**
- 45–60 seconds

**Benefits**
- Strengthens and stabilizes the upper, middle, and lower back

**Caution**
- Shoulder issues

**Annotation Key**
* indicates deep muscles

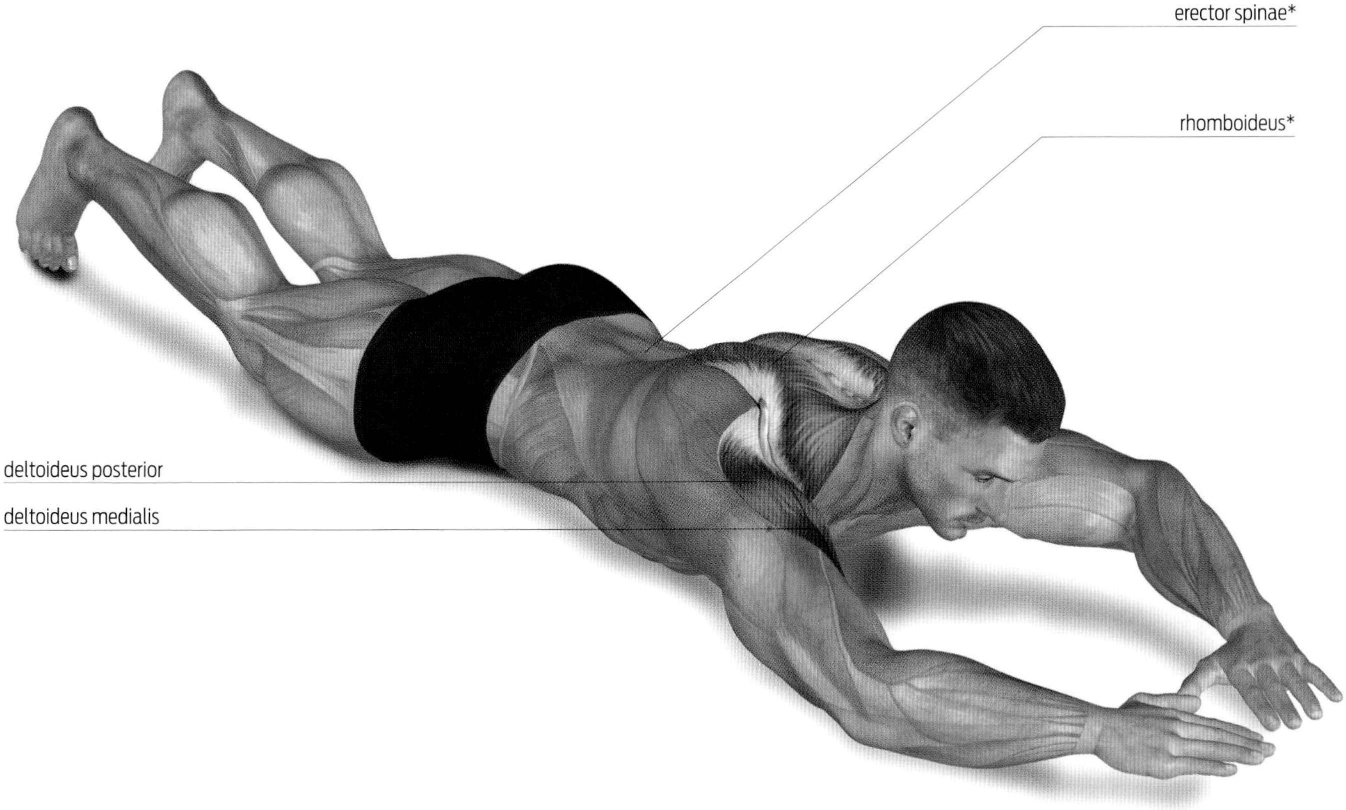

erector spinae*

rhomboideus*

deltoideus posterior

deltoideus medialis

# One-Arm Dumbbell Row

A great combination move, the One-Arm Dumbbell Row strengthens your upper body and stabilizes your core. This is an advanced exercise that can also be performed by walking the dumbbell forward or backward as in the Alligator Crawl (pages 128–129). Make sure to use dumbbells with a flat edge so that they remain stationary.

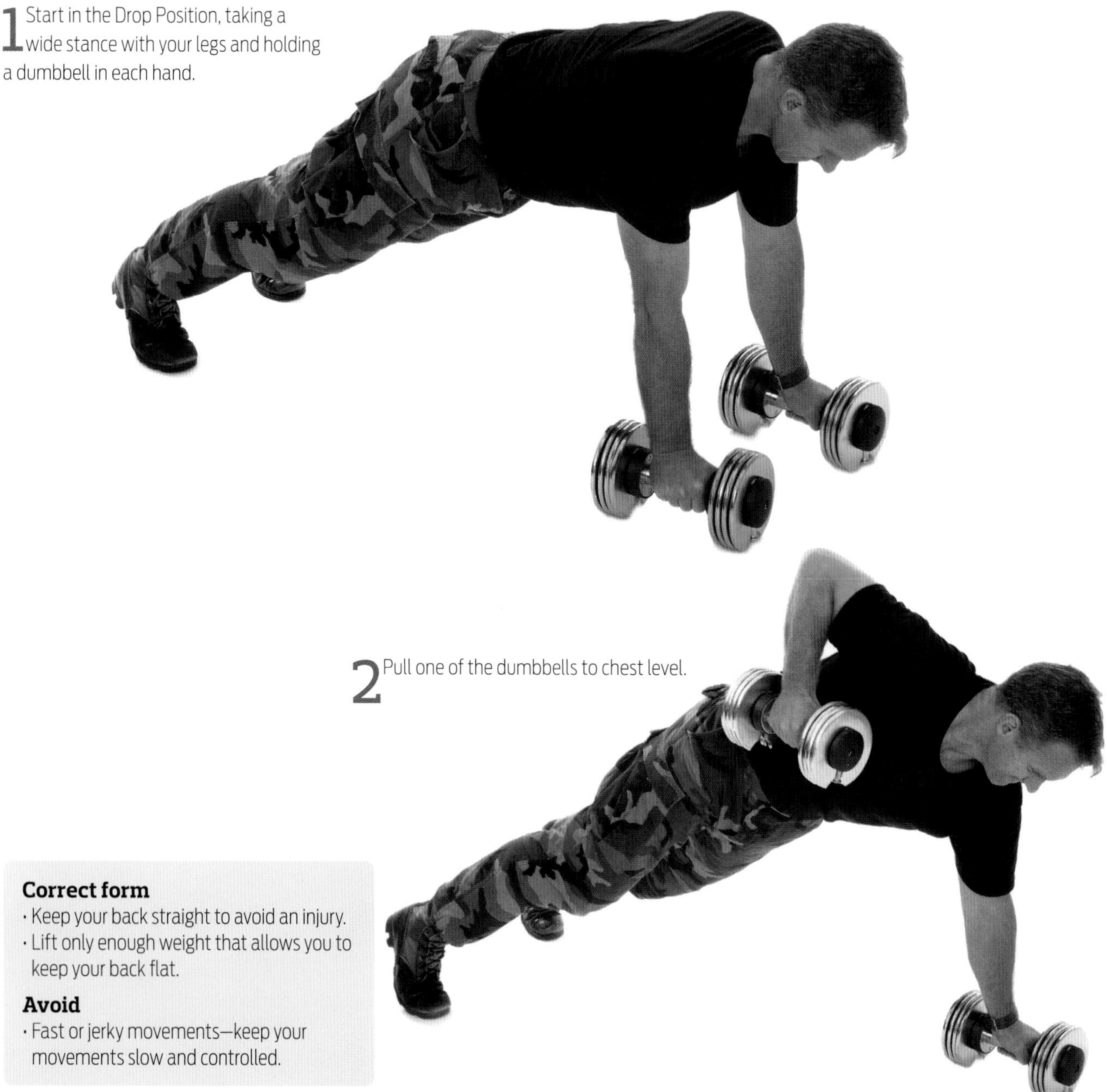

1 Start in the Drop Position, taking a wide stance with your legs and holding a dumbbell in each hand.

2 Pull one of the dumbbells to chest level.

**Correct form**

- Keep your back straight to avoid an injury.
- Lift only enough weight that allows you to keep your back flat.

**Avoid**

- Fast or jerky movements—keep your movements slow and controlled.

3 Slowly lower the weight back to the floor to return to the Drop Position. Repeat with the other arm to complete one repetition. Perform 15 reps.

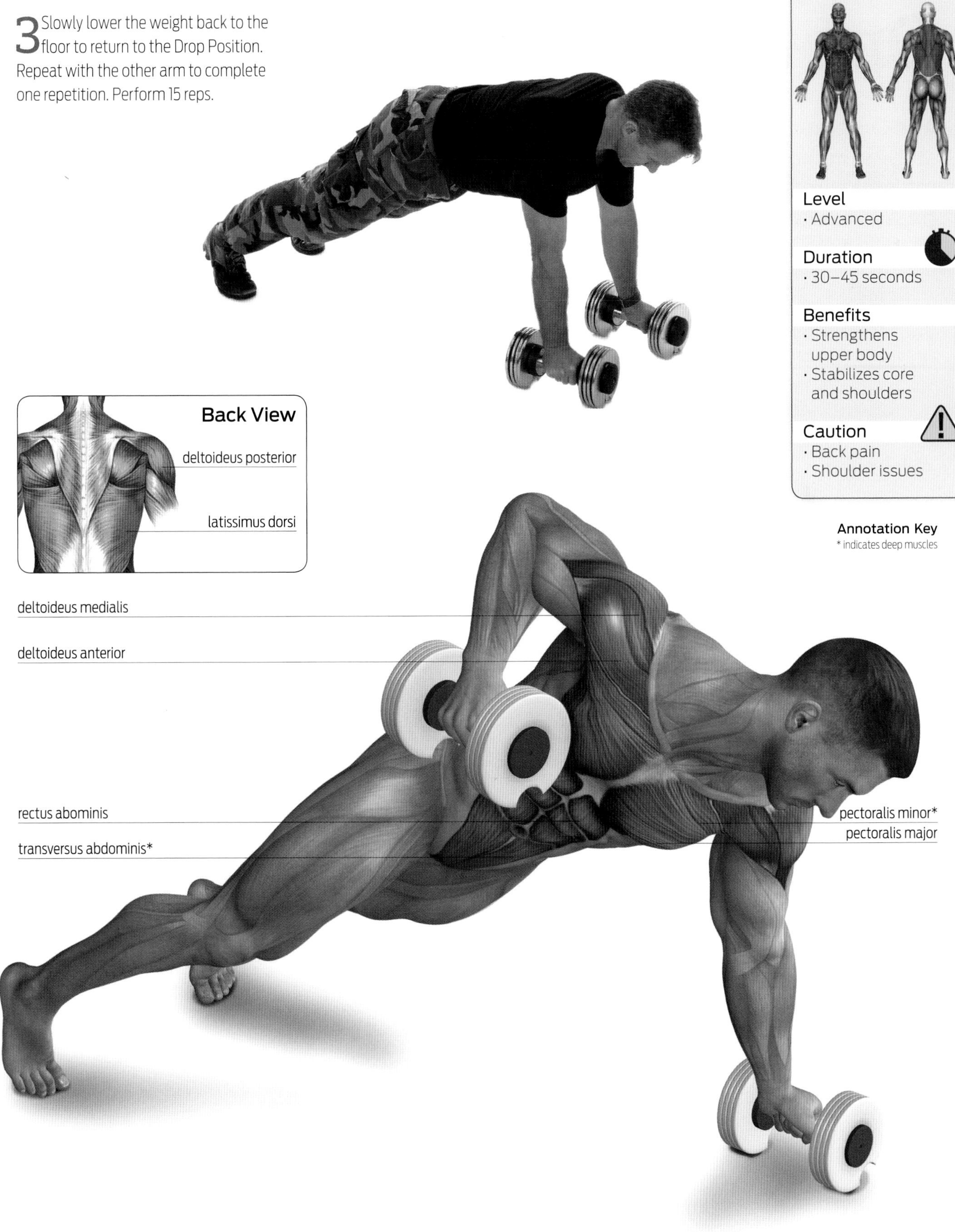


**Level**
- Advanced

**Duration**
- 30–45 seconds

**Benefits**
- Strengthens upper body
- Stabilizes core and shoulders

**Caution**
- Back pain
- Shoulder issues

**Annotation Key**
* indicates deep muscles

# One-Arm T-Row

The One-Arm T-Row is a tough exercise that builds both strength and stability in the core and upper body. Only use enough weight so you that can maintain proper form. As with the One-Arm Dumbbell Row (pages 138–139), be sure to use dumbbells with a flat edge so that they don't roll to the side.

1 Start in the Drop Position, taking a wide stance with your legs and holding a dumbbell in each hand.

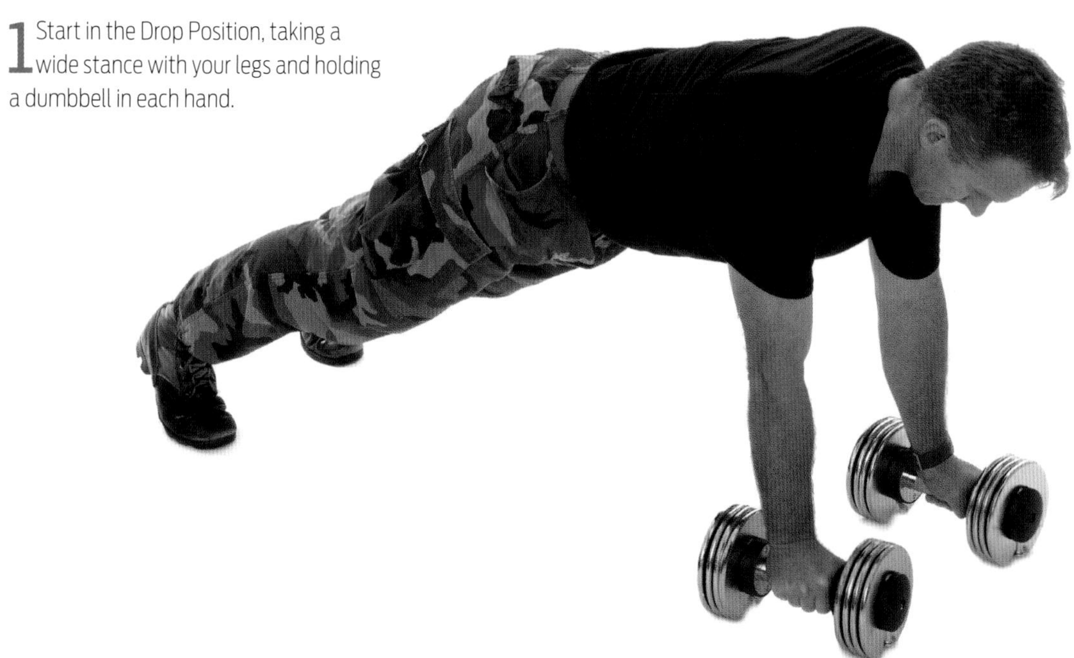

2 Pull one of the dumbbells to chest level.

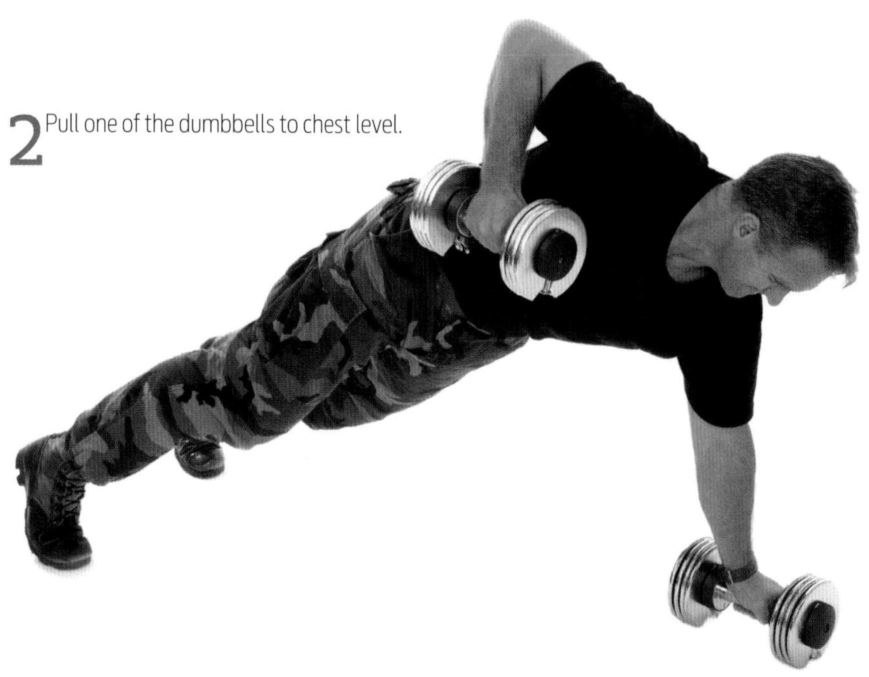

**Correct form**

- Open your stance as wide as possible for stability.
- Move the weight slowly, so as not to knock you off balance.

**Avoid**

- Using a weight heavier than you can comfortably lift over your head.
- Attempting this movement before you can perform the High Plank (pages 118–119) and One-Arm Dumbbell Row (pages 138–139) exercises without pain.

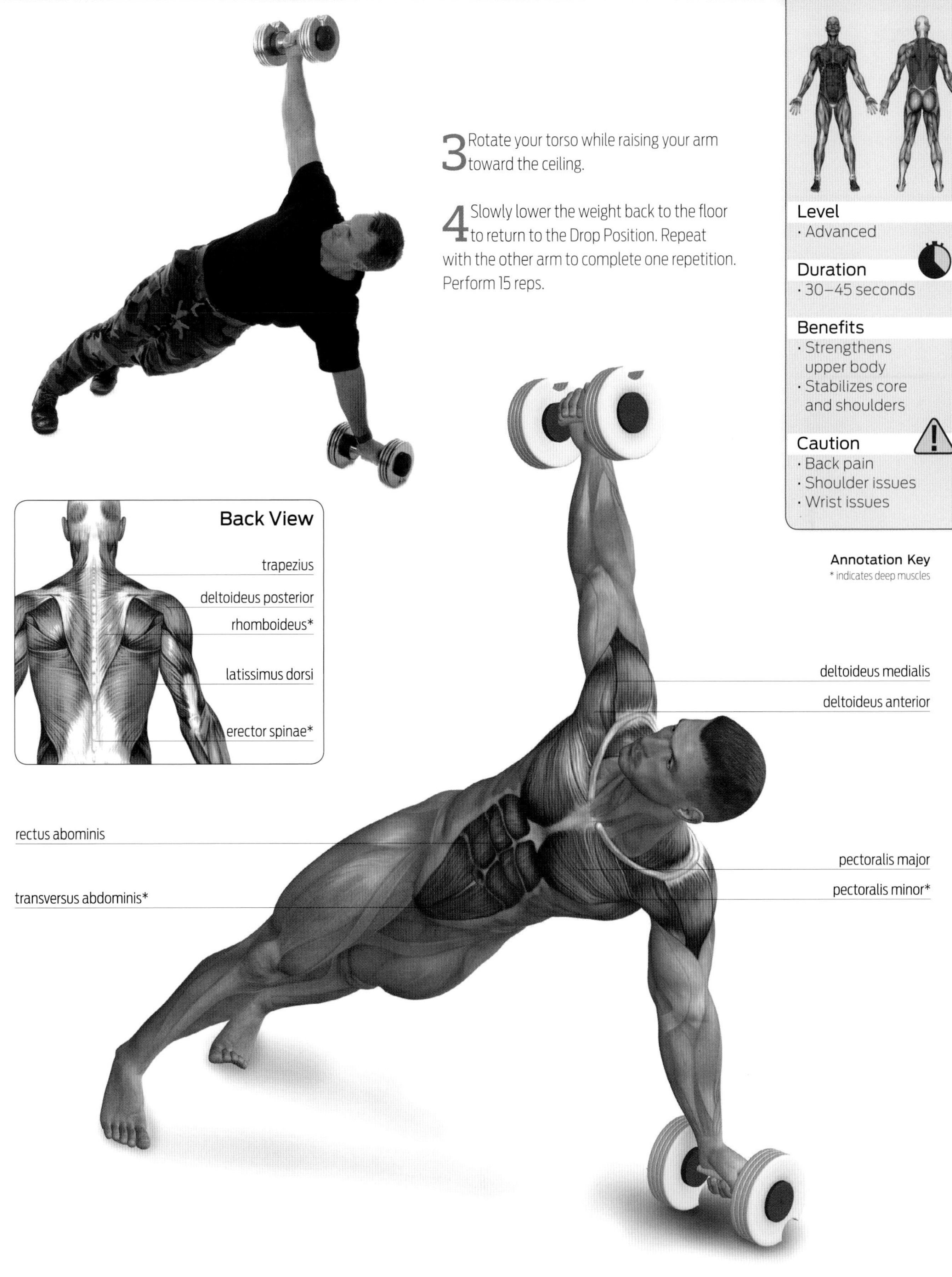


3 Rotate your torso while raising your arm toward the ceiling.

4 Slowly lower the weight back to the floor to return to the Drop Position. Repeat with the other arm to complete one repetition. Perform 15 reps.

**Level**
- Advanced

**Duration**
- 30–45 seconds

**Benefits**
- Strengthens upper body
- Stabilizes core and shoulders

**Caution**
- Back pain
- Shoulder issues
- Wrist issues

# Skip Rope

Skip Rope is a great exercise to perform as a rest between other exercise sets to recover your heart rate. This calorie burner works mainly on your calf muscles, while strengthening your bones and improving your balance and coordination. If you are just starting an exercise program, choose a heavy PVC rope, which will make you jump more slowly.

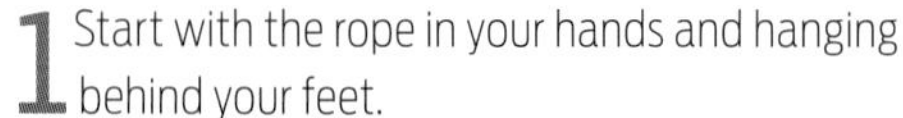

1 Start with the rope in your hands and hanging behind your feet.

2 Swing the rope around your body and jump over it. Keep your arms as straight as you can during the movement, and land with both feet together on the floor. Perform for 2 minutes.

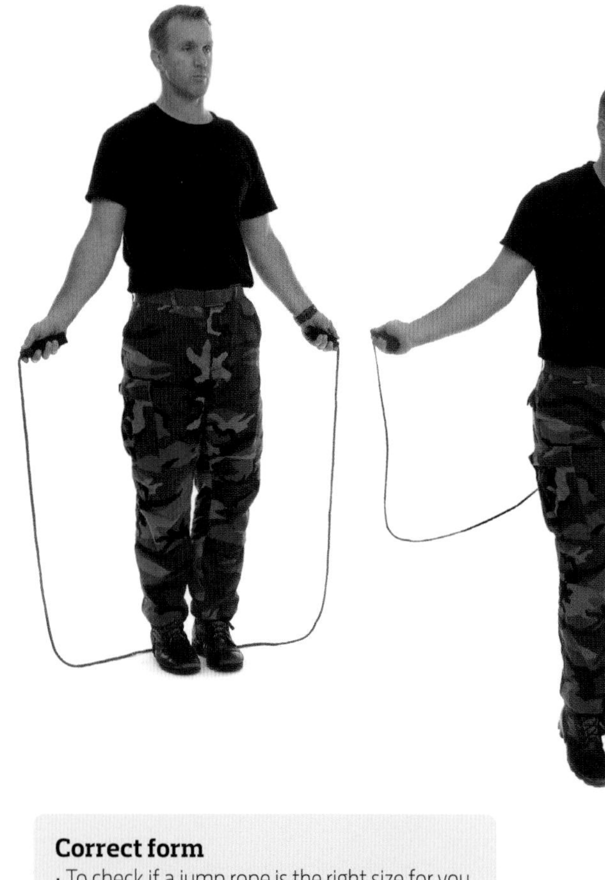

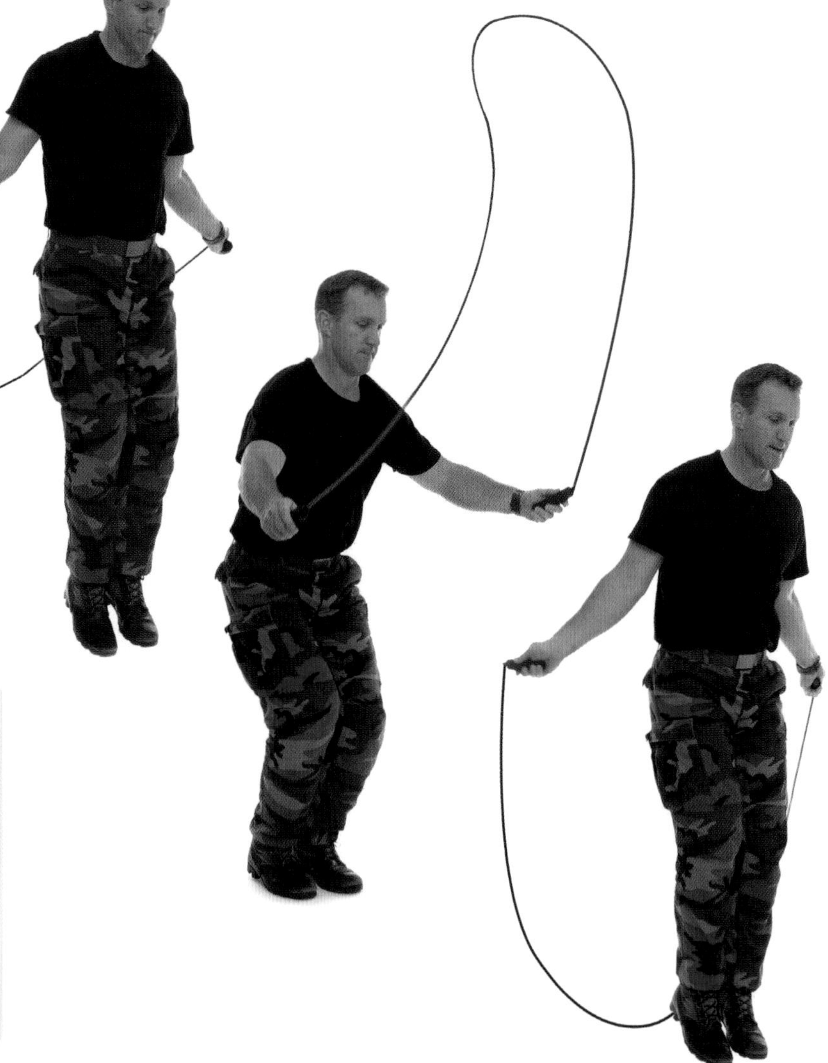

**Correct form**

- To check if a jump rope is the right size for you, place one foot in the center of the rope, and then lift the handles—they shouldn't reach higher than your armpits.
- Land on the balls of your feet.

**Avoid**

- Bending your elbows.
- Landing flat on your feet, which can compact the knee.

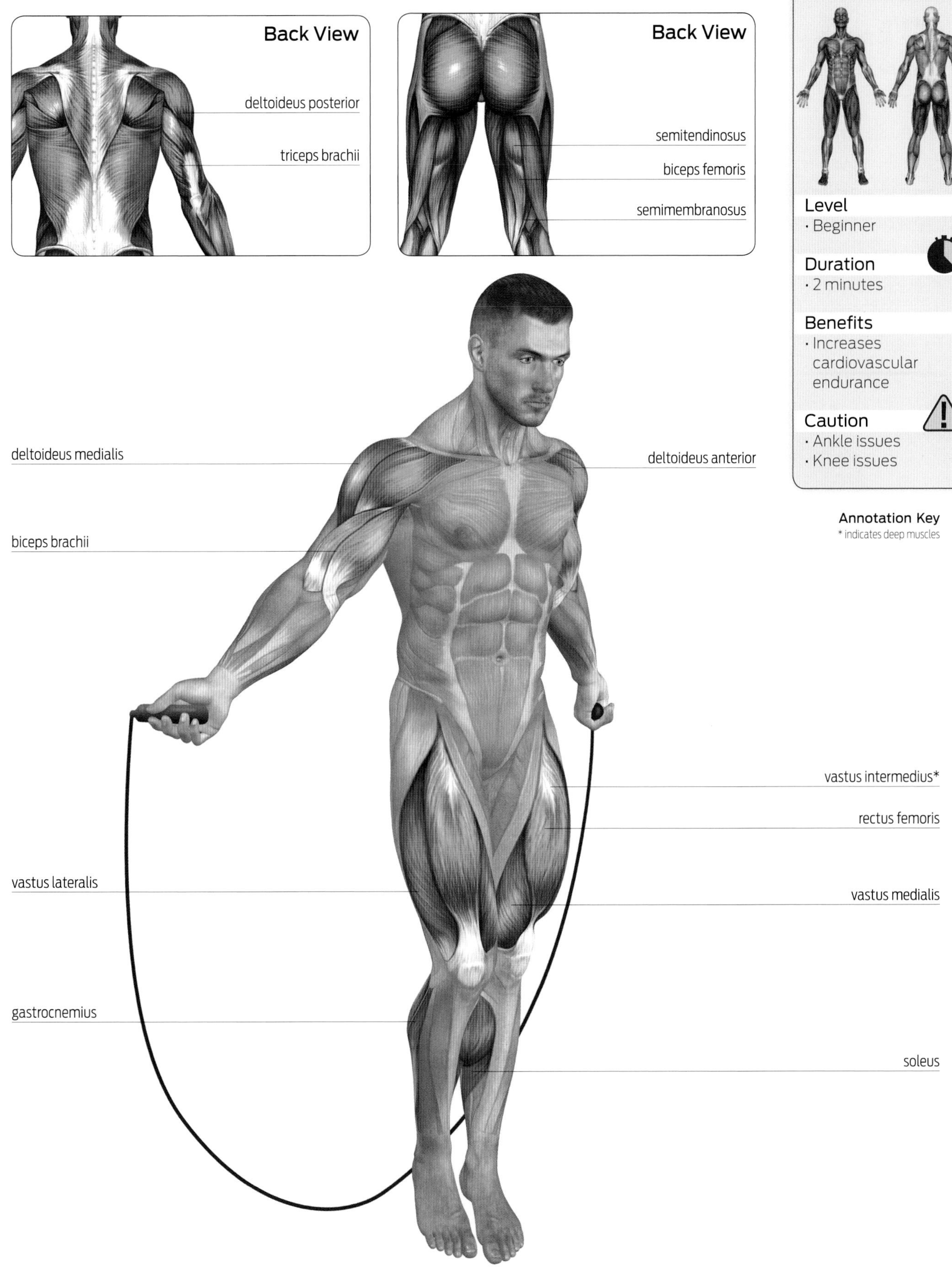


**Level**
- Beginner

**Duration**
- 2 minutes

**Benefits**
- Increases cardiovascular endurance

**Caution**
- Ankle issues
- Knee issues

**Annotation Key**
* indicates deep muscles

# Slalom Skier

The Slalom Skier is an intense move that revs up your cardiovascular system while strengthening the muscles of your chest, shoulders, arms, and legs. In the military, the term *gut check* means "a test of determination, will, and character." When performed with Mountain Climber (pages 146-147), Slalom Skiers make a great gut check. You don't need to go to this extreme, but if you perform them correctly, you might feel as if you are going to throw up before you've completed your reps.

1 Start in the Drop Position.

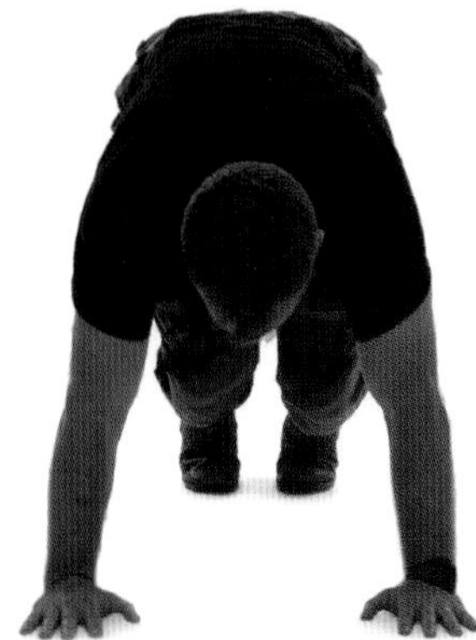

2 Jump both feet together to the left so that both feet land outside your left arm. Tuck your knees toward your chest while you jump.

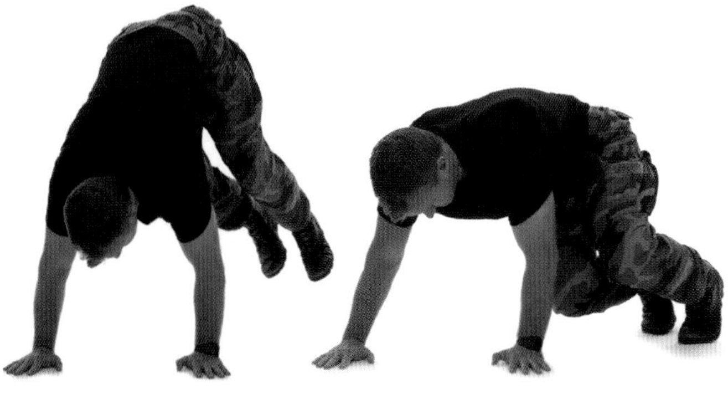

3 Jump your feet back to the leaning rest position, and then jump both feet back across your body to the right, landing with both feet outside your right arm and both knees bent toward your chest.

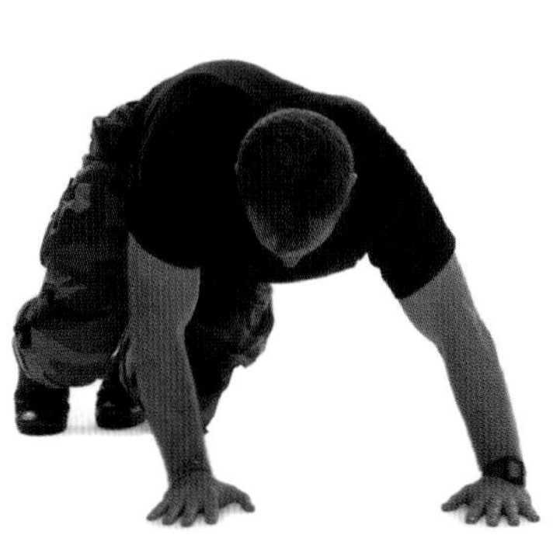

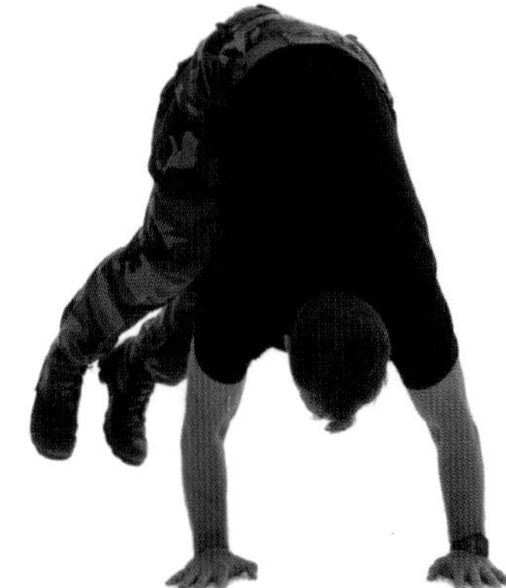

4 Immediately jump back to the left, and continue alternating sides. Both left and right equal one repetition. Perform 10 reps.

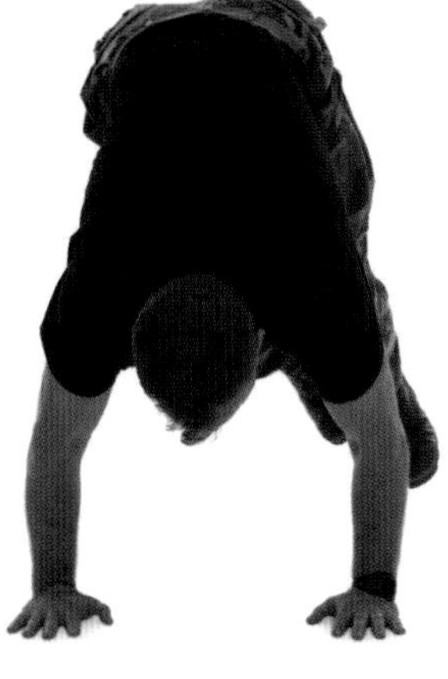

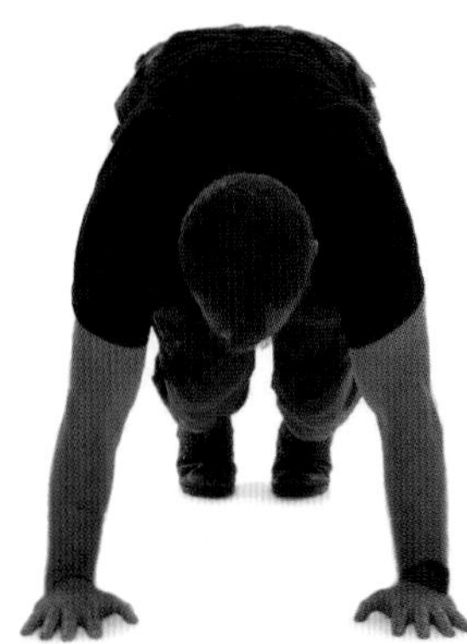

**Correct form**
- When you jump your feet, bend your knees as though they were coming to your chest.

**Avoid**
- Jumping your feet too high, which places all of your body weight on your wrists.

## Back View

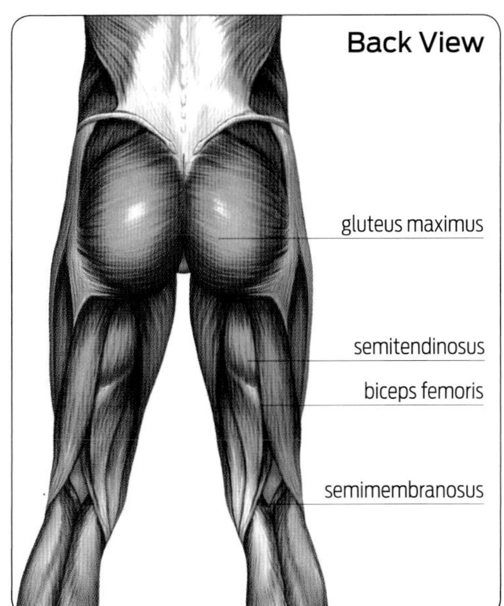


## Front View

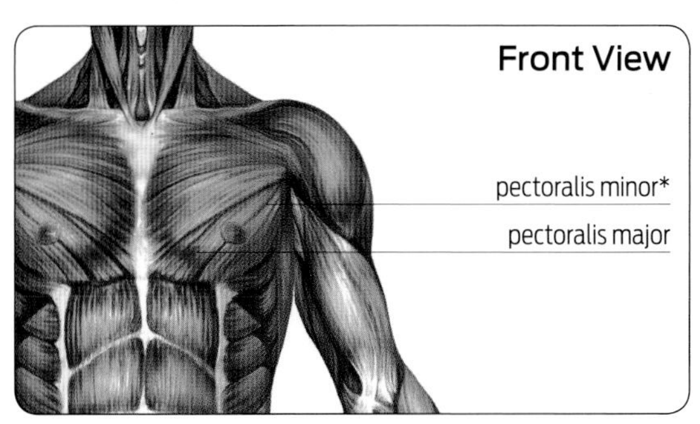


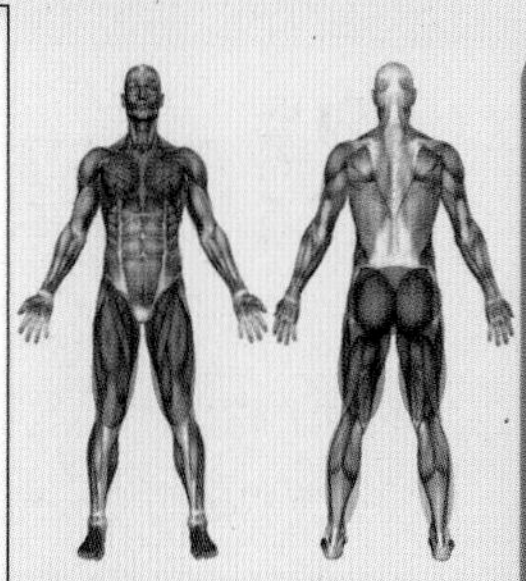

**Level**
- Intermediate

**Duration** 
- 30–45 seconds

**Benefits**
- Strengthens upper body and core
- Increases agility
- Improves coordination
- Increases cardiovascular endurance

**Caution** 
- Wrist issues

**Annotation Key**
* indicates deep muscles

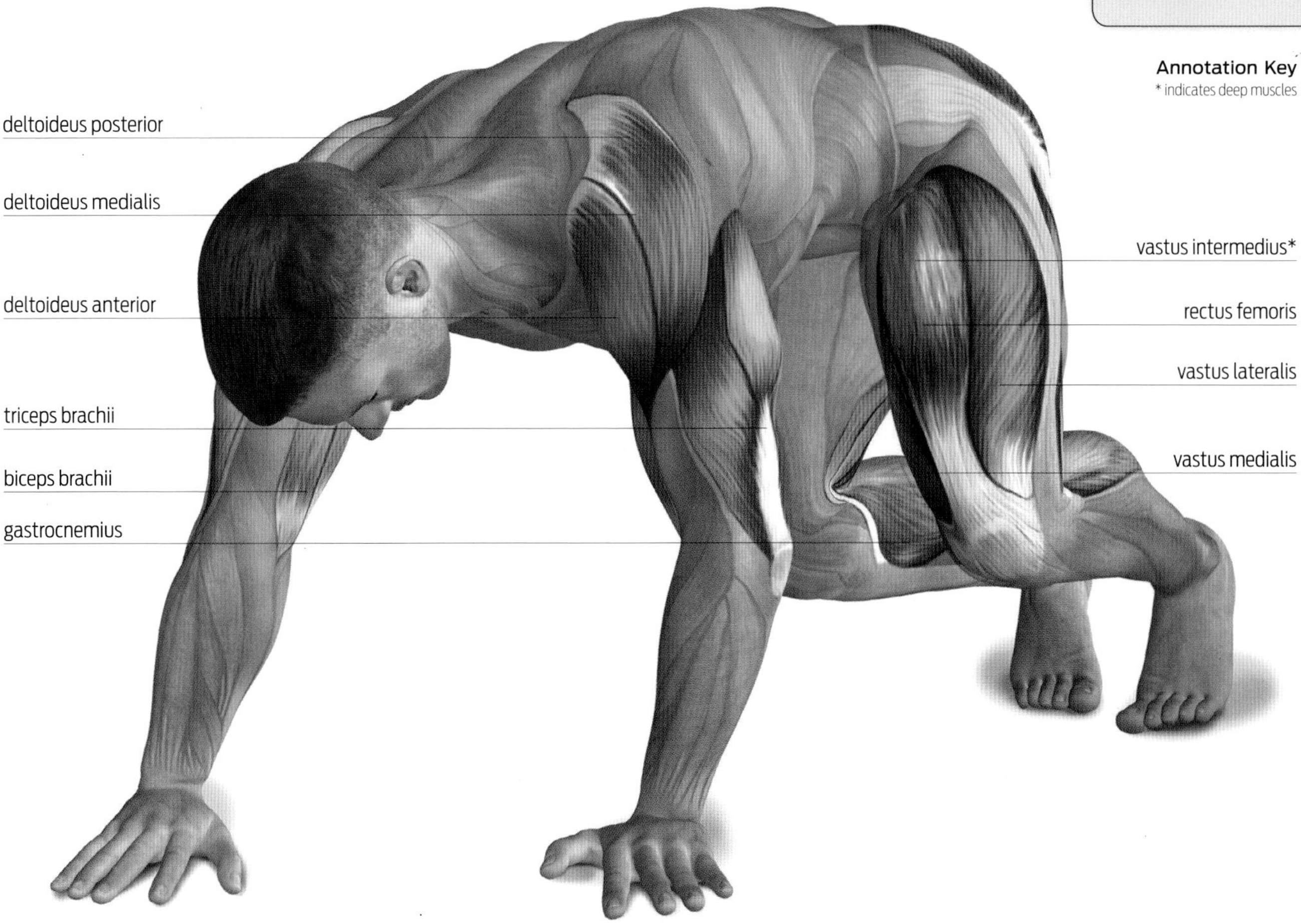

deltoideus posterior
deltoideus medialis
deltoideus anterior
triceps brachii
biceps brachii
gastrocnemius
vastus intermedius*
rectus femoris
vastus lateralis
vastus medialis

# Mountain Climber

Mountain Climber is a great way to build upper-body strength while giving your cardiovascular system an intense workout. Also known as Rabbit Chasers, this anaerobic exercise is performed to a 4-count rhythm.

1 Start in the Drop Position. Bring your right knee to your chest for count 1.

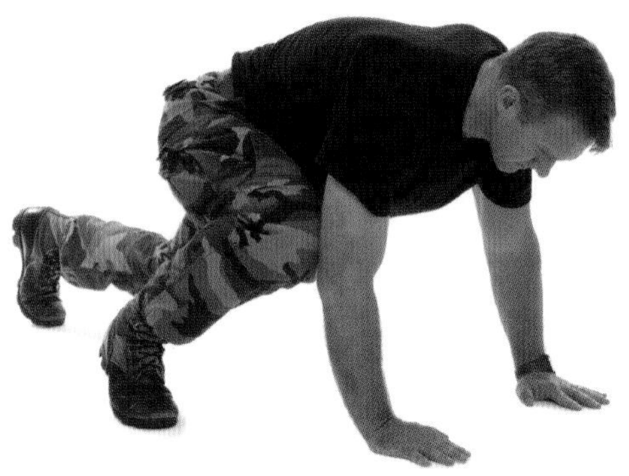

2 Jump, and bring your left knee to your chest for count 2.

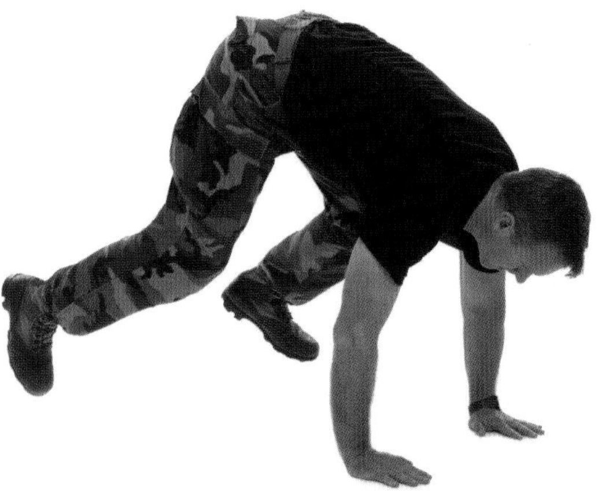

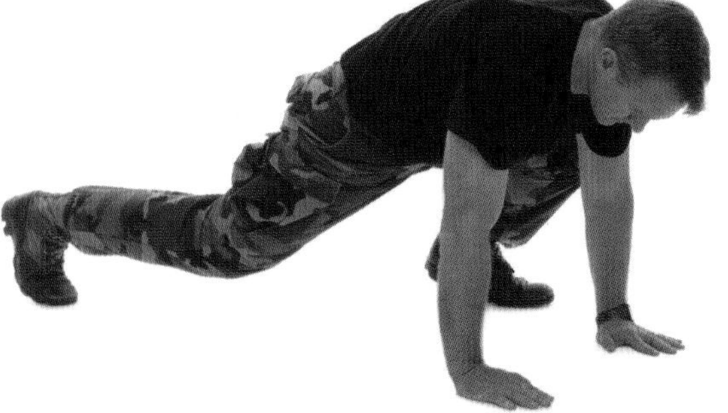

3 Jump, and bring your right knee to your chest for count 3.

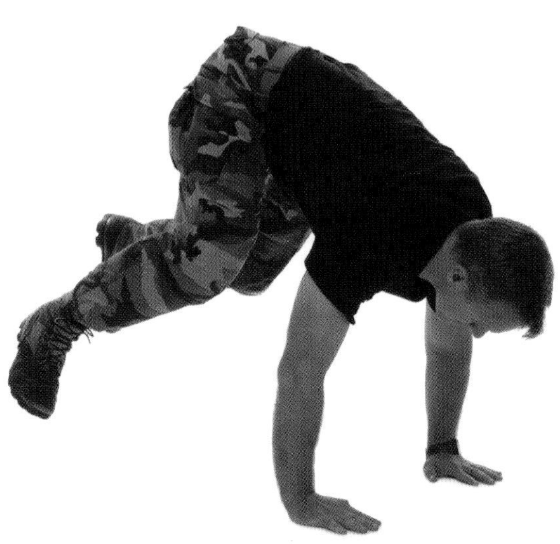

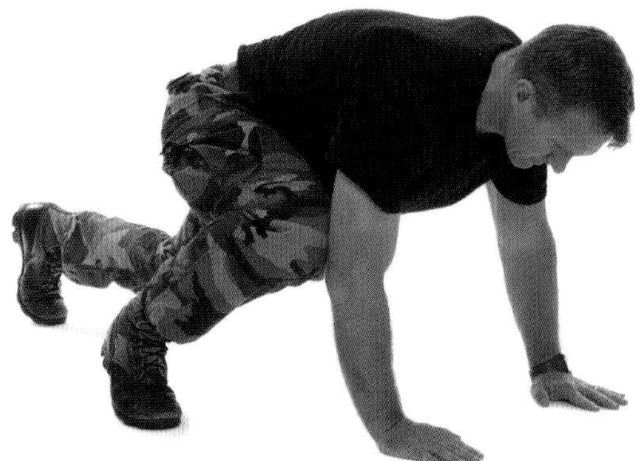

**Correct form**

- Keep your back straight.
- Flare your hands out to ease shoulder stress.

**Avoid**

- Making small movements with your legs; attempt to bring each knee to your chest for each count.

4 Jump, and bring your left to knee to your chest for count 4. Each 1-to-4 count equals one repetition. Perform 10 reps.

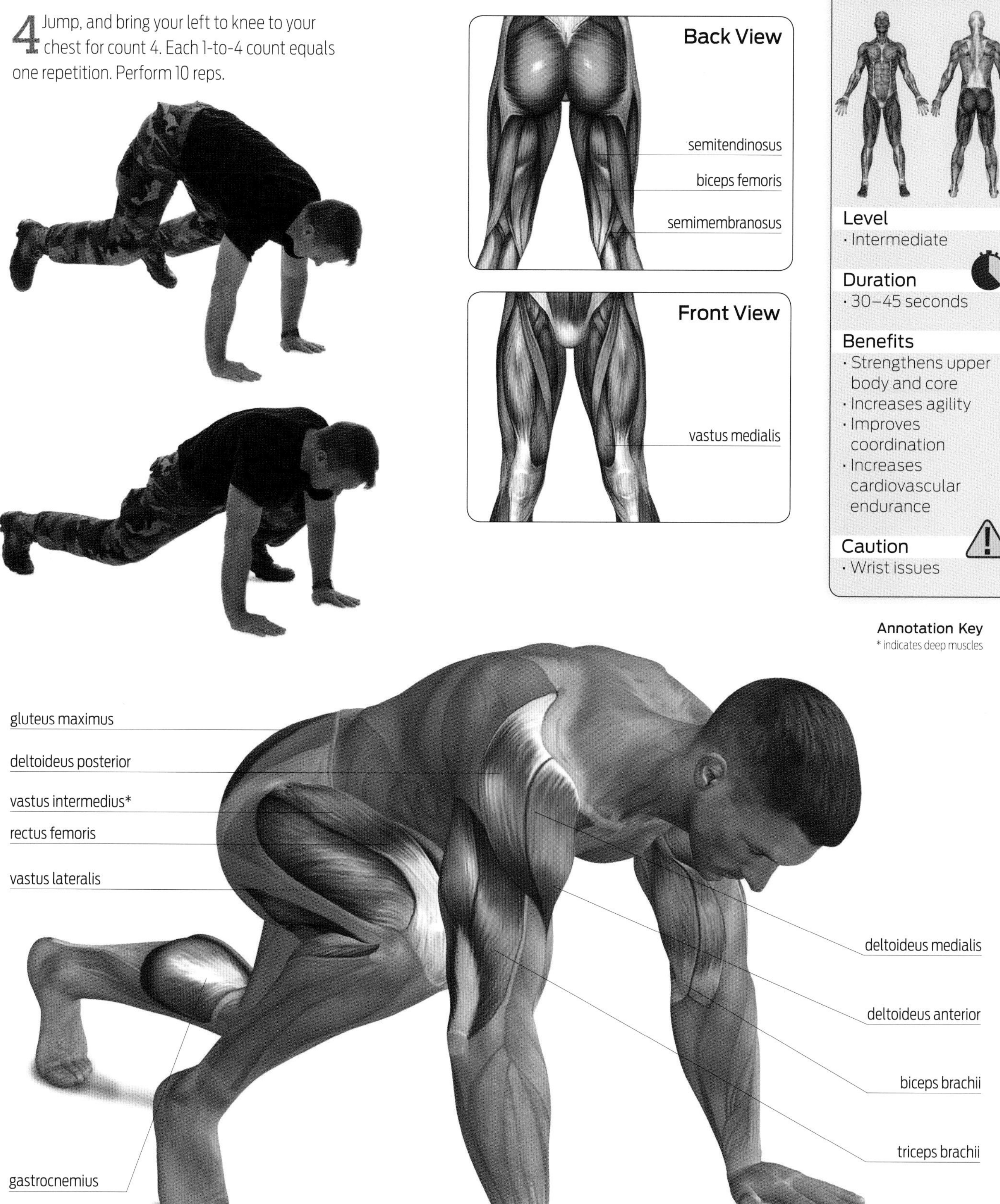


**Level**
- Intermediate

**Duration**
- 30–45 seconds

**Benefits**
- Strengthens upper body and core
- Increases agility
- Improves coordination
- Increases cardiovascular endurance

**Caution**
- Wrist issues

**Annotation Key**
* indicates deep muscles

# Up–Down

The Up-Down exercise gets your blood pumping and the fat burning. This multiphase exercise is meant to tax your cardiovascular system by using almost all of your muscles, and it has the added benefit of increasing your coordination and agility.

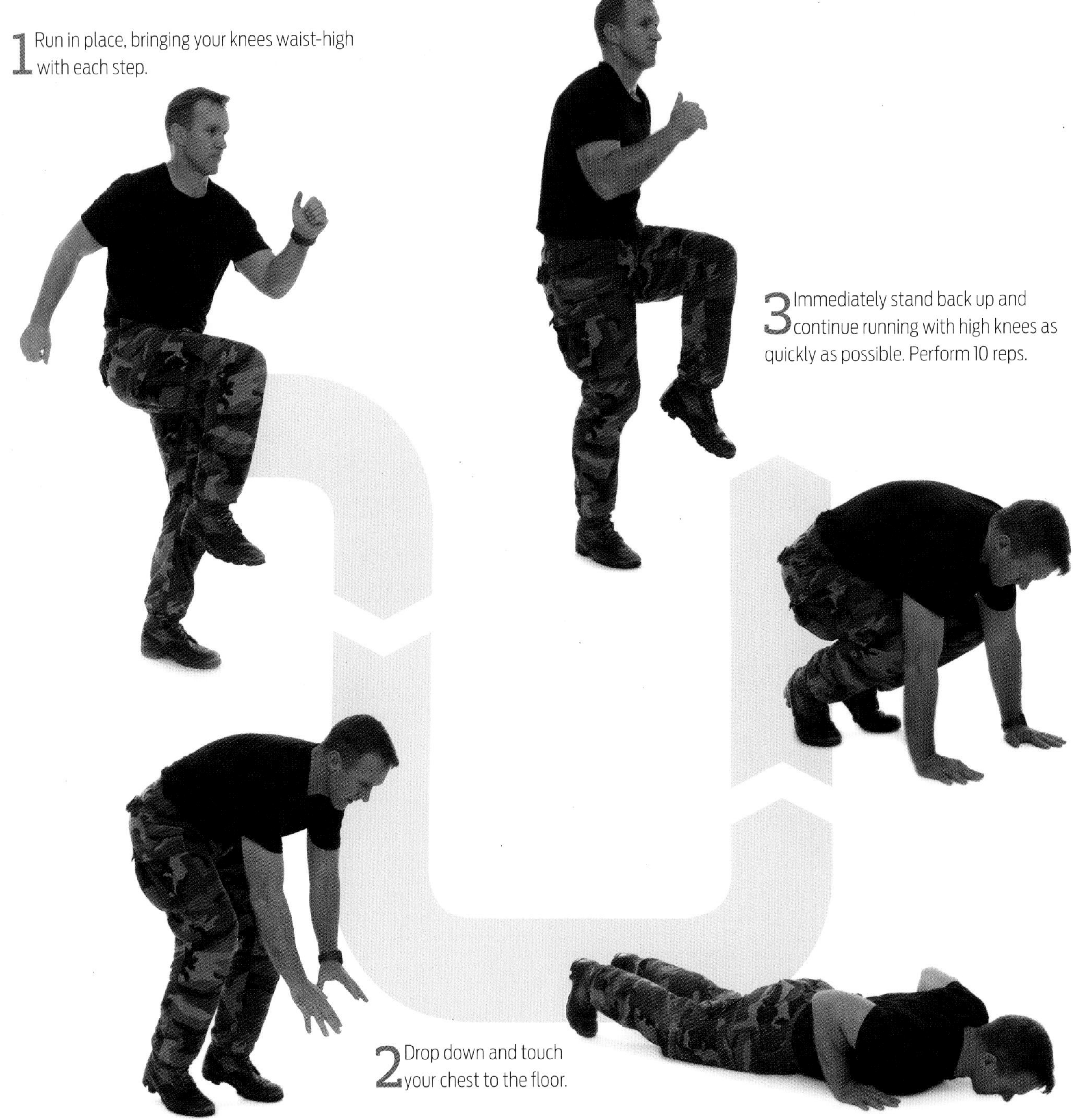

1 Run in place, bringing your knees waist-high with each step.

2 Drop down and touch your chest to the floor.

3 Immediately stand back up and continue running with high knees as quickly as possible. Perform 10 reps.

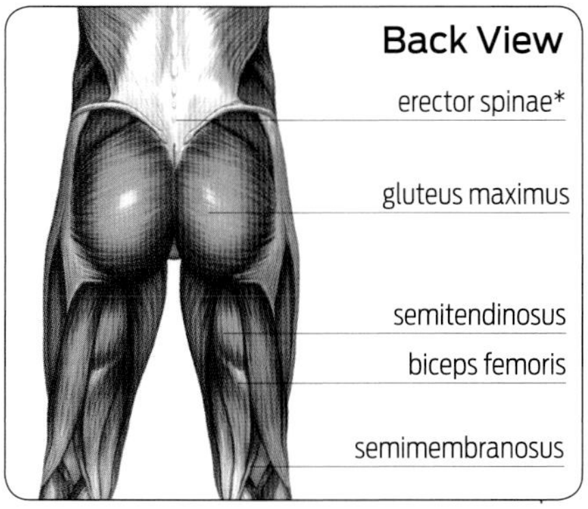

**Back View**

erector spinae*
gluteus maximus
semitendinosus
biceps femoris
semimembranosus

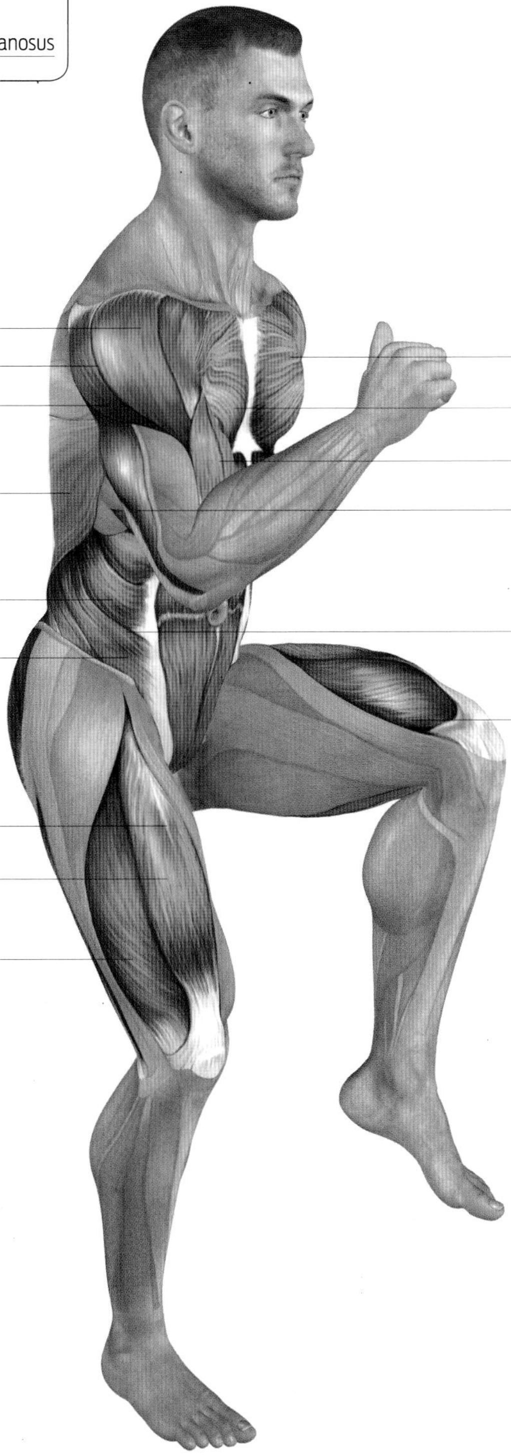

deltoideus anterior
deltoideus medialis
deltoideus posterior
latissimus dorsi
rectus abdominis
obliquus externus
vastus intermedius*
rectus femoris
vastus lateralis

pectoralis minor*
pectoralis major
biceps brachii
triceps brachii
obliquus internus*
vastus medialis

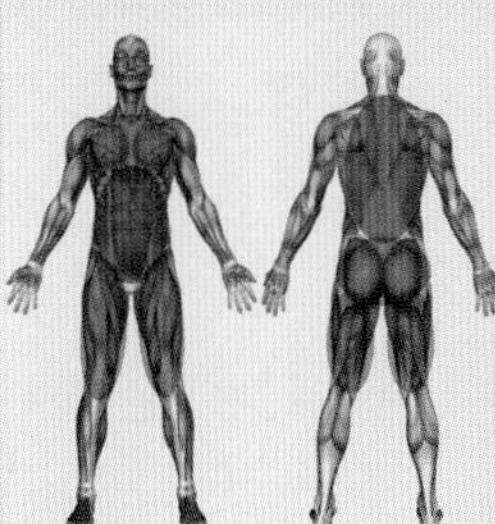

**Level**
· Advanced

**Duration** 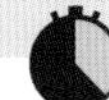
· 45–60 seconds

**Benefits**
· Strengthens upper body and core
· Increases agility
· Improves coordination
· Increases cardiovascular endurance

**Caution** 
· Wrist issues

**Annotation Key**
* indicates deep muscles

## Correct form

- Keep your knees at waist level while running in place.

## Avoid

- Landing on your chest—allow your hands to contact the floor first, and then lower onto your chest.
- Flopping on to the floor—move with control.

# Up-Down with Push-Up

The Up-Down with Push-Up adds another element of upper-body conditioning to the Up-Down. While working multiple muscle groups, you'll also get a challenging cardio workout. Sport teams and military personnel rely on this exercise to develop agility and speed.

1 Run in place, bringing your knees waist-high with each step.

2 Drop down and touch your chest to the floor.

3 Perform a Push-Up.

4 Immediately jump back up to your feet.

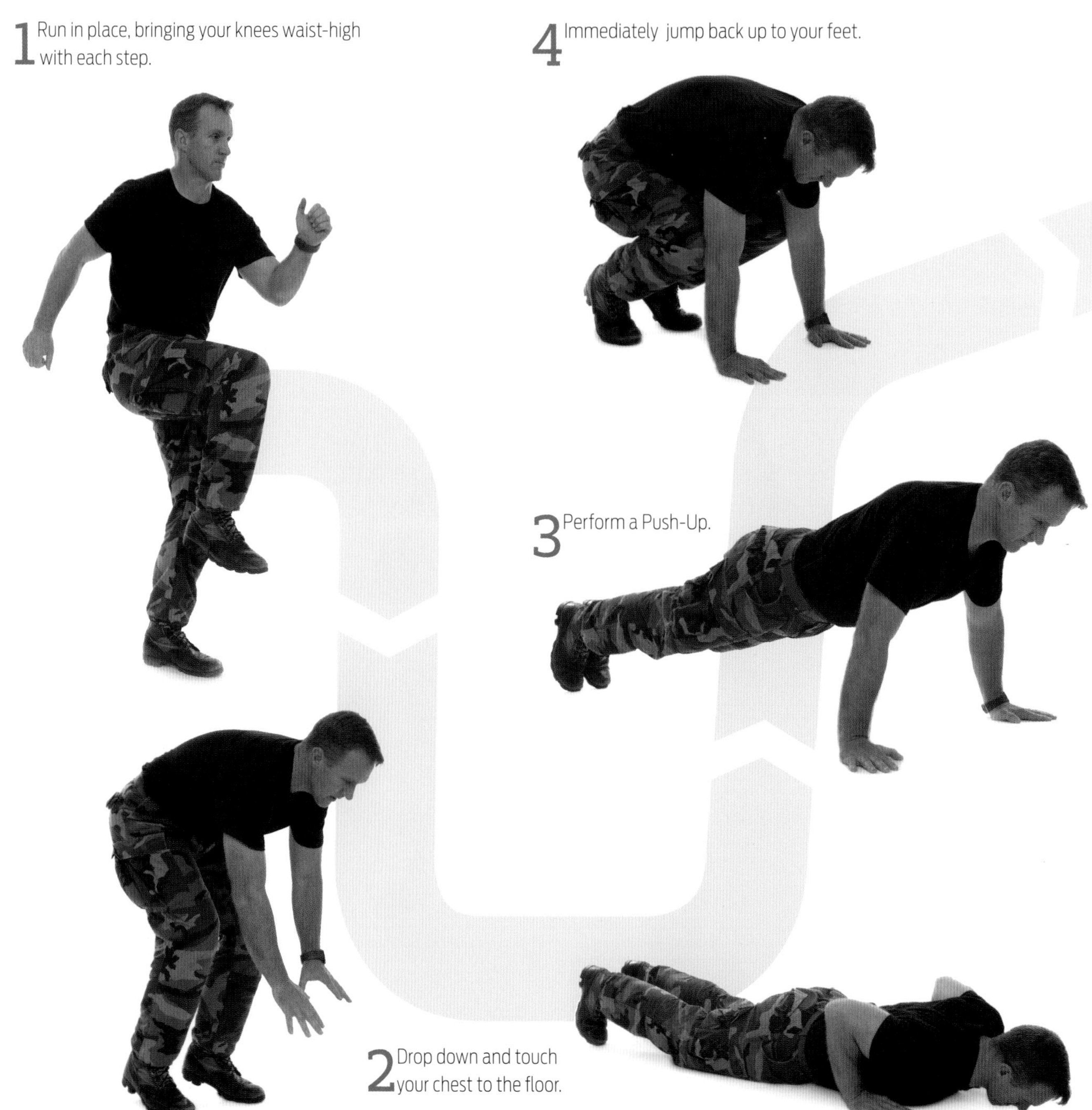

5 Continue running with high knees as quickly as possible. Perform 10 reps.

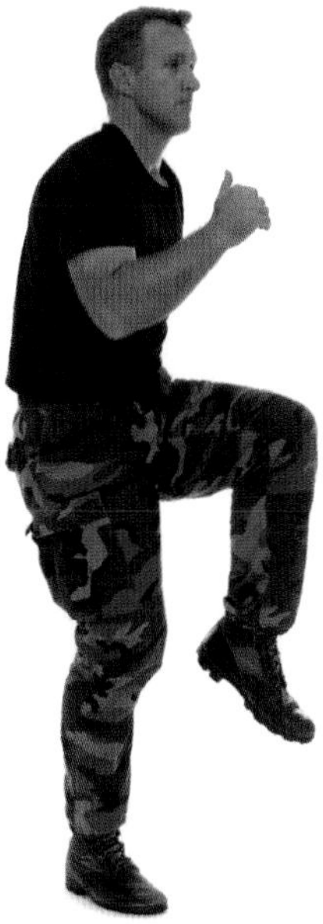

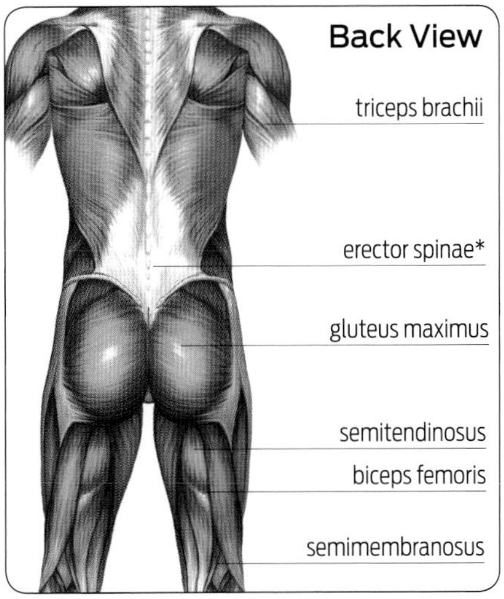

**Back View**

triceps brachii
erector spinae*
gluteus maximus
semitendinosus
biceps femoris
semimembranosus

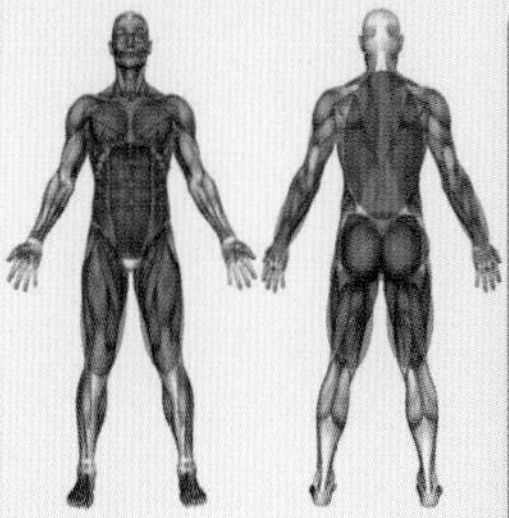

## Level
· Advanced

## Duration
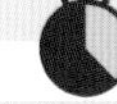
· 45–60 seconds

## Benefits
· Strengthens upper body and core
· Increases agility
· Improves coordination
· Increases cardiovascular endurance

## Caution

· Wrist issues

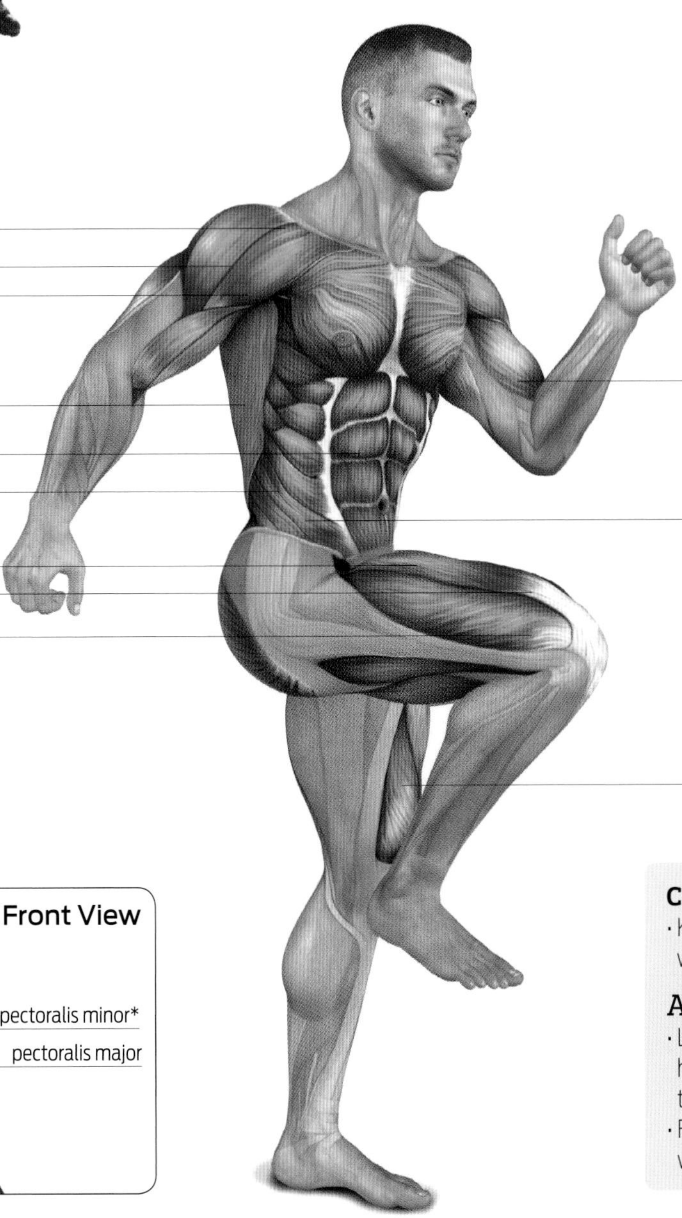

deltoideus posterior
deltoideus medialis
deltoideus anterior
latissimus dorsi
rectus abdominis
obliquus externus
vastus intermedius*
rectus femoris
vastus lateralis

**Annotation Key**
* indicates deep muscles

biceps brachii
obliquus internus*
vastus medialis

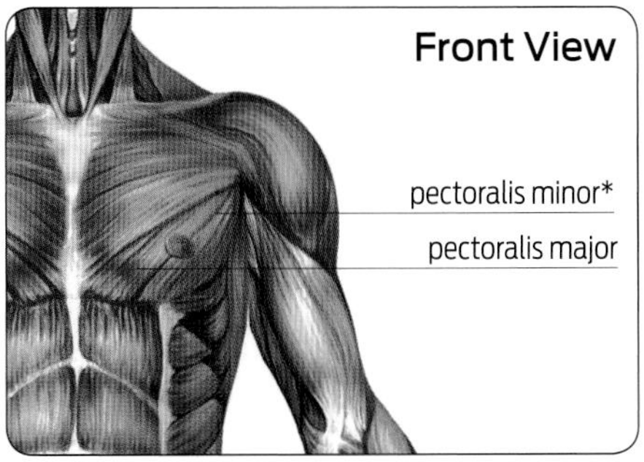

**Front View**

pectoralis minor*
pectoralis major

## Correct form
· Keep your knees at waist level while running in place.

## Avoid
· Landing on your chest—allow your hands to contact the floor first, and then lower onto your chest.
· Flopping on to the floor—move with control.

## Contents

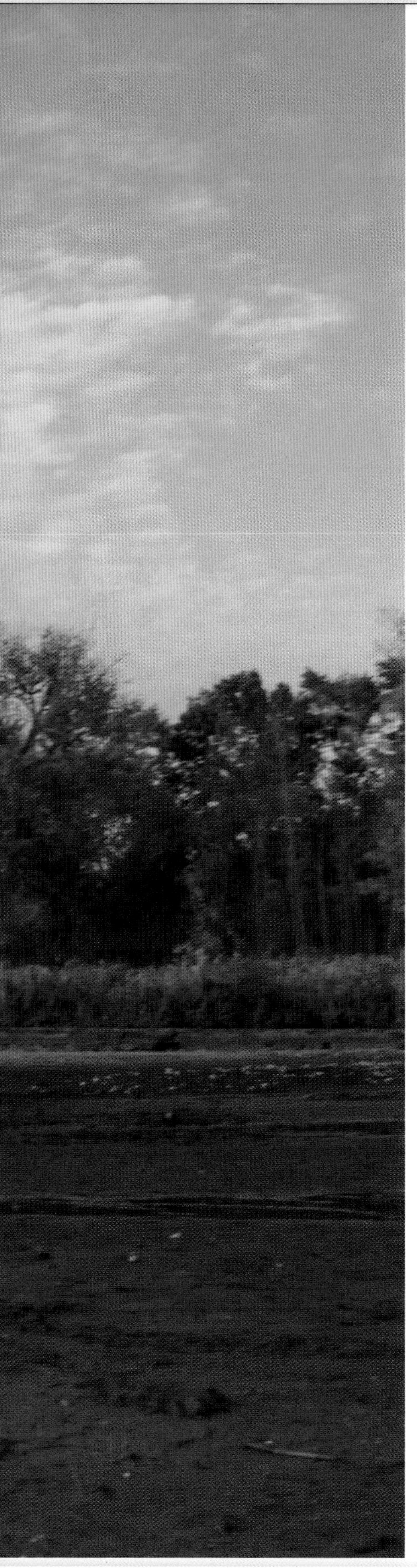

# Swimming & Running

Swimming and running are major components of special forces fitness, with both activities part of the stringent qualification tests for new recruits.

Special forces operatives must be expert swimmers. The Navy SEALs, for example, are most well known for their ability to operate in a maritime environment. The Underwater Demolition Teams of World War II, from which the SEALs developed, were tasked with blowing up underwater obstacles and preparing the beaches for landing craft during the Normandy invasion. Today, the SEALs and special forces teams from around the world continue to excel at these tough assignments.

Whether you are new to swimming, just seeking tips for improvement, or acquiring specialized skills like combat or rescue swimming, you must learn proper form. The following pages give you tips on perfecting your own form, along with instructions for three of the most common swim strokes used in the special forces.

Much like anyone can jump in a pool and attempt laps, anyone can put on sneakers and attempt to run. Running, however, also requires careful attention to proper form, or injuries are likely. This section will introduce you to the basic running form, from how the foot hits the ground, to gaining speed from foot rate, to force production and efficiency. Armed with this knowledge, you can hit the trail, gaining the greatest benefits from your running routine.

# Swimming

Special forces team members must become expert swimmers, but swimming is a near-perfect exercise for anyone, and it can be done at any age.

What makes swimming near perfect is that it uses all the muscles of the body (only cross-country skiing uses more) and is highly aerobic because water creates resistance around each muscle. It's also been proven to lower blood pressure, cholesterol levels, and resting heart rates as well as reducing body fat. No matter what your current fitness level, medical condition, body-fat percentage, age, or gender, you can learn proper form and become fit by using the water for resistance.

## Quality over quantity

Many swim coaches will tell you to not worry about form—eventually, if you perform enough laps, your stroke will become efficient and smooth. This approach, however, is backward. Swimming is a skill sport, and, as with any skill, learning the correct form or technique comes first. A pitcher does not develop his form by throwing a high number of pitches, and a weight lifter does not learn proper squat form by doing endless reps. Swimming is the same.

The by-product of learning proper swimming form is fitness. Learning proper swimming form is much more difficult, however, than learning a tennis swing, pitching technique, or squat form due to the number of muscles involved. With time and practice, you will increase your endurance and become able to swim for long periods, improving your aerobic capacity and efficiency of stroke.

## Efficiency of stroke

To learn proper swim form, you must first understand the concept of "efficiency." The best swimmers take the fewest strokes. This means that they are able to grab the most water with their arms, legs, and torso, with each stroke propelling them through the water. Their strokes become long, and they glide through the water.

Velocity in the water is determined by the formula V = SL x SR, where SL means "stroke length" and SR means "stroke rate." This means that how far you travel per stroke times the number of strokes you take will determine your speed. This formula is the foundation for developing speed through efficiency and is used within SEAL training to learn speed. Learning to take long strokes is the main way to gain efficiency in the water.

SL is a skill to be worked on using mind energy, while SR is just hard work using muscles and the lungs. Work on SL first, as that helps increase SR while also addressing body drag. Drag is the resistance of water on a body moving through it. Streamline your body in the water, and you will glide with less drag. SR will then follow with much less effort. Increasing SR first just burns energy, but offers little in propulsion. As you gain efficiency via proper technique by increasing your SL, you will get faster without getting more tired. This is when your fitness level will take off, and SR will become easy. You will find yourself swimming longer and faster while remaining relaxed in the water.

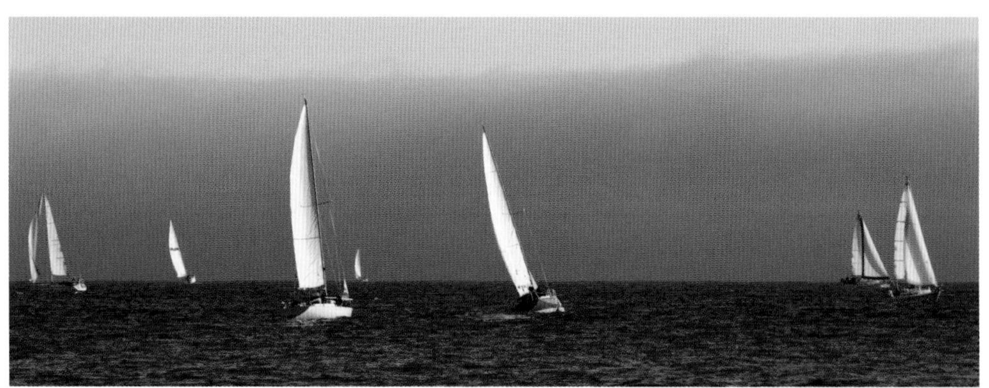

### Swim like a sailboat

Think of a sailboat and a tugboat. A tugboat is wide and built for power. A sailboat is long and built for speed. Do you think it would be best to swim like a tugboat or sailboat to gain SL? A sailboat rolls side-to-side to gain speed, while a tug just churns through the water. Rolling side-to-side like a sailboat creates speed.

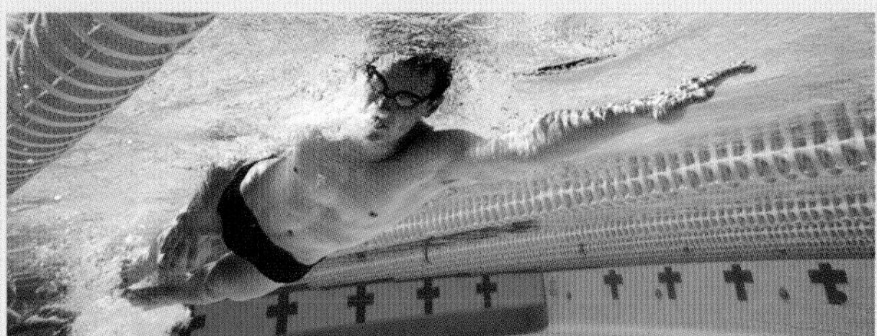

When you move through water, water pushes back, resulting in drag. The splashes and bubbles created by your arms and legs pushing through water show drag in action.

### What is drag?

There are three main types of drag: form, wave, and frictional.

**Form drag** is the resistance caused by your body's shape and profile as it moves through the water. It varies according to body type. Large, wide bodies create more drag than smaller, narrow ones.

**Wave drag** is resistance caused by the turbulence of your body moving through the water. The faster you swim, the more waves you create, but you can create fewer waves by making your strokes smoother. Your hands and feet will make fewer splashes, enabling you to mover faster.

**Frictional drag** is the resistance caused by an object's surface texture as it moves through a fluid. The clothes you wear create this friction, which is why professional swimmers wear swim caps and smooth, form-fitting bathing suits, and even shave all body hair.

## SL acceleration and deceleration

Many swimmers accelerate and decelerate during their stroke, meaning that they speed up and slow down as their arms or head are out of the water. An efficient SL does not speed up and slow down. Instead, the torso is used for SL when the head and arms are out of the water, creating propulsion that allows the body to continue at a constant speed.

Rotating the torso side-to-side creates speed. Therefore, as you take your arm out of the water to recover and breathe, you should be on one side, and as your hand enters the water to stroke, you must roll onto your opposite side to pull the opposite hand out of the water. Rolling from side-to-side is how the torso is used to produce speed when the arm or head is out of the water creating drag. Side swimming while keeping the head straight and in line with the body allows the torso to create speed and decrease drag.

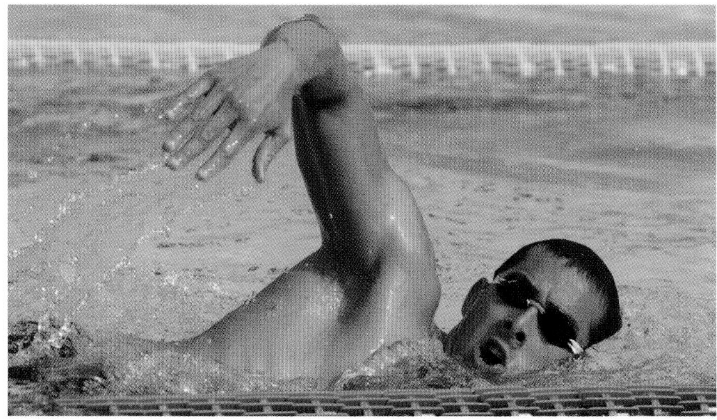

Rotating your torso allows you to take a breath as you lift your arm out of the water. You should then roll to the opposite side as your hand lowers back to the water to complete a stroke.

## Balance and body length

Along with moving your torso side-to-side, balance and body length make a difference to SL. Balance is created by keeping your head in line with your body. If you lift your head out of the water, your feet automatically drop. Dropping your feet places your body in an uphill position that creates drag in your torso. While swimming, picture your spine as a steel rod that cannot bend—your head and torso are one unit.

Rolling your body on its side without lifting your head to breathe keeps your head in line with your body, creating a balanced, horizontal body position.

Your chest also contributes to balance. Your lungs act like a buoy in your chest. Pressing your "buoy" into the water while rolling side-to-side keeps your head in line with your spine and balances your feet with your torso.

Making your body longer in the water uses what is referred to as "front quadrant swimming." Our natural tendency is to swim with our arms in opposition: one arm is forward and the other arm backward. If an arm is always in the front quadrant, that arm is breaking the water's drag. If both arms are simultaneously below the shoulders (lower quadrants) then the head and shoulders are creating drag. In front quadrant swimming, one arm or hand is always in front of your body.

To try this style, as you swim, reach above your head with one arm to grab as much water as possible while lying on your side. As you pull that arm through the water, roll onto the opposite side, and replace the front quadrant hand with the other hand, which will decrease drag while you roll onto the opposite side.

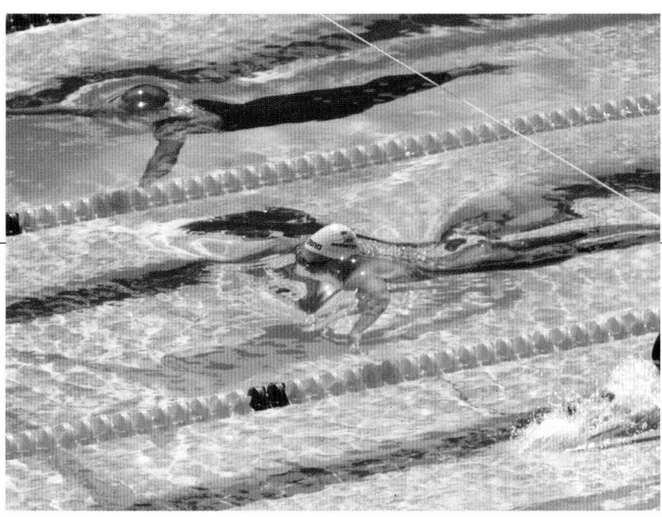

Rival swimmers during a 200-meter breaststroke competition keep their bodies long and streamlined to reduce drag.

## Swim strokes

The freestyle stroke, or front crawl, is the basic stroke used by most swimmers and is a good one to practice as you learn proper form and efficient stroke technique. SEAL teams rely on two other strokes: breaststroke and combat sidestroke. These two strokes are efficient and allow a low profile in the water for tactical situations.

### *Freestyle*

The front crawl, often called the freestyle stroke, is the fastest swim stroke. When performing the freestyle, keep in mind the efficiency of your stroke, your balance, and your body length.

- Begin in a squat position against the wall of the pool, and then push off, staying streamlined with your arms extended forward and your biceps close to your ears. Point your fingers forward and extend your legs backward, keeping your toes pointed. Look downward while keeping your head in line with your torso.
- Alternate drawing giant circles with each arm, sweeping it down, then back toward your feet, then up toward your hip, and then out of the water to its starting position.
- At the same time as you move your arms, kick up and down from your hips, keeping your legs long and straight and your ankles relaxed. You should feel both the tops and bottoms of your feet pushing the water.

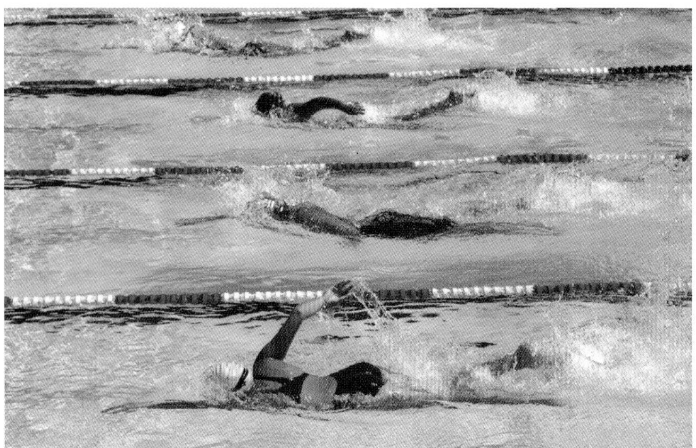

Swimmers in a freestyle race demonstrate how to move swiftly through the water while kicking with straight legs.

### *Breaststroke*

The breaststroke is a favorite with recreational swimmers because it is a stable move that keeps the head out of the water for much of the time. Unlike other strokes, your limbs work simultaneously and symmetrically. For SEALs and lifeguards teams, it is particularly useful because the eyes remain above the water, which allows a rescuer to approach without losing sight of a victim.

- Begin in a squat position against the wall of the pool, and then push off, staying streamlined with your arms extended forward and your biceps close to your ears. Point your fingers forward and extend your legs backward, keeping your toes pointed. Look downward while keeping your head in line with your torso.
- Rotate your hands outward, separating your arms so that your body forms a Y shape.
- When your arms are about 2 feet apart, flex your elbows and continue to move your hands backward and also downward, while starting to flex your knees, drawing your feet toward your butt.
- When your hands have moved past your shoulders, move them toward each other until they meet below your chest. Your torso will rise above water and your feet will continue to move toward your butt.
- Kick your feet backward and apart while extending your arms forward underwater. Your chest and your head will again drop in the water.
- When your legs are completely extended, bring them together, and glide forward. As the momentum of the glide wanes, start a new cycle.

## *Combat sidestroke*

Developed by the SEALs, the combat sidestroke (CSS) is an extremely efficient, low-energy stroke that reduces the body's profile in the water, making a swimmer harder to spot during combat operations. Both hands remain submerged at all times, using what is known as the "underwater recovery arm." In this method, two arm pulls are used: the pull arm and the paddle arm. As the pull arm comes off the side to meet the paddle arm at the chest, it remains underwater, with the hand staying very close to the torso. This decreases drag and removes any splashing or profile in the water.

The cadence of this stroke and body position also make it a favorite among tactical athletes. The same principles as the freestyle stroke apply: efficiency of stroke, balance, and body length.

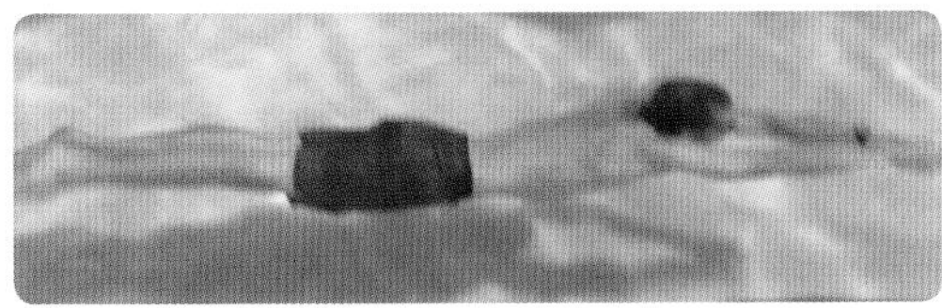

- Begin with your body flat and both arms overhead, palms facing downward. One arm will be your pull arm, and the other will be the paddle arm.

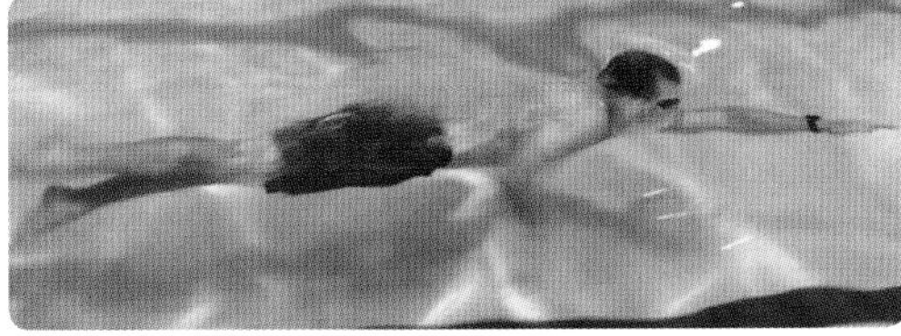

- Pull your pull arm from overhead until it rests on your side and rolls your body to the side. Your paddle arm will still be overhead.

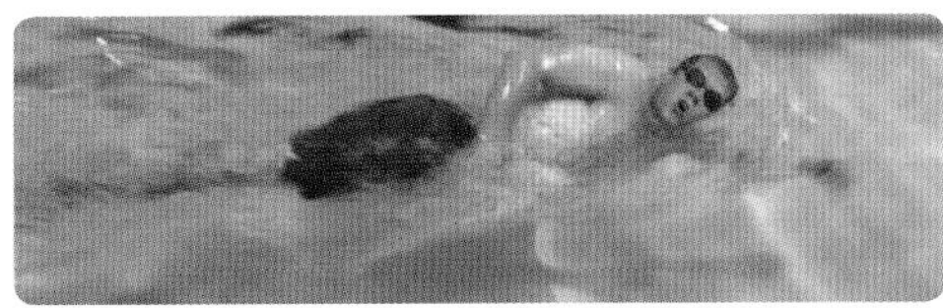

- Make a circle with your paddle arm, lowering your hand to chest level. As your hand nears your chest, move the hand of your pull arm in front of your body, meeting both hands together. Your body position now is on your side with both hands at your chest, palms facing you.
- Scissor kick from your hips, with your legs long and straight and your ankles relaxed, and move both arms overhead with hands on top of each other. Your body is now in an arrow position, with arms perfectly straight overhead, hands on top of each other, biceps on ears, "buoy" down, back and legs straight, and feet pointed and together. This decreases drag and allows the body to glide and float to the surface.
- When you tire on one side, switch to the other.

### The 500m swim

The first requirement in the Navy SEAL PST is the 500m swim. Many BUD/S candidates wear themselves out during the swim due to inefficient form. This leaves little energy for the Push-Up, Sit-Up, Pull-Up, or run. Learning proper swim form before taking the PST helps SEAL wannabes become active operatives.

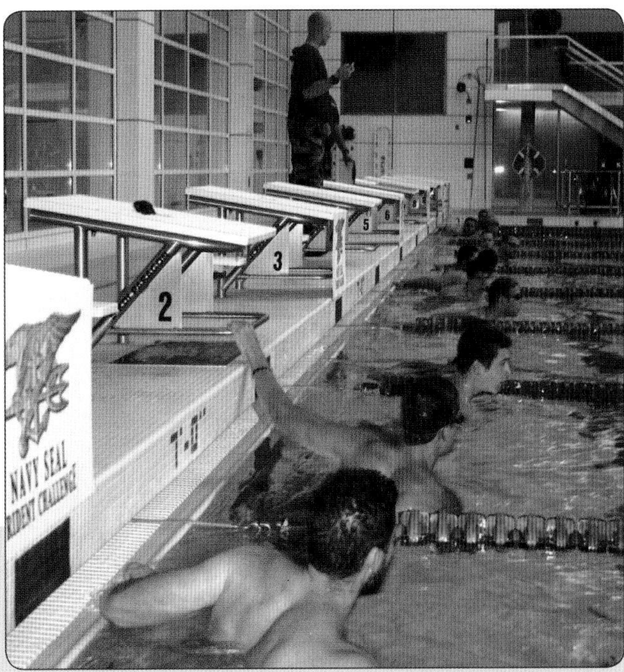


Navy SEAL hopefuls compete in a Trident Challenge to see if they have what it takes to make it in the special forces.

# Running

Running is the most common form of exercise. It is also one of the easiest because it is a very natural movement—essentially an extension of walking.

For humans, running is as natural as walking, and just as necessary. Running is also a form of sport. And much like swimming, biking, weight-lifting, or team sports, running requires proper technique.

Running is both an aerobic and anaerobic exercise. Aerobic running is determined by heart rate. Distance events like marathons are long and are performed at an aerobic heart rate. Anaerobic, or high-heart rate, running includes events like sprinting.

## A multipurpose sport

The majority of runners do so to lose fat and keep it off. These days, however, competitive running is on the rise. Mud runs, distance events, adventure racing, and triathlons are increasing in popularity. But whatever the reason you decide to run, learning the correct technique will let you run faster, farther, and with fewer injuries. As you practice the swimming form, you will discover that you become faster with less effort. Running is the same. As you practice the techniques outlined below, your speed will increase and you will expend less effort.

## The mechanics of running

You must start with the basic mechanics of running to understand how they apply to sport, exercise, and tactical purposes. Runners must be able to produce force quickly and continue the force over time from the foot, leg, and core muscles. The amount of force produced from each running step is a function of muscle endurance, strength, and the ability to coordinate movement in a rhythmic pattern. Once you have mastered proper foot strike, stride length, cadence, posture, and arm swing, you can run for speed, agility, endurance, and tactical training.

## *Foot strike*

How your foot contacts the ground will determine your running form. To determine your foot strike, pay attention to how your forward foot lands as you run. If it is landing near your toes, it is a forefoot strike. Landing between your heel and toes is a midfoot strike. If you are landing on your heel and then rolling to your toes, it is a heel strike. Each of these running forms has a different effect on muscles, joints, and tissues.

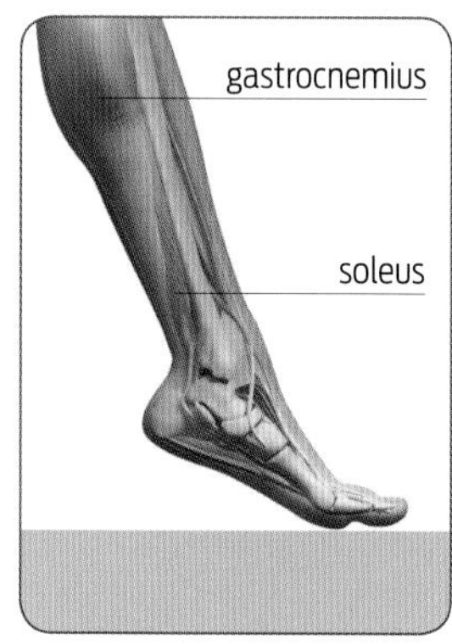

Forefoot strike

Forefoot running relies on supination, which means that the foot rolls inward to stay rigid. A rigid foot allows for increased propulsion and speed, which is good for sprinters. For most runners, though, a forefoot strike places excessive stress on a part of the foot that is not designed to handle a lot of force. Further, because it mainly uses the gastrocnemius and soleus, these muscles of the calf must be strong. Weak muscles can result in muscle strain or Achilles tendinitis, a condition that produces pain and sometimes swelling of the heel and tendon.

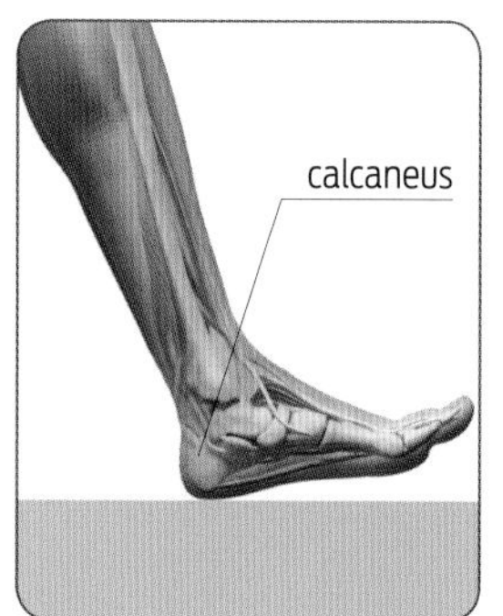

Heel strike

Heel strike is the most common pattern. The large calcaneus bone of the heel is designed to absorb impact, and as the foot flattens in a motion called pronation, it continues to absorb the force of hitting the ground.

### Weight training for runners

Weight-lifting can add another level to your running program. Runners who train at low intensities (light weights and low reps only 1 to 2 days per week) can improve their running endurance. The muscle strength gained by lifting weights allows the runner to have more energy left in the final lap or mile and to also recover more quickly.

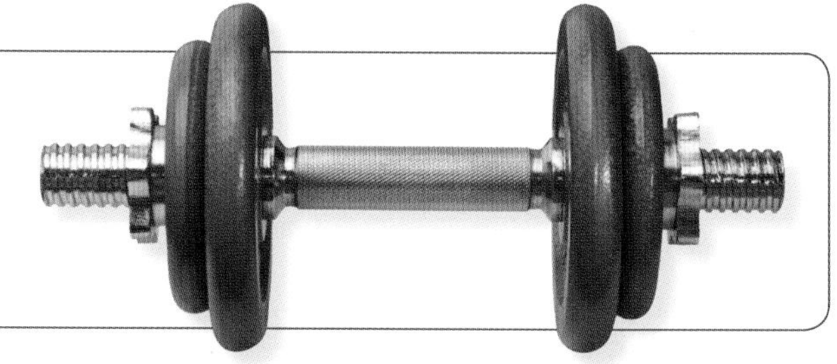

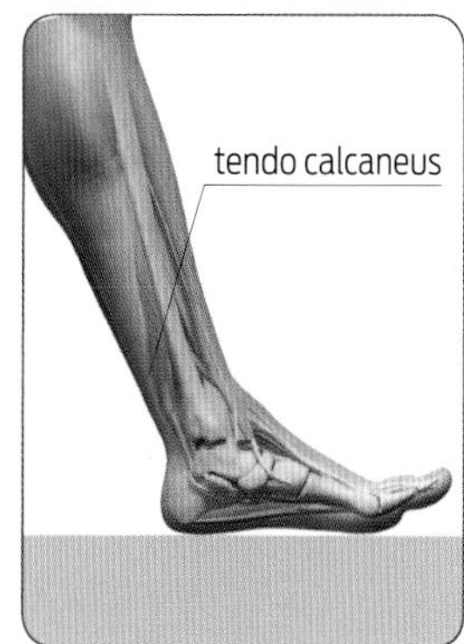

Midfoot strike

A midfoot strike absorbs force more evenly than a heel strike, so it is less jarring. It also doesn't rely as heavily on the calf muscles, relieving strain on the Achilles tendon (tendo calcaneus) reducing the chance of Achilles tendinitis. Still, form is essential—to maintain shock absorption, the foot must pronate efficiently, so that the arch doesn't just collapse without control. Without control, a runner can suffer fatigue in the foot muscles. This can lead to lead to knee, hip, and lower-back pain.

## *Stride length*

For optimum endurance running, shorter is better. Fluid and energy-efficient forward motion results from slight knee lift, quick leg turnover, and short stride. To make sure that you are running at your ideal stride length, land with your feet directly underneath your body, and, as your foot strikes the ground, slightly flex your knee so that it can bend naturally on impact. If your lower leg extends out in front of your body, your stride is too long.

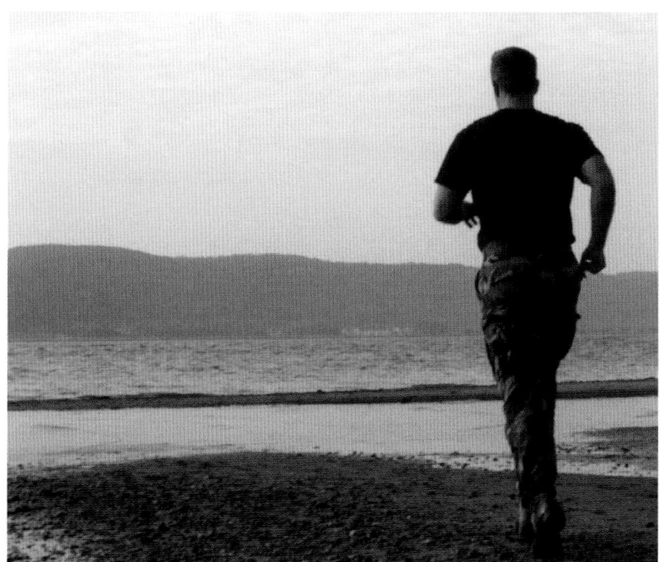

Proper running form includes attention to your upper body. Lean slightly forward and pump your arms behind your torso.

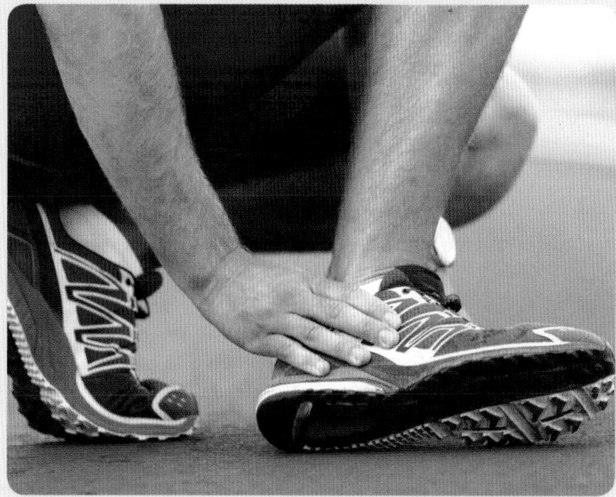

### Heel strike and overuse injuries

Overuse injuries are the result of too much force over a period of time. The heel may be designed to absorb shock, but many runners using the heel strike still suffer overuse injuries, mainly due to overstride, insufficient hip extension of the leg, or shoes that are too heavy. To avoid these injuries, concentrate on landing with a midfoot strike at a cadence of 180 strides per minute. Wear light shoes with a low angle from the heel to the midfoot and be mindful of fully extending the rear leg.

## *Cadence*

Cadence is the amount of strides you take per minute. Cadence is most easily determined on a treadmill with varying levels of difficulty. To establish your cadence, begin running on a treadmill at warm-up pace, and then adjust the level to one that mimics your usual running style—easy, marathon, uphill, etc. After a minute, count your steps for 30 seconds and multiply the number by two. This is your baseline cadence.

Research has shown that 180 is about the ideal cadence. To achieve that number, work on upping your cadence gradually, aiming for 5 percent increases until you hit 180. For example, if your easy cadence was 160, aim for 168. After you have comfortably achieved that, work on hitting 176.

## *Posture and arm swing*

Upper-body posture is important when running. Torso form should be upright with a slight forward lean. Allowing your body to lean forward gives you momentum during the run. A slight forward lean also allows for proper arm swing. Your arms should be bent at 90 degrees and swing behind your torso. To get a sense of this, imagine holding a hammer in your hands and pounding a nail in the wall behind you.

## Speed

Speed is necessary for virtually all athletic and tactical environments. Running speed is a series of repetitive falling forward movements determined by stride frequency and stride length. Stride frequency, or how rapidly your feet hit the ground, is the most important element of speed generation. The higher the frequency, the greater the speed.

## Agility

Agility is the ability to maintain a velocity while changing direction. This includes reacting to a stimulus like a gunshot or a whistle, or moving laterally to stop a ground ball. Balance, coordination, and explosive power are necessary to achieve maximum agility. Many exercises found in this book serve to help with agility. The 8-Count Body Builder (pages 86–87), DFRB (pages 114–115), and Alligator Crawl (pages 128–129) are examples of exercises using body weight that help you gain coordination and explosive power of the body.

In a tactical environment, a soldier's uniform often contains a flak jacket, Kevlar helmet, water, ammunition, med pack, weapon, and rucksack. This uniform can add up to 180 pounds. Training requires the resistive techniques that build agility so the soldier can move quickly and maintain a heart rate low enough for fine motor coordination. Often military personnel will train in uniform, performing the exercises in this book to gain agility for the tactical environment.

To acclimate themselves to the rough terrain they may encounter on active duty, BUD/S recruits and other spec ops trainees run in boots and on unstable surfaces. Running on soft sand adds new challenges to the ankles, knees, and hips.

The most common injury among tactical athletes is outside knee pain—it is so common in SEAL Training that it is called "BUD/S knee." Soft sand or other unstable surfaces can cause the knee joint to shift, which irritates the outside of the knee and the iliotibial band (the tough group of fibers that run along the outside of the thigh). Exercises like Good Morning, Darling (pages 72–73) and Speed Skater (pages 110–111) target the inner and outer thighs, which help to stabilize them and prevent common injuries, such as iliotibial band syndrome, which causes stinging or pain in the knees and thighs.

Recruits are trained in a technique that helps keep them stable in soft sand—landing a foot toe-first inside a footprint already compacted by another runner. This lessens the impact and shifting of the knee.

### Resistance running

Special forces teams must often run against resistance—dragging a sled or parachute, pushing a car, running in water, wearing a heavy vest or boots, or running up hills. You can add resistance running to your routine, which works to increase stride frequency when running without resistance. Essentially, your body adjusts to moving quickly while carrying heavy loads, so that once the load is removed, you are able to run faster. Try wearing heavier clothes or strapping a rucksack on your back, but be sure not to increase your body weight by more than 10 percent.

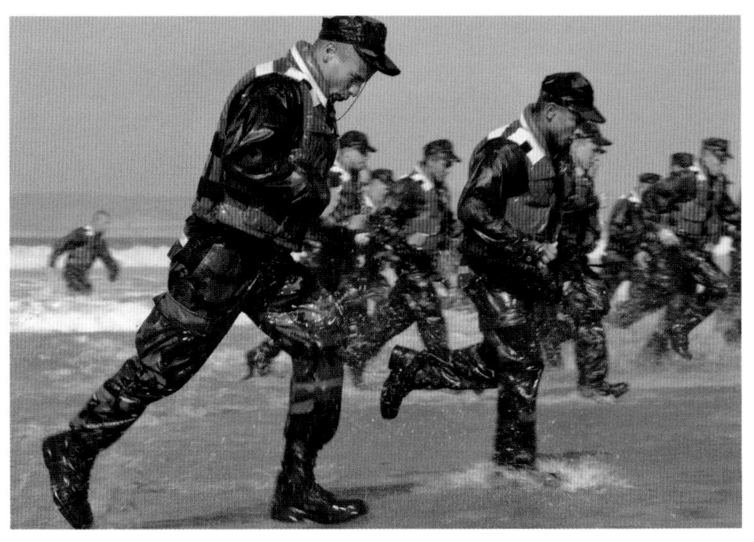

Students at the Naval Amphibious Base Coronado participate in a surf passage exercise, which calls for them to run in water wearing full gear. This is part of the first phase of BUD/S training.

## Running programs

In designing a running program, there are five different run types to consider.

- *LSD (long slow duration) training:* These are aerobic runs of 45 minutes to 2 hours, geared toward fat loss and muscle endurance.
- *Pace/tempo training:* The purpose of pace/tempo training is to improve both aerobic and anaerobic ability while pacing your speed during a run or cardio session. You run at maximal intensity for about 20 to 30 minutes, usually with brief periods of recovery taken when you can no longer stay at the same speed. Recovery will be an easy-paced jog.
- *Interval training:* This is similar to pace/tempo, but rather than jog to recovery, you walk to recovery. You should sprint from 30 seconds to 5 minutes, and then walk an equal amount of time (1:1 work:rest ratio). This is done to enhance anaerobic capacity and should only be done by those with a solid aerobic running base.
- *REPS (repetition training):* In REPS training, you sprint at maximum intensity for 30 to 90 seconds, and then rest five times as long (1:5 work:rest ratio). There are multiple benefits of this type of running: increased speed, efficiency, and anaerobic capacity. For competitive runners, it helps them give an extra push at the end of a race.
- *Fartleks:* This is a combination run of the other techniques. Jog with interval sprints for short and longer times, and take interval rests at 1:1 and 1:5 ratios.

**Sample training program for marathon running**

| | RUN TYPE | DURATION |
|---|---|---|
| SUNDAY | Rest | |
| MONDAY | Fartleks | 45 minutes |
| TUESDAY | LSD | 1/8 mile sprint |
| WEDNESDAY | Interval | 45 minutes |
| THURSDAY | Run at race pace over hills and flats | 60 minutes |
| FRIDAY | REPS | 45 minutes |
| SATURDAY | LSD | 120 minutes |

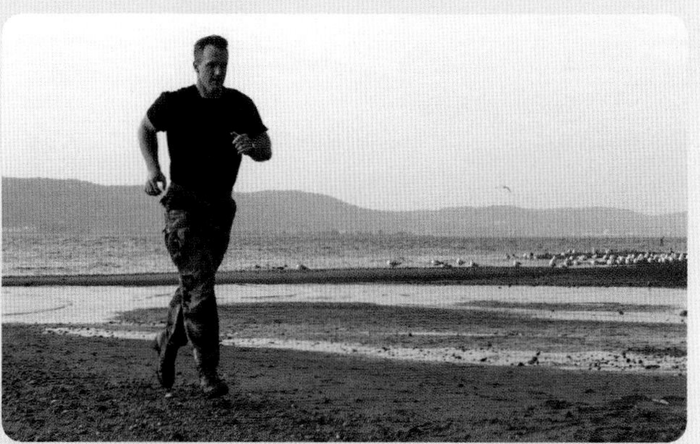

### Stew Smith's 3-Mile Workout

To prepare them for the SEAL PST, former SEAL Stew Smith trains potential recruits using this 3-mile track workout—a pace/tempo variation that builds speed and endurance. This plan calls for run distances of 1.5 miles, with a separate 4-mile timed run. As it is often done in the military, most of it is done to cadence. The basic fitness cadence is an 8-minute-mile pace, which means that the number of strides you take per minute will cover a mile in 8 minutes. If you are seeking special operations level performance, then a cadence well below an 8-minute-mile pace is mandatory. During this running interval workout, you recover during the jog, but there should not be any walking.

**3-mile track workout**

| JOGGING DISTANCE | CADENCE PACE | SPRINT DISTANCE |
|---|---|---|
| 1-mile jog | (7–8 minutes pace) | 1/4 mile sprint |
| 1/4-mile jog | (7–8 minutes pace) | 1/4 mile sprint |
| 1/4-mile jog | (7–8 minutes pace) | 1/8 mile sprint |
| 1/8-mile jog | | 1/8 mile sprint |
| 1/8-mile jog | | 1/8 mile sprint |
| 1/8-mile jog | | 1/8 mile sprint |
| 1/8-mile jog | | |

## Combination training

You don't have to stick to one type of running program. Choose the one that fits your needs, or combine them to get the results you want. Marathon runners, for example, benefit from a mix of training types (see chart at left).

## Make a plan

You must first begin to determine why you are running. What is your goal? You now have the basics to get started, so set micro goals and map out a plan to achieve it. This information will take you far in preparation when you use and practice it. You will gain efficiency, fitness and athletic ability using these principles. Swimming may be the most perfect exercise, but running is the one most utilized for all athletics, including tactical.

## Contents



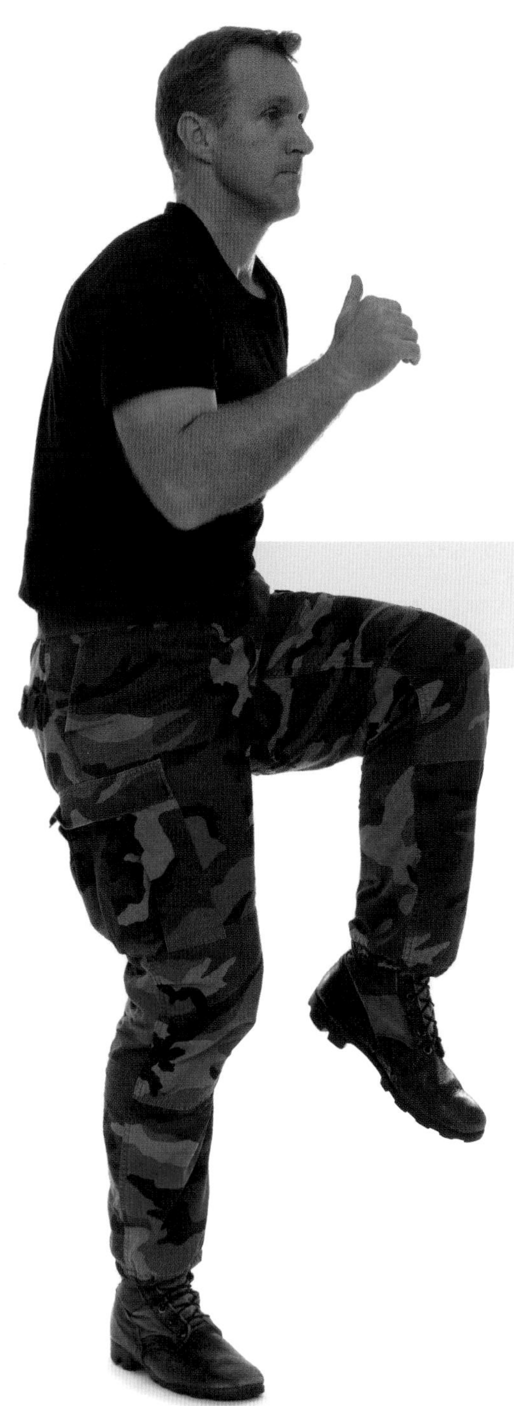

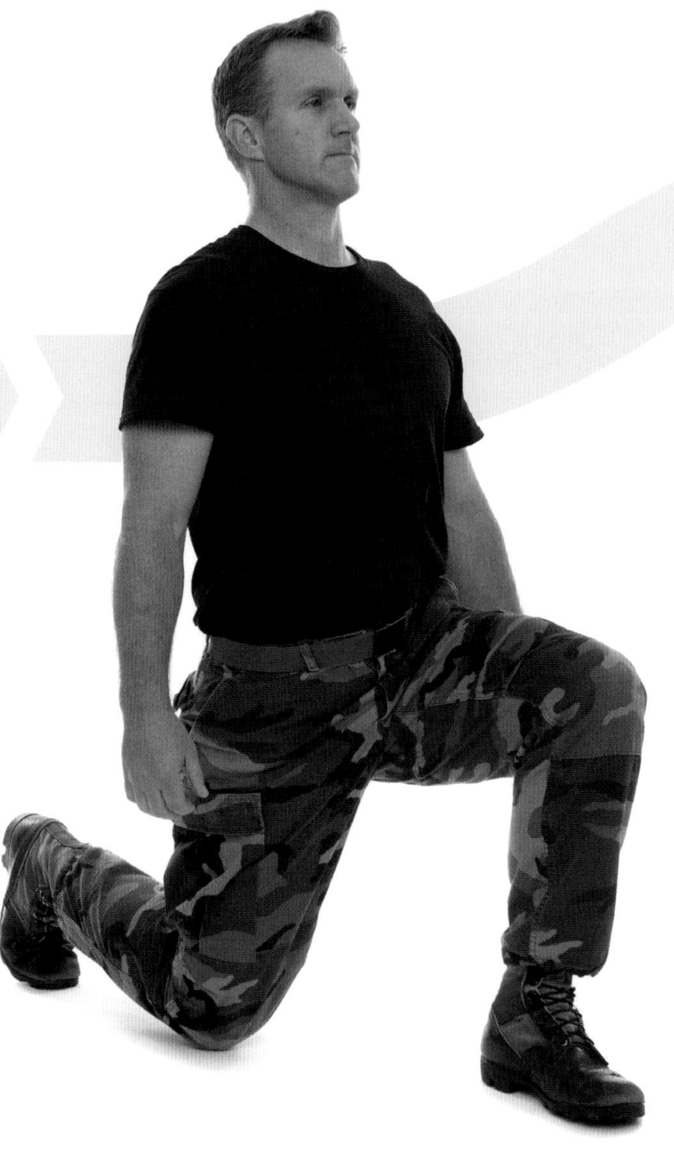

# Workouts

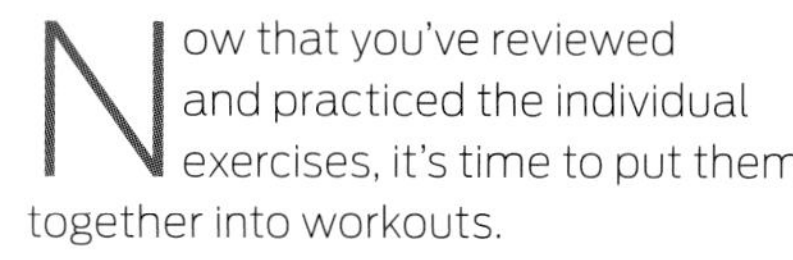

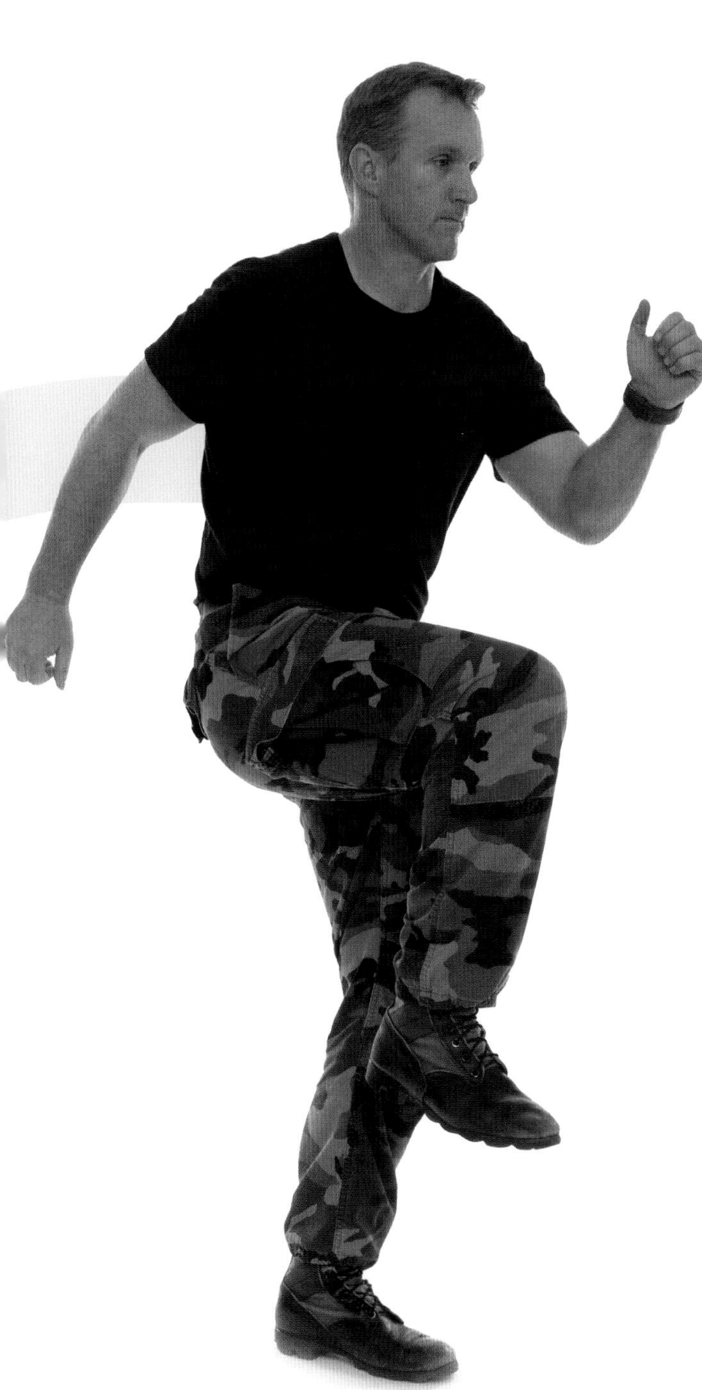

Now that you've reviewed and practiced the individual exercises, it's time to put them together into workouts.

Begin with the Phase I Workout, which is equivalent to a SEALs Phase I training routine. As your level of fitness increases, move on to the more challenging Phase II workouts, practicing them regularly until you are proficient at executing the recommended reps with optimal form.

When you are ready to advance further, the Phase III workout will really put you through your paces—it is equivalent to a special forces workout for those at the highest level of training.

You can also craft your own workouts, choosing to focus either on muscle endurance or a combination of endurance and cardiovascular training.

- A muscle endurance workout is one that concentrates on one body part at a time; for example, performing Push-Ups with minimal rest between sets targets your upper-body muscles. You could then move on to a series of exercises that target the abdominals. Feel free to add in any running and swimming into these workouts.
- A combination cardiovascular and endurance workout moves between various body parts, causing the heart to shift blood to different muscle groups, which elevates your breath and heart rate. How high you elevate your heart rate will determine whether you are working aerobically or anaerobically. Both aerobic and anaerobic exercise is very important if you seek ultimate fitness levels similar to those serving in the special forces.

# Phase I Workout

This workout is equivalent to a SEAL Phase I workout, and it is also the kind of workout performed at special forces training camps around the world. It will familiarize you with the movements necessary to achieve the fitness level of a special forces operative.

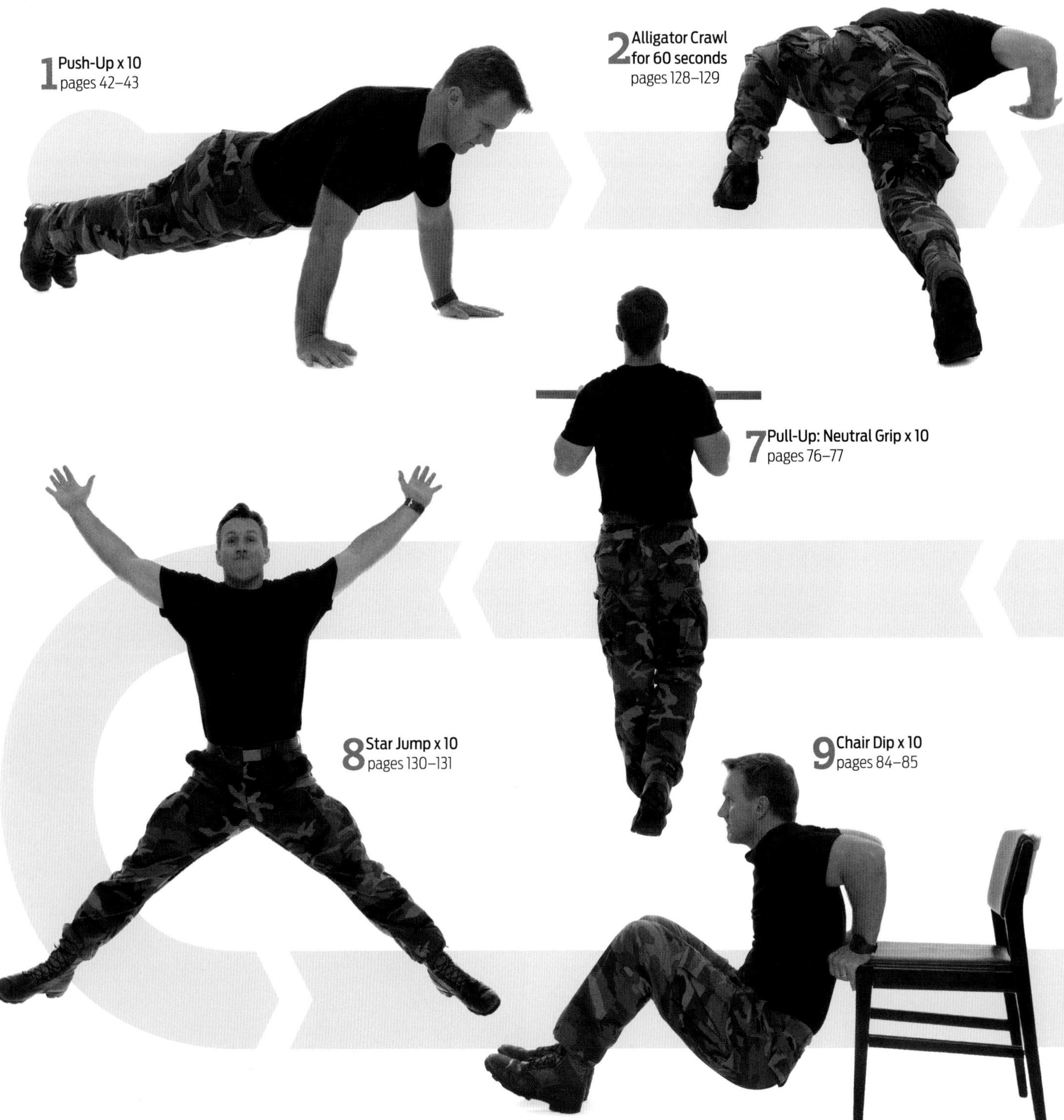

1 Push-Up x 10
pages 42–43

2 Alligator Crawl for 60 seconds
pages 128–129

7 Pull-Up: Neutral Grip x 10
pages 76–77

8 Star Jump x 10
pages 130–131

9 Chair Dip x 10
pages 84–85

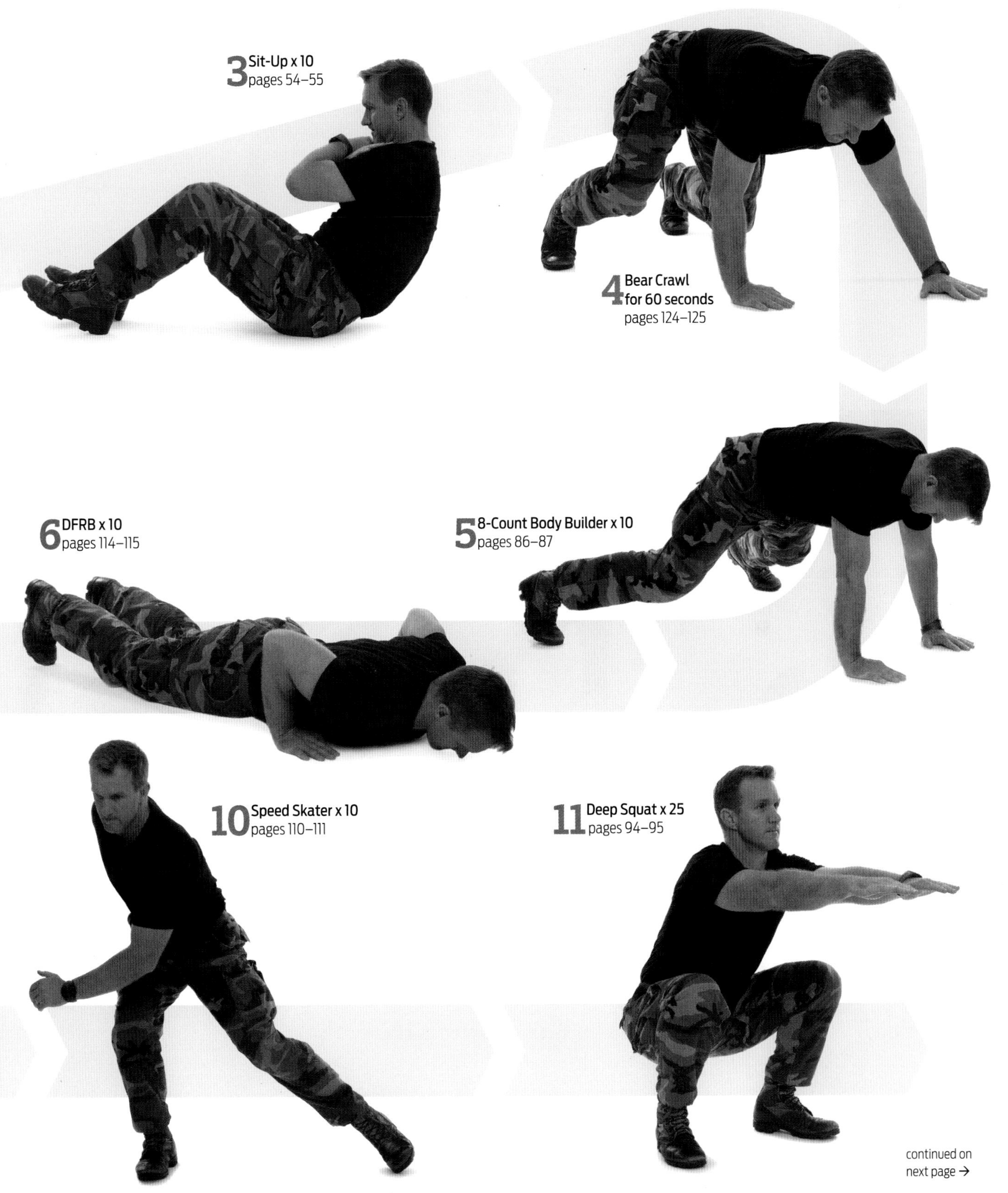


continued on next page →

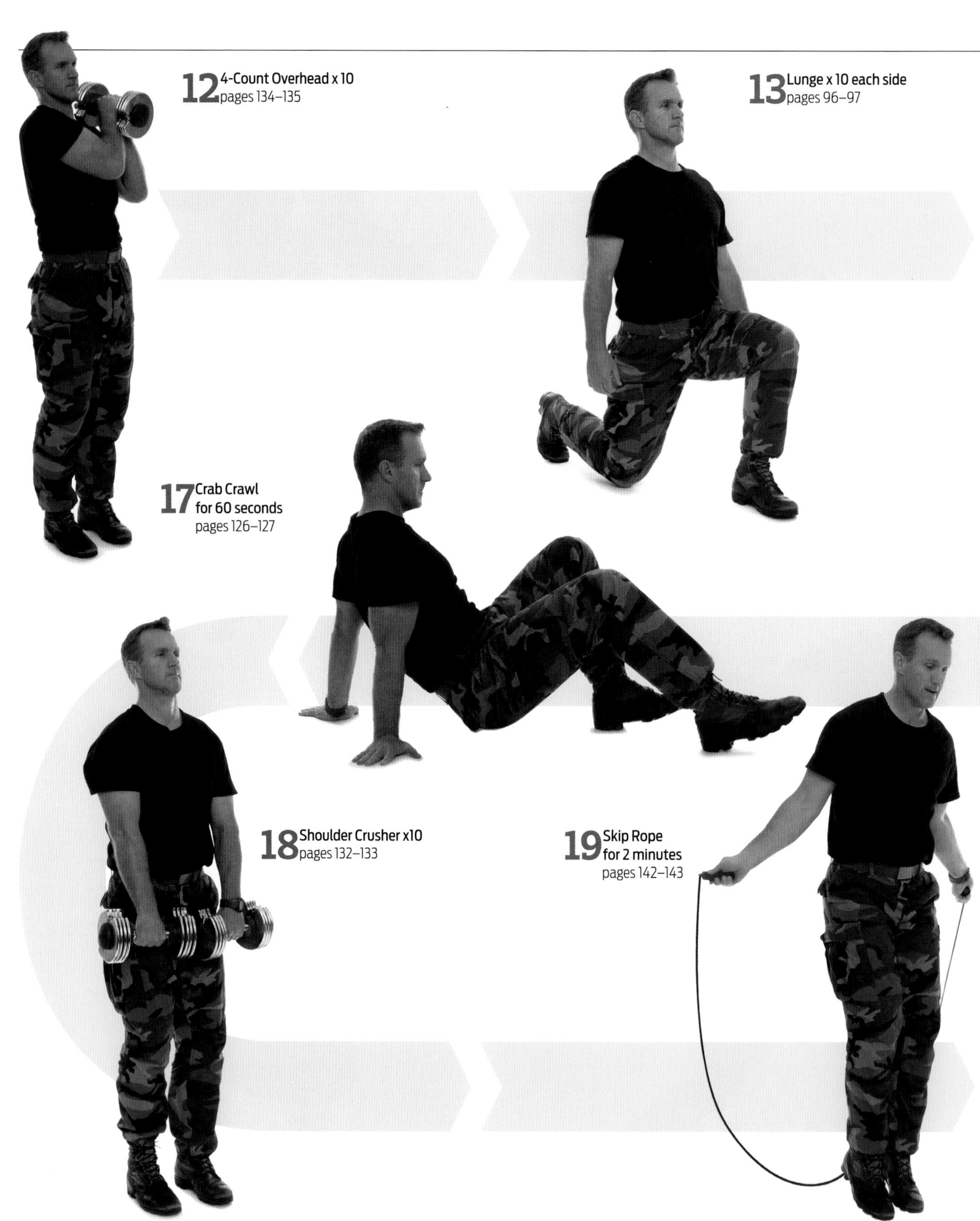
12 4-Count Overhead x 10
pages 134–135
13 Lunge x 10 each side
pages 96–97
17 Crab Crawl
for 60 seconds
pages 126–127
18 Shoulder Crusher x10
pages 132–133
19 Skip Rope
for 2 minutes
pages 142–143

**14** Switch Lunge x 10 each side
pages 98–99

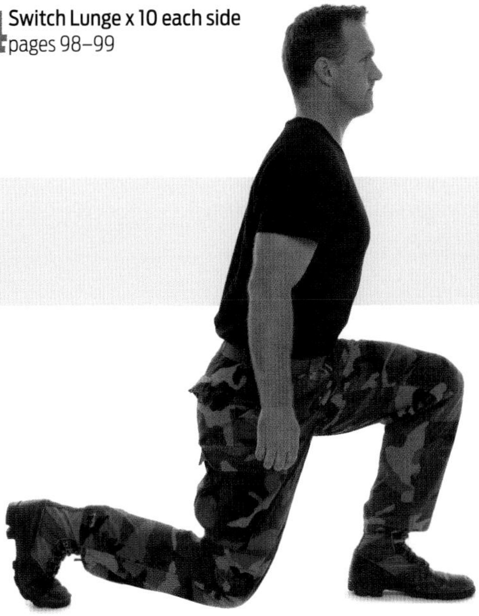

**15** Up-Down x 10
pages 148–149

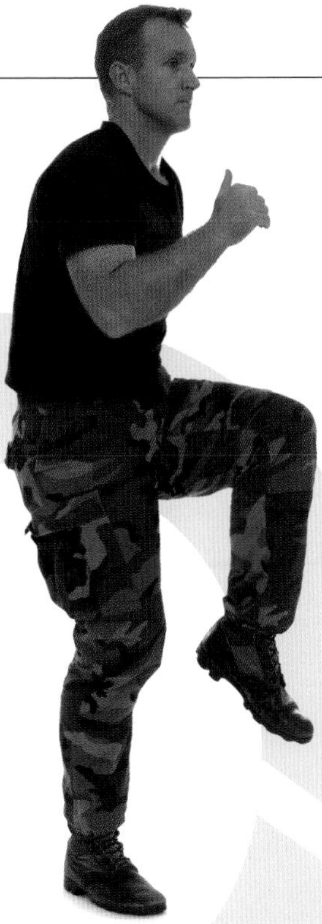

**16** Turtle Shell for 60 seconds
pages 62–63

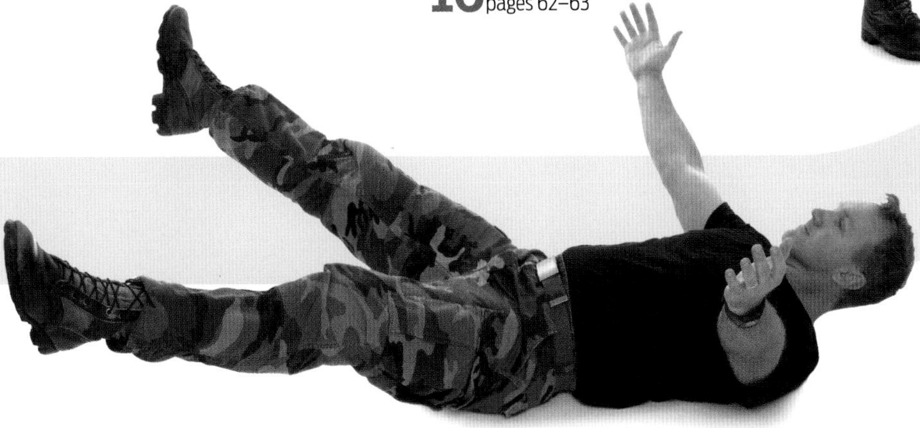

**20** Mountain Climber x 10
pages 146–14

**21** Slalom Skier x 10 each side
pages 144–145

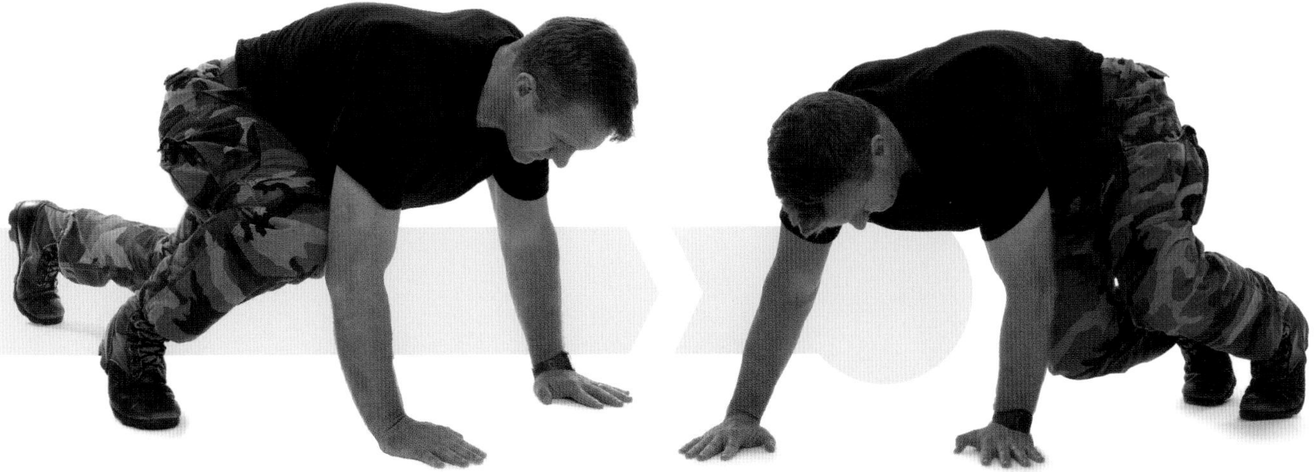

# Phase II Workout

Once you have reached a stage at which you can comfortably perform the 21 exercises that form the Phase I Workout (pages 164–166), it is time to push yourself to the next level. Using the same 21 exercises, the following workout forms a Phase II challenge composed of seven sets. Each set is a superset, meaning that you perform the entire group without stopping to rest. Work on performing all of the exercises in each set as quickly as you can with perfect form, adding sets until you can complete all seven consecutively. To recover between sets, you should perform Skip Rope. Attempt to beat your previous time every time you work out.

**SET 1**
- Push-Up x 25 + Mountain Climber x 25 + Slalom Skier x 25
- Skip Rope until recovered.

**1** Push-Up
pages 42–43

**2** Mountain Climber
pages 146–147

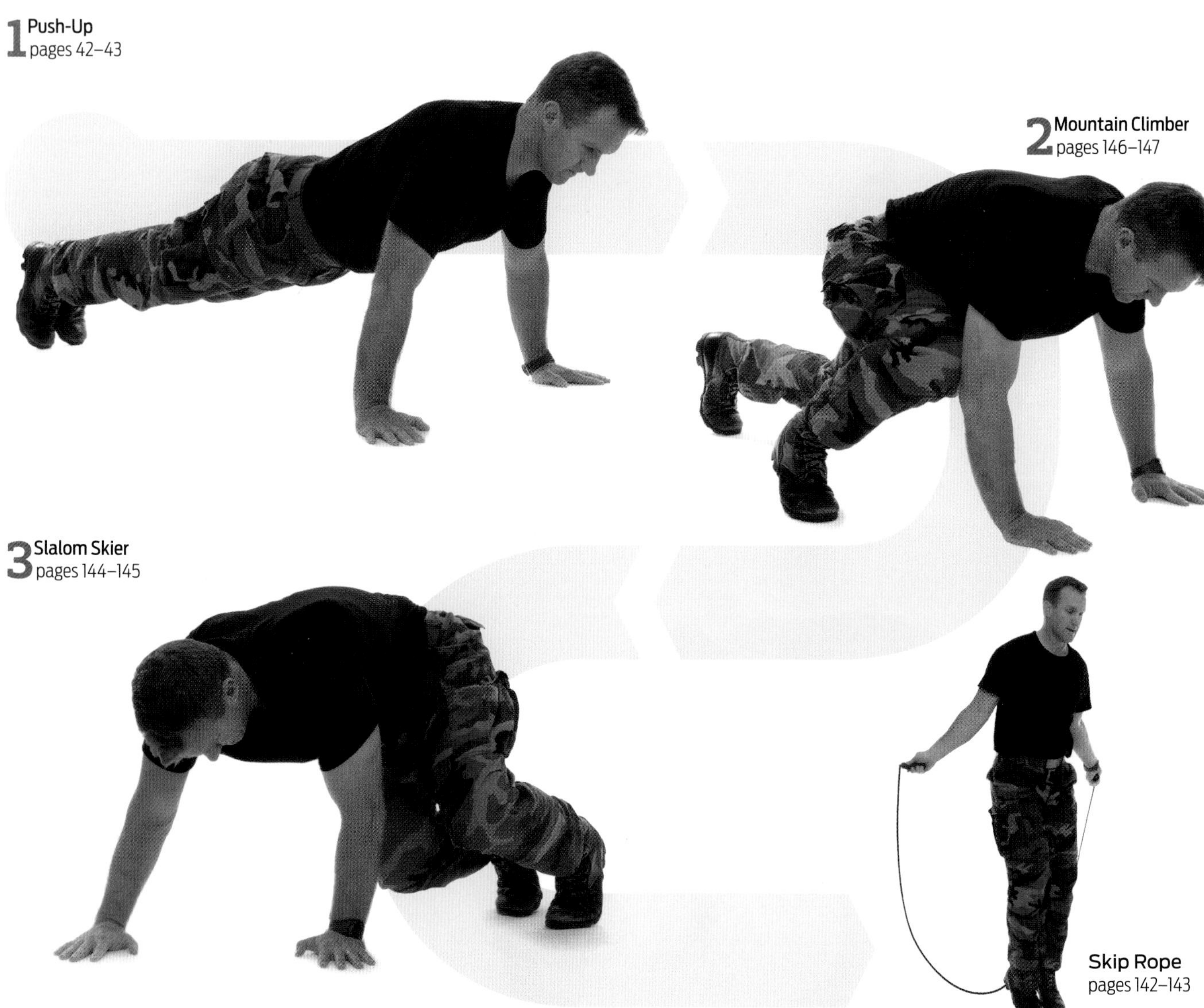

**3** Slalom Skier
pages 144–145

Skip Rope
pages 142–143

**SET 2**

- Alligator Crawl for 60 seconds + Bear Crawl for 60 seconds + Crab Crawl for 60 seconds
- Skip Rope until recovered.

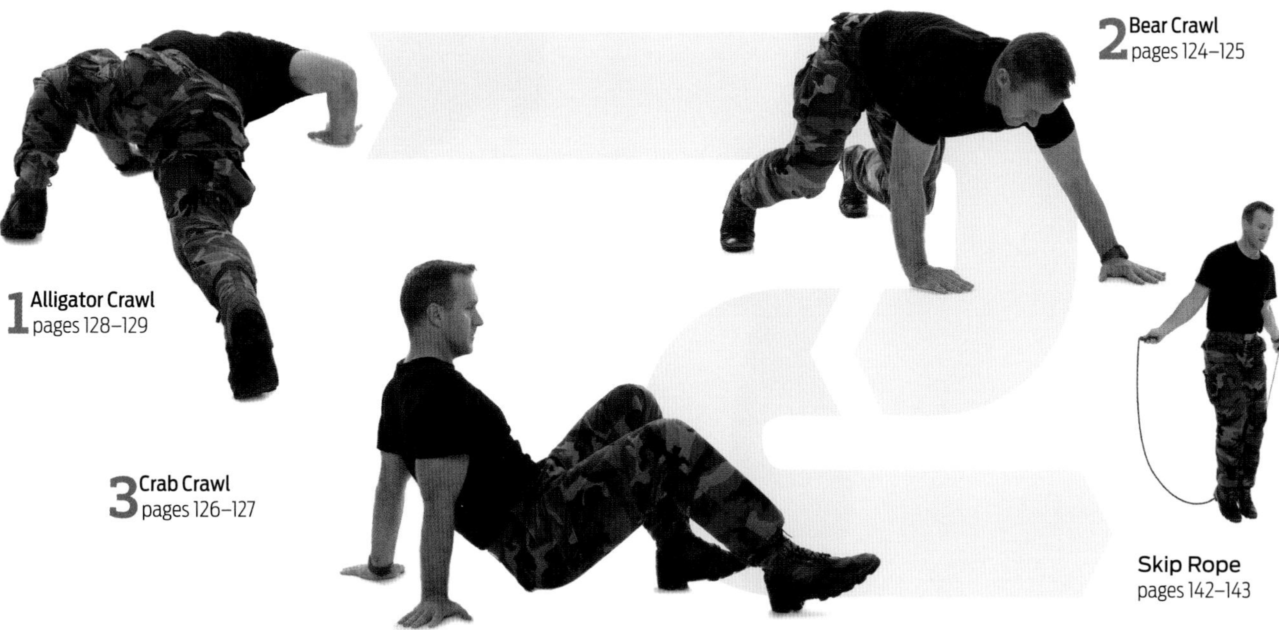

1 Alligator Crawl
pages 128–129

2 Bear Crawl
pages 124–125

3 Crab Crawl
pages 126–127

Skip Rope
pages 142–143

**SET 3**

- 8-Count Body Builder x 1 + Pull-Up: Neutral Grip x 5 = 1 repetition. Perform 10 reps.
- Skip Rope until recovered.

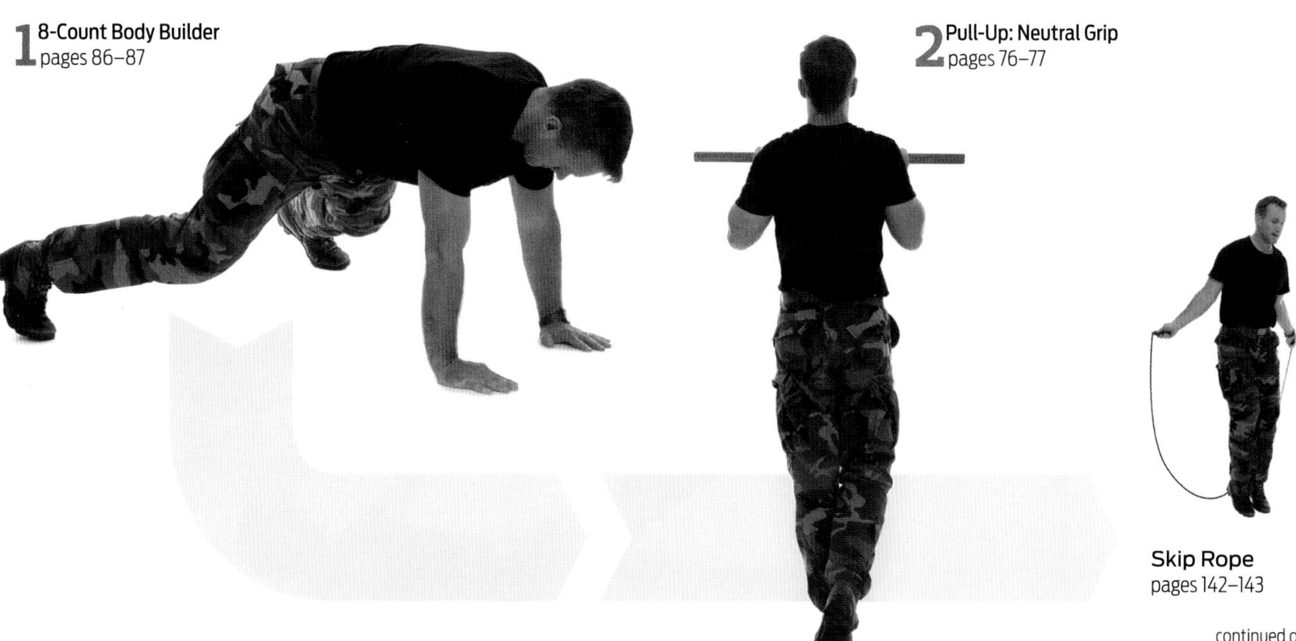

1 8-Count Body Builder
pages 86–87

2 Pull-Up: Neutral Grip
pages 76–77

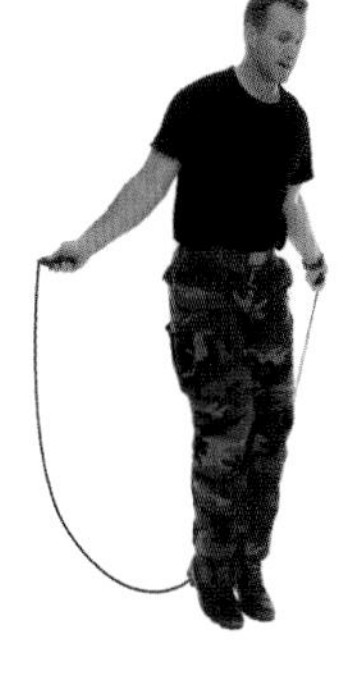

Skip Rope
pages 142–143

continued on next page →

**SET 4**
- Shoulder Crusher x 10 + 4-Count Overhead x 10 + DFRB x 10
- Skip Rope until recovered.

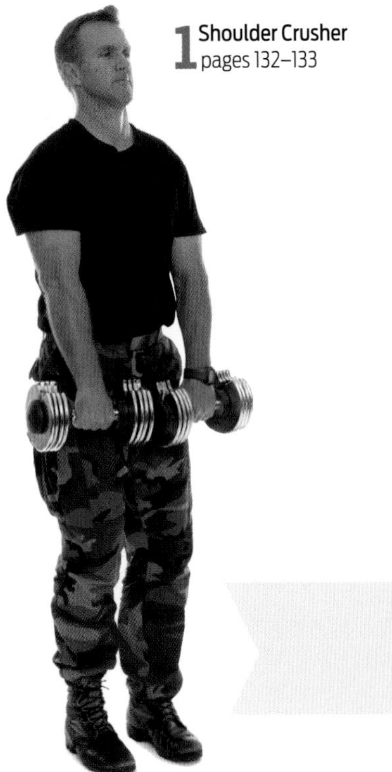

1 Shoulder Crusher
pages 132–133

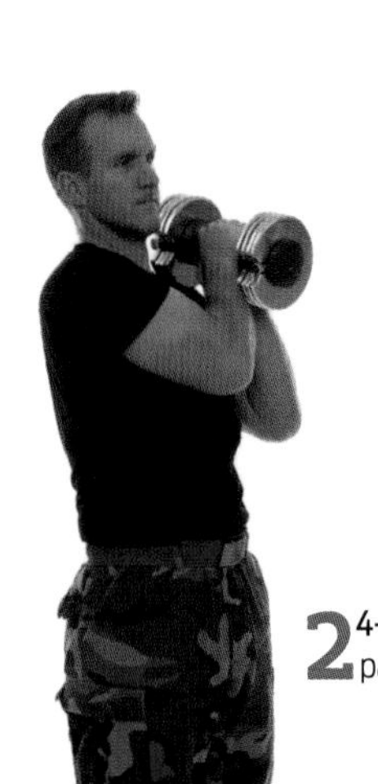

2 4-Count Overhead
pages 134–135

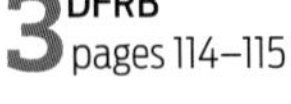

3 DFRB
pages 114–115

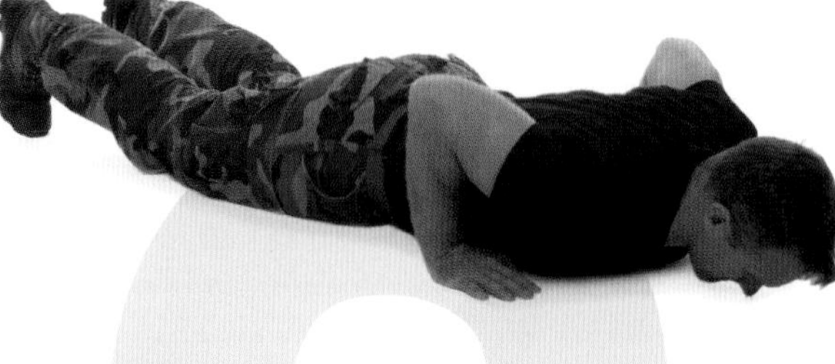

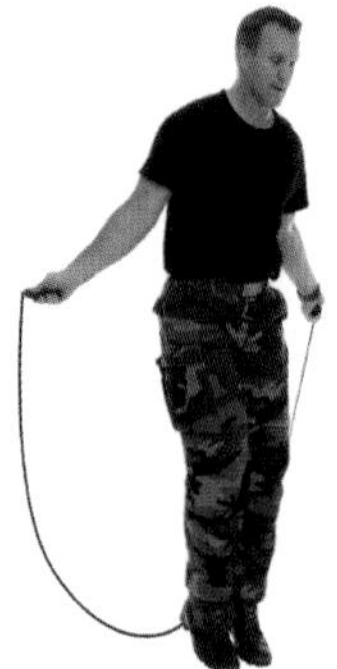

Skip Rope
pages 142–143

**SET 5**
- Sit-Up x 10 + Turtle Shell for 60 seconds = 1 repetition. Perform 3 reps.
- Skip Rope until recovered.

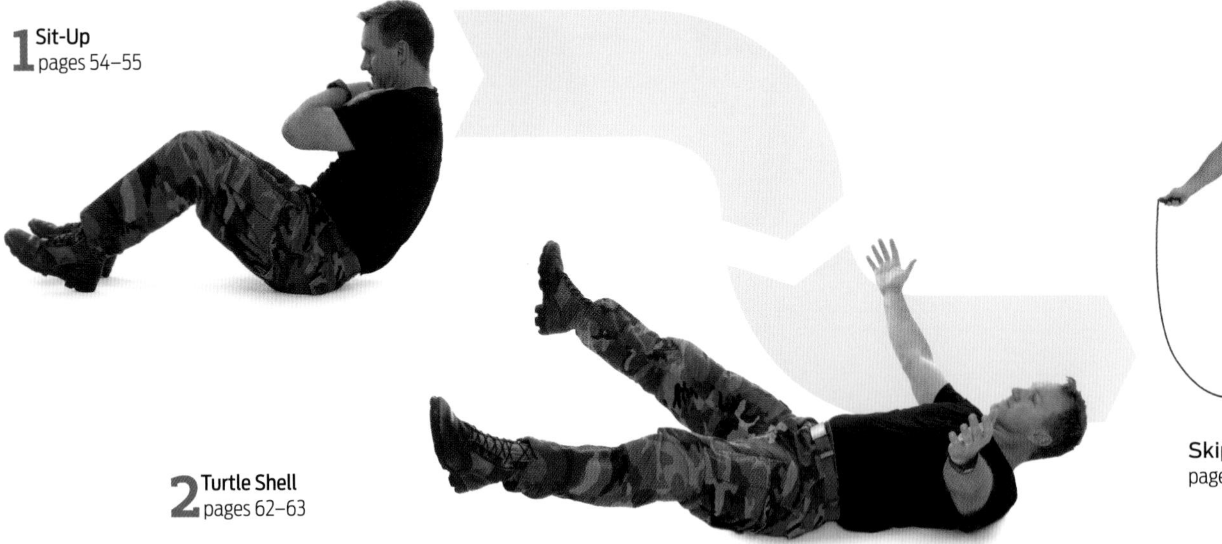

1 Sit-Up
pages 54–55

2 Turtle Shell
pages 62–63

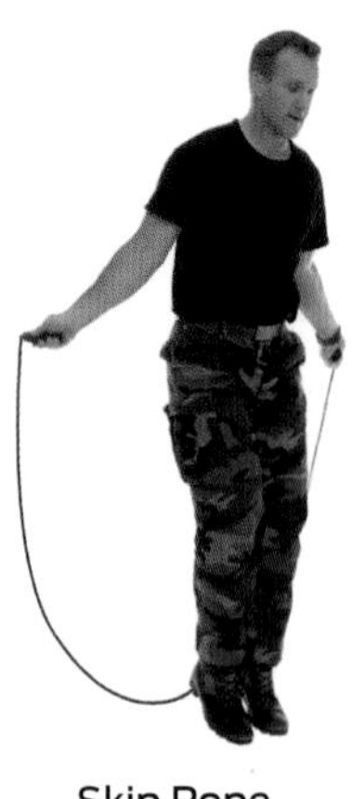

Skip Rope
pages 142–143

**SET 6**

· Deep Squat x 25 + Star Jump x 10 + Speed Skater x 15 + Lunge x 10 + Switch Lunge x 10
· Skip Rope until recovered.

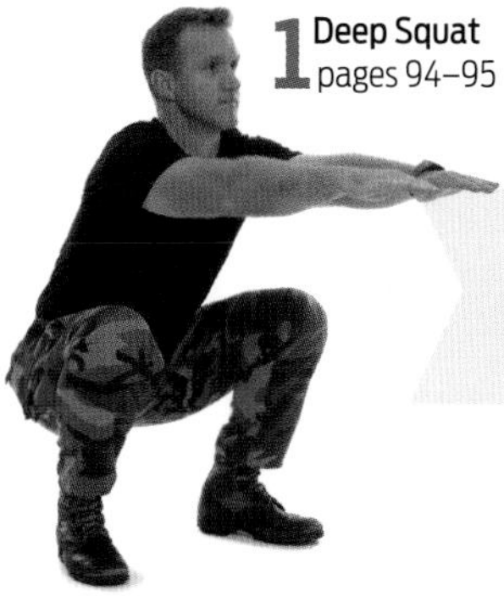

1 Deep Squat
pages 94–95

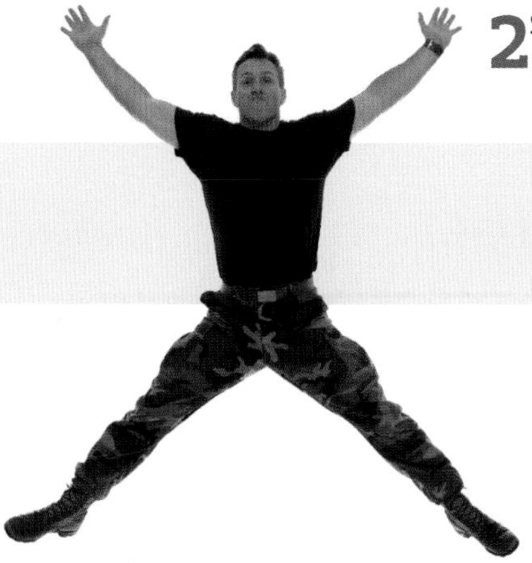

2 Star Jump
pages 130–131

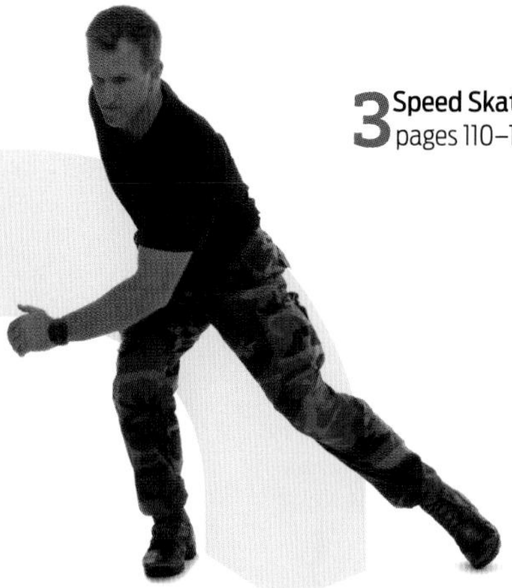

3 Speed Skater
pages 110–111

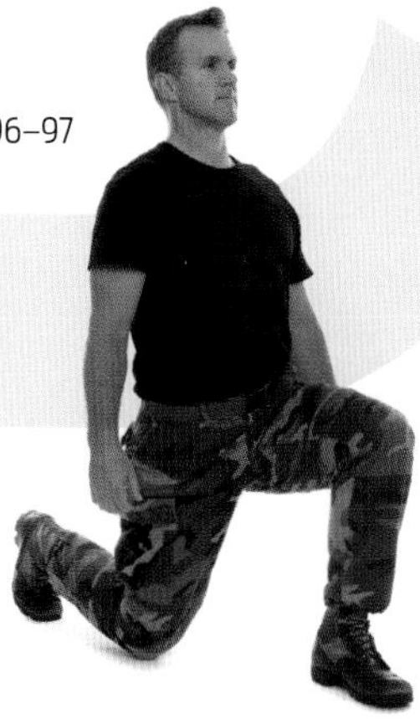

4 Lunge
pages 96–97

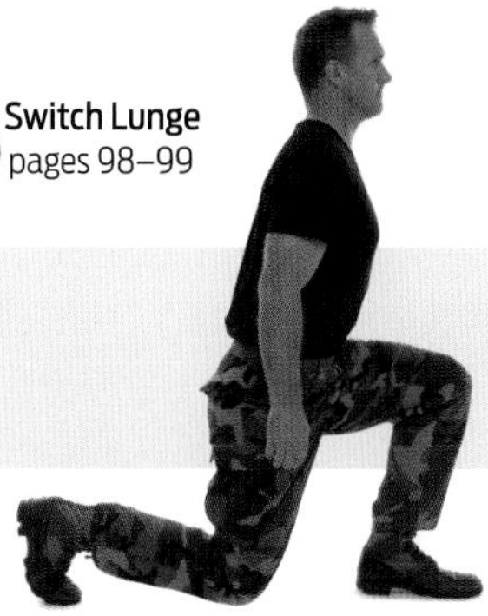

5 Switch Lunge
pages 98–99

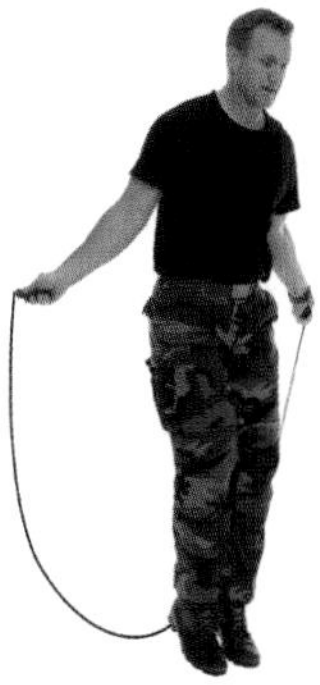

Skip Rope
pages 142–143

**SET 7**

· Up-Down x 10 + Chair Dip x 15 = 1 repetition. Perform 3 reps.
· Skip Rope until recovered.

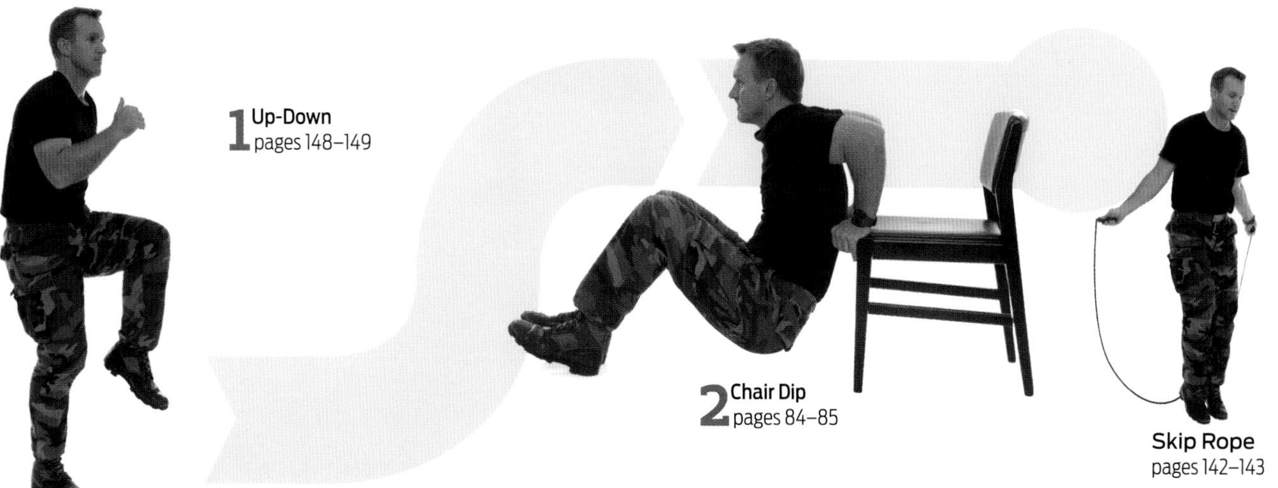

1 Up-Down
pages 148–149

2 Chair Dip
pages 84–85

Skip Rope
pages 142–143

# Phase II Focus Workout

This muscle-endurance workout concentrates on one body part at a time. Your heart rate will not get as high as a more-advanced Phase III workout, but it will make your muscles very sore, so be careful and pace yourself. You can begin by working on one or two groups at a time, building stamina and strength. As you become stronger, add another group until you can perform the entire workout in one session.

**FOCUS: ABDOMINALS**

- V-Up
- Bicycle Crunch
- Obliques
- Penguin Crunch
- Turtle Shell
- Sit-Up

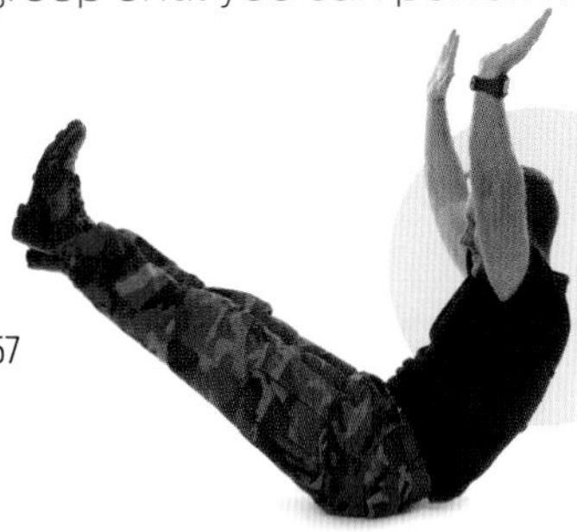

1 V-Up
pages 56–57

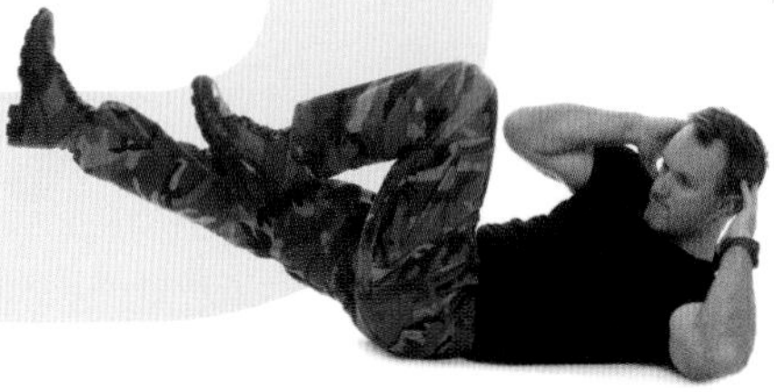

2 Bicycle Crunch
pages 58–59

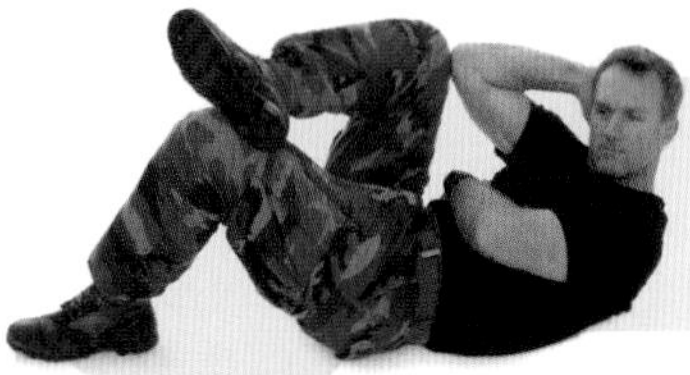

3 Obliques
pages 64–65

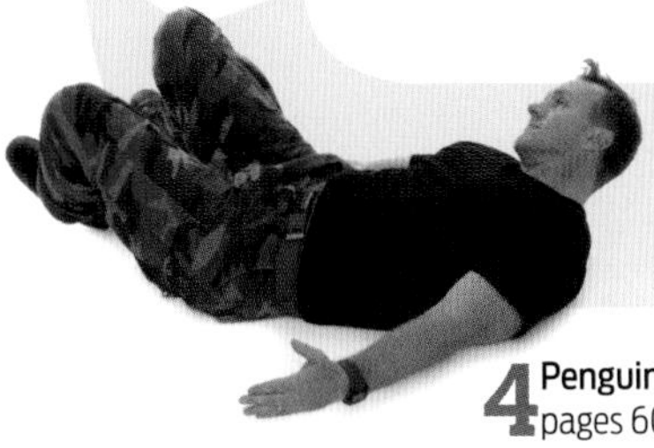

4 Penguin Crunch
pages 60–61

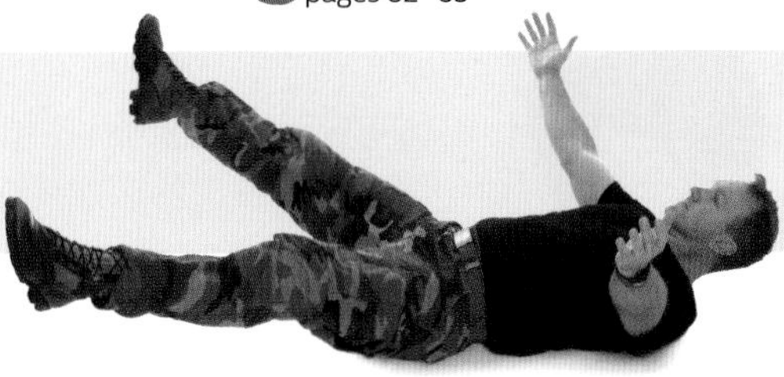

5 Turtle Shell
pages 62–63

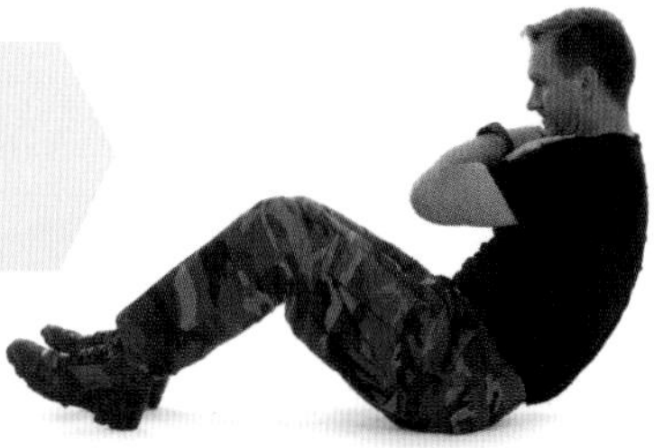

6 Sit-Up
pages 54–55

**FOCUS: CHEST**

Performing each exercise in this section equals one set. Attempt to perform 3 to 5 sets. 15 seconds rest is recommended for recovery between each exercise.

- Push-Up
- Triceps Push-Up
- Decline Push-Up
- Wide Push-Up
- Sprawl Push-Up
- Dive Bomber

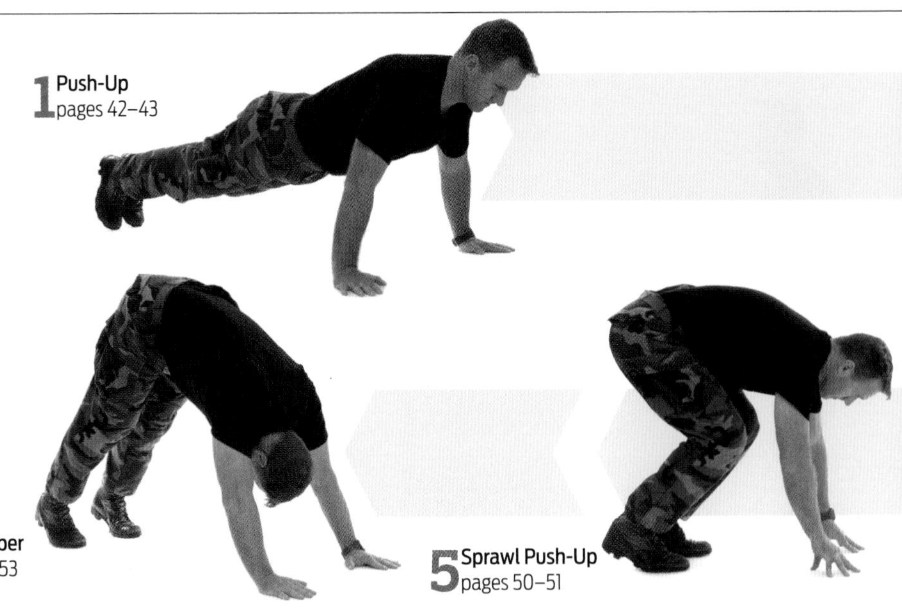

1 Push-Up
pages 42–43

6 Dive Bomber
pages 52–53

5 Sprawl Push-Up
pages 50–51

**FOCUS: LEGS**

- Deep Squat
- Lunge
- Straight-Leg Skater
- Lateral Lunge with Squat
- Walking Lunge
- Switch Lunge
- Speed Skater

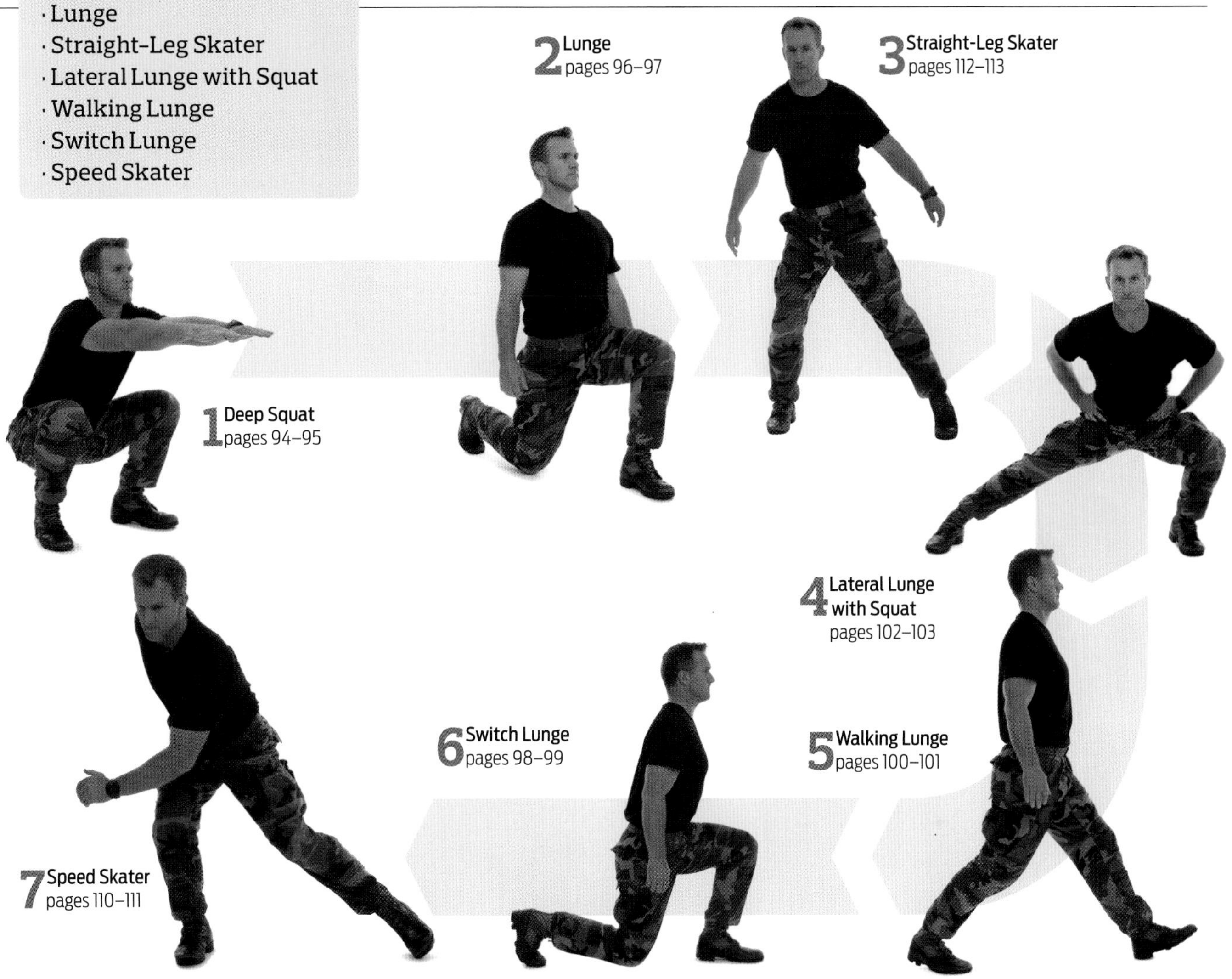

1 Deep Squat pages 94–95

2 Lunge pages 96–97

3 Straight-Leg Skater pages 112–113

4 Lateral Lunge with Squat pages 102–103

5 Walking Lunge pages 100–101

6 Switch Lunge pages 98–99

7 Speed Skater pages 110–111

2 Triceps Push-Up pages 44–45

3 Decline Push-Up pages 46–47

4 Wide Push-Up pages 48–49

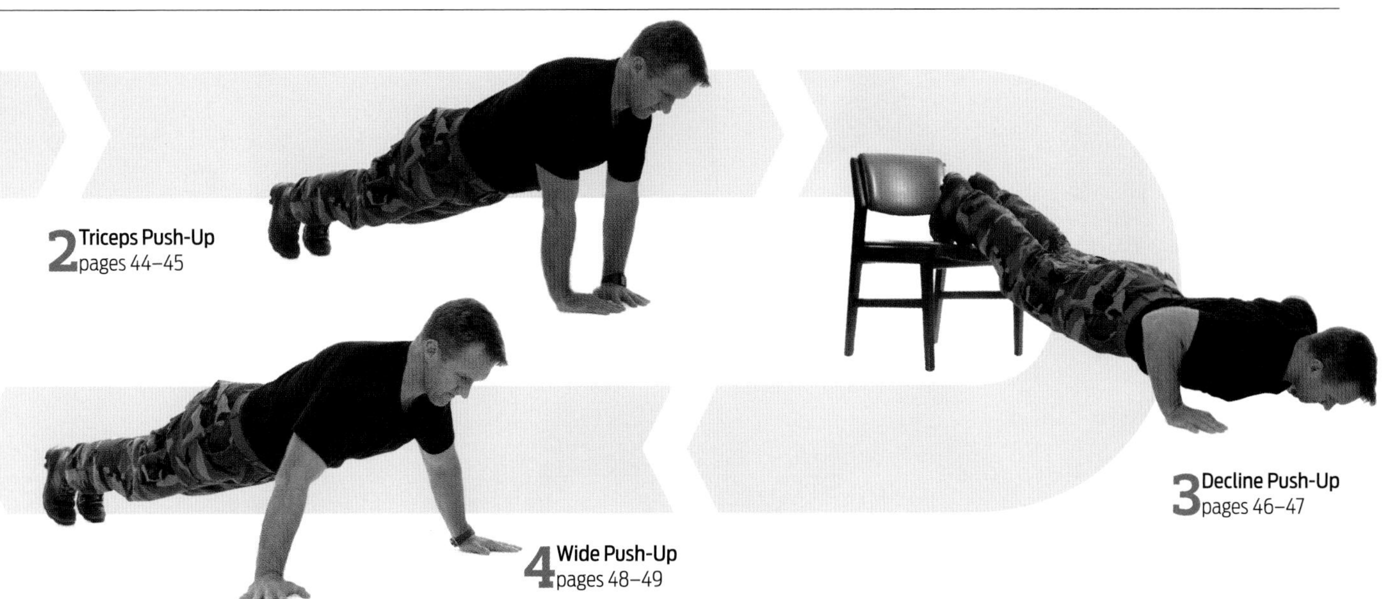

**FOCUS: AGILITY**

- Crab Crawl
- Burpee with Pull-Up
- Alligator Crawl
- Mountain Climber
- Up-Down
- Skip Rope
- DFRB
- 10-Count Body Builder
- 12-Count Body Builder
- Star Jump
- Burpee
- Slalom Skier
- Bear Crawl
- Up-Down with Push-Up

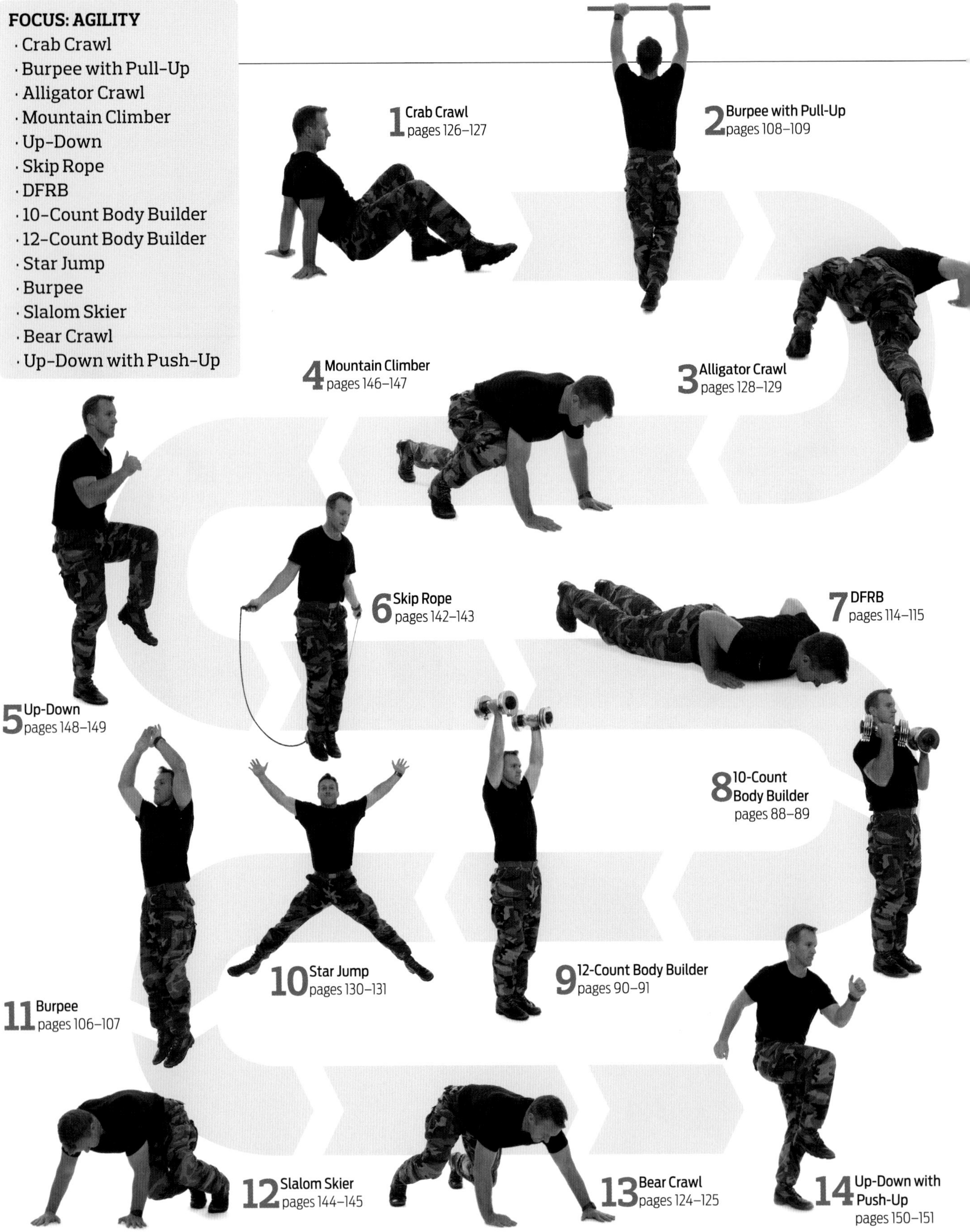

1 Crab Crawl
pages 126–127

2 Burpee with Pull-Up
pages 108–109

3 Alligator Crawl
pages 128–129

4 Mountain Climber
pages 146–147

5 Up-Down
pages 148–149

6 Skip Rope
pages 142–143

7 DFRB
pages 114–115

8 10-Count Body Builder
pages 88–89

9 12-Count Body Builder
pages 90–91

10 Star Jump
pages 130–131

11 Burpee
pages 106–107

12 Slalom Skier
pages 144–145

13 Bear Crawl
pages 124–125

14 Up-Down with Push-Up
pages 150–151

**FOCUS: PULL-UP**

Perform five consecutive sets of each grip variation listed below. The entire Pull-Up workout is 150 reps. Between grips, take as much time as you need to recover.

Pull-Up: Neutral Grip
- Set 1: x 2 + 15-second rest
- Set 2: x 4 + 30-second rest
- Set 3: x 6 + 45-second rest
- Set 4: x 8 + 60-second rest
- Set 5: x 10

Pull-Up: Close Grip
- Set 1: x 2 + 15-second rest
- Set 2: x 4 + 30-second rest
- Set 3: x 6 + 45-second rest
- Set 4: x 8 + 60-second rest
- Set 5: x 10

Pull-Up: Mountain-Climber Grip
- Set 1: x 2 + 15-second rest
- Set 2: x 4 + 30-second rest
- Set 3: x 6 + 45-second rest
- Set 4: x 8 + 60-second rest
- Set 5: x 10

Pull-Up: Reverse Grip
- Set 1: x 2 + 15-second rest
- Set 2: x 4 + 30-second rest
- Set 3: x 6 + 45-second rest
- Set 4: x 8 + 60-second rest
- Set 5: x 10

Pull-Up: Wide Grip
- Set 1: x 2 + 15-second rest
- Set 2: x 4 + 30-second rest
- Set 3: x 6 + 45-second rest
- Set 4: x 8 + 60-second rest
- Set 5: x 10

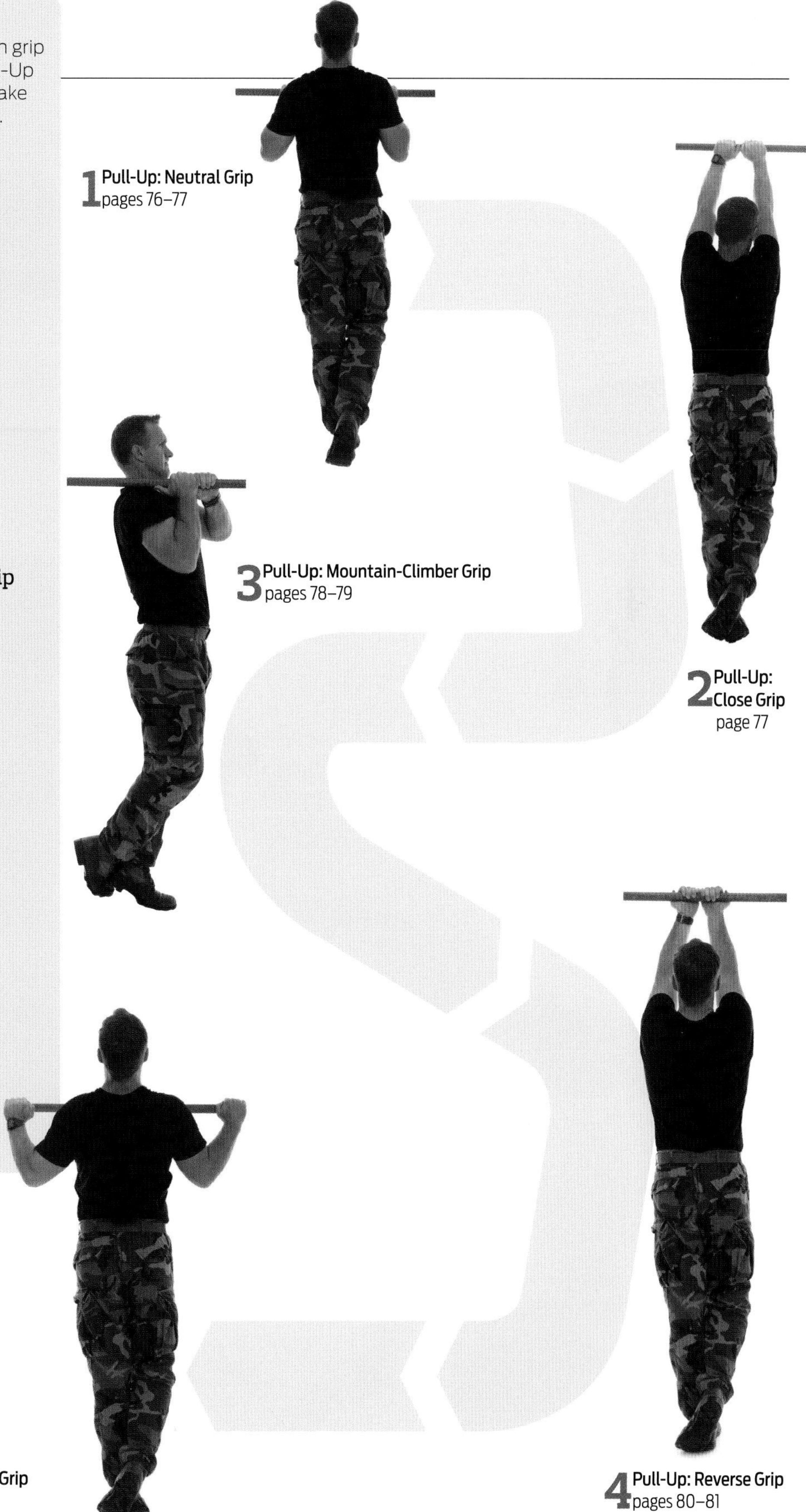

1 Pull-Up: Neutral Grip pages 76–77

2 Pull-Up: Close Grip page 77

3 Pull-Up: Mountain-Climber Grip pages 78–79

4 Pull-Up: Reverse Grip pages 80–81

5 Pull-Up: Wide Grip pages 82–83

**FOCUS: CORE**
- Lower-Back Extension
- Plank
- Bird Dog
- High Plank
- Arm Hauler
- Side Plank

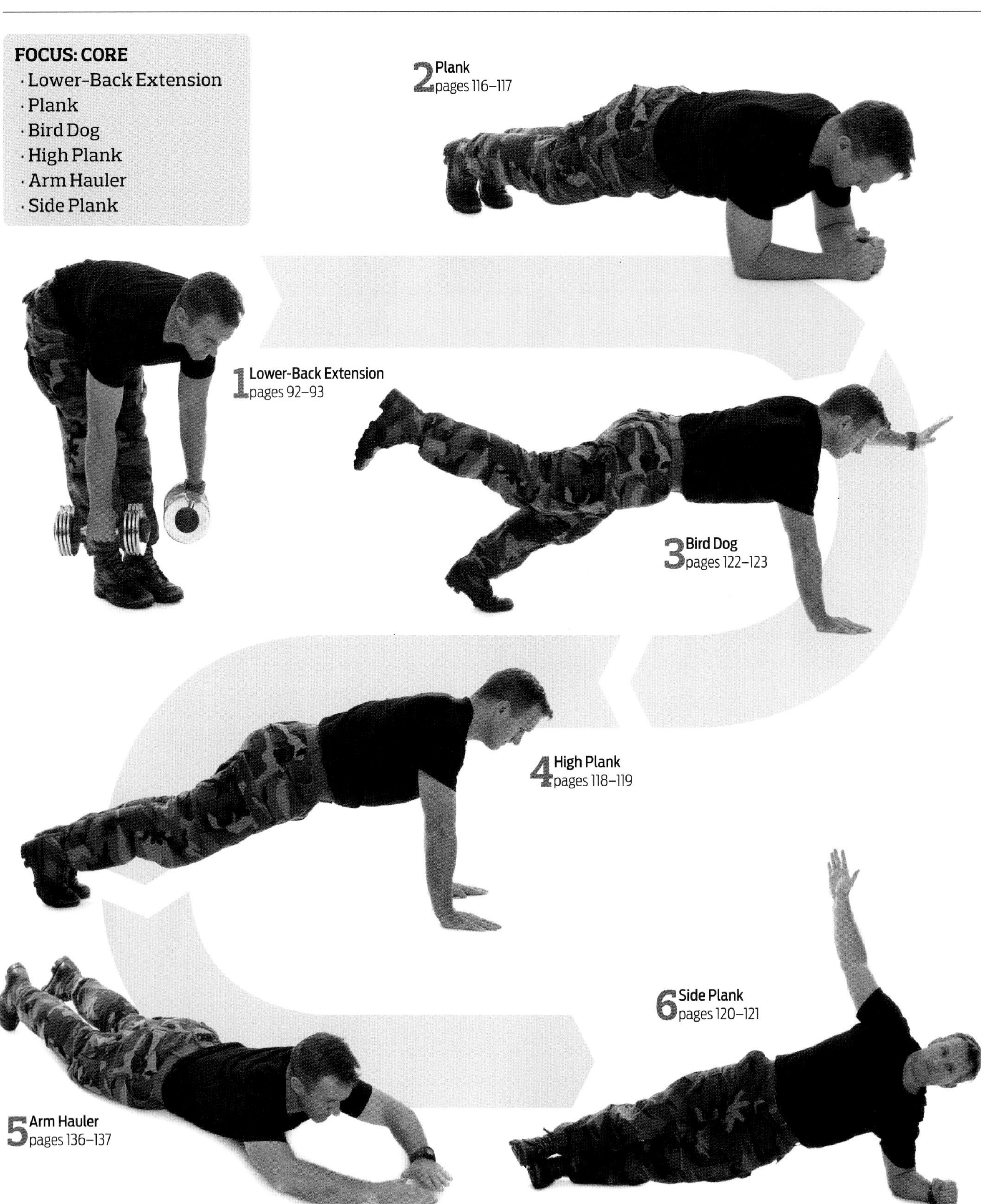

**FOCUS: UPPER BODY**

- 4-Count Overhead
- One-Arm Dumbbell Row
- Chair Dip
- Shoulder Crusher
- One-Arm T-Row
- Shoulder Flex ing

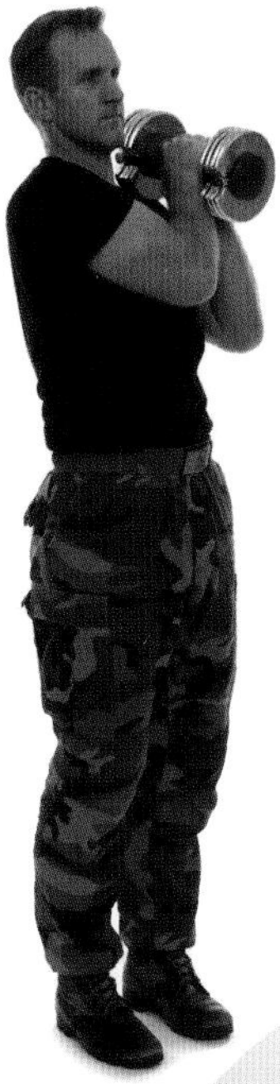

**1** 4-Count Overhead
pages 134–135

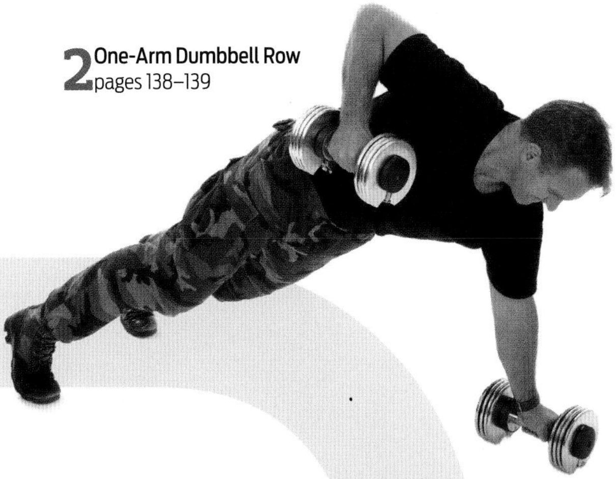

**2** One-Arm Dumbbell Row
pages 138–139

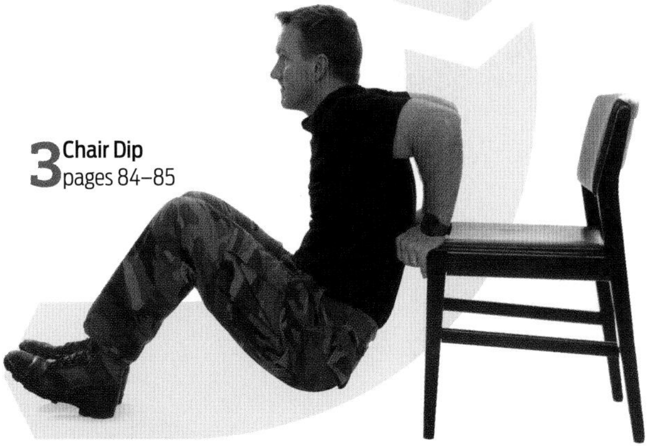

**3** Chair Dip
pages 84–85

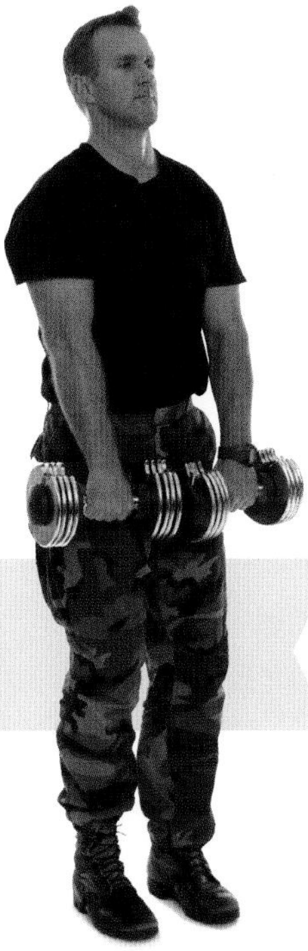

**4** Shoulder Crusher
pages 132–133

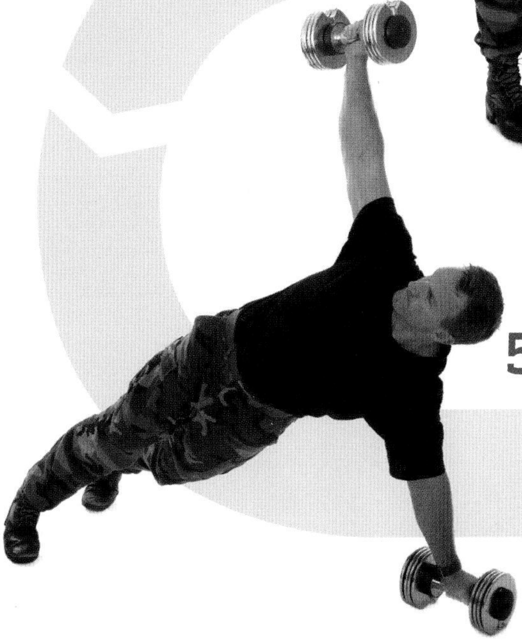

**5** One-Arm T-Row
pages 140–141

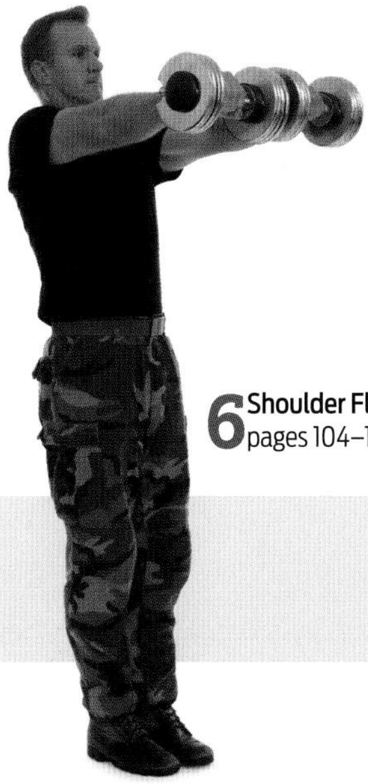

**6** Shoulder Flexing
pages 104–105

# Phase III Workout

The Phase III Workout is the ultimate challenge, taking you through two circuits that combine endurance and cardiovascular exercises. Perform all the exercises shown for both the Alpha and Bravo circuits in the order they appear, resting between circuits until recovery.

**CIRCUIT ALPHA**

- Plank for 30 seconds
- High Plank for 30 seconds
- Side Plank for 15 seconds per side
- Sit-Up x 15
- Bicycle Crunch x 15 each side
- Flutter Kick x 15
- Leg Levelers x 15
- 6-90 x 15
- Push-Up x 15
- Decline Push-Up x 15
- Deep Squat x 15
- Lunge x 15 each leg
- 4-Count Overhead x 10
- Chair Dip x 15
- Mountain Climber x 10
- Burpee x 5
- Up-Down x 10
- Pull-Up: Neutral Grip x 10
- Pull-Up: Reverse Grip x 10

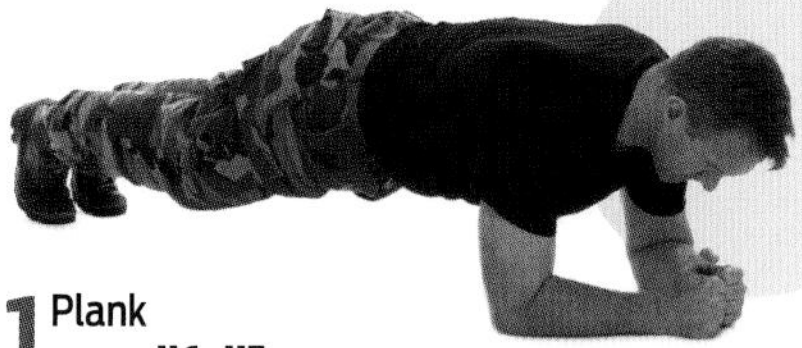

**1** Plank pages 116–117

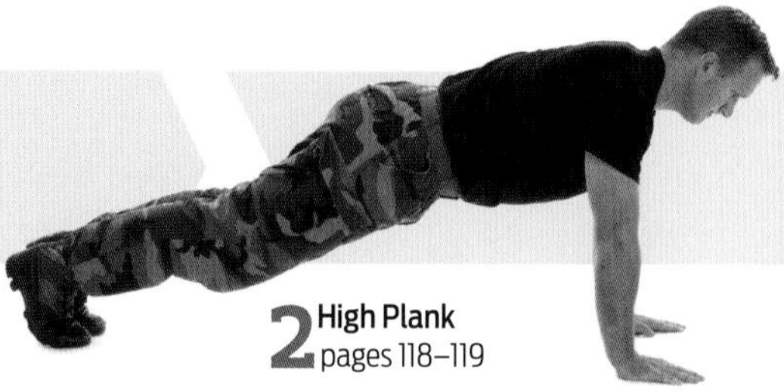

**2** High Plank pages 118–119

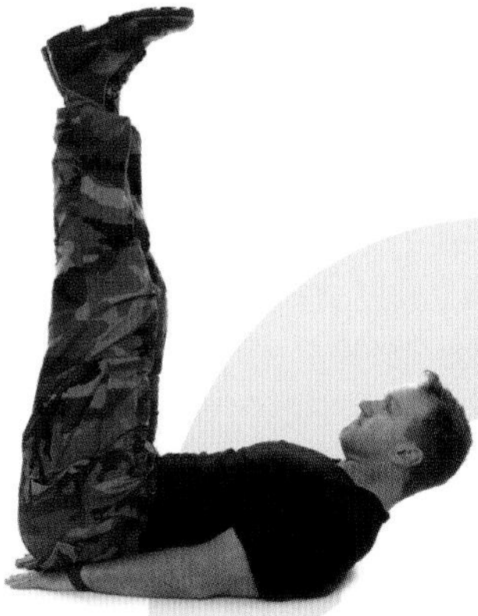

**8** 6-90 pages 70–71

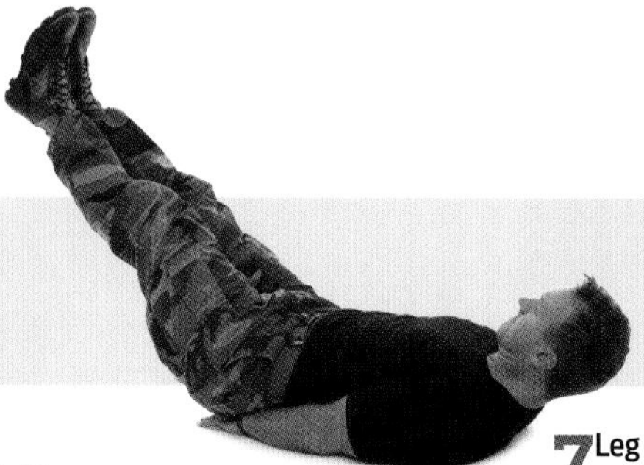

**7** Leg Levelers pages 74–75

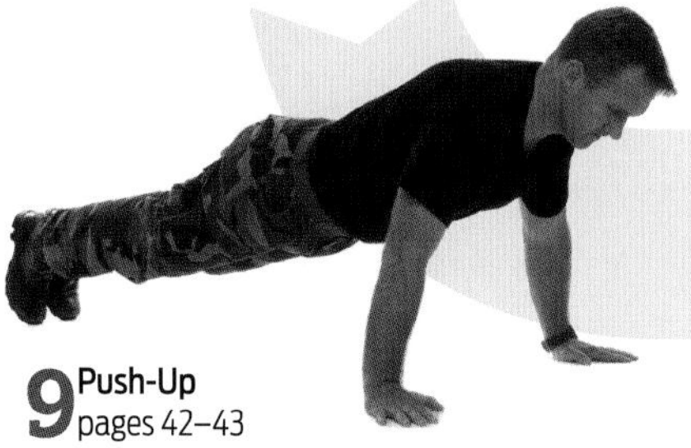

**9** Push-Up pages 42–43

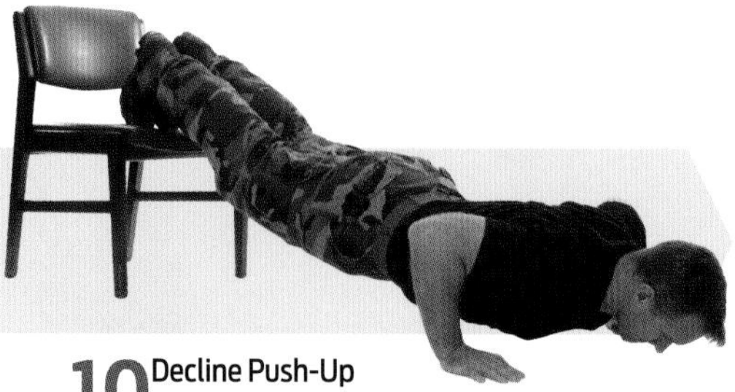

**10** Decline Push-Up pages 46–47

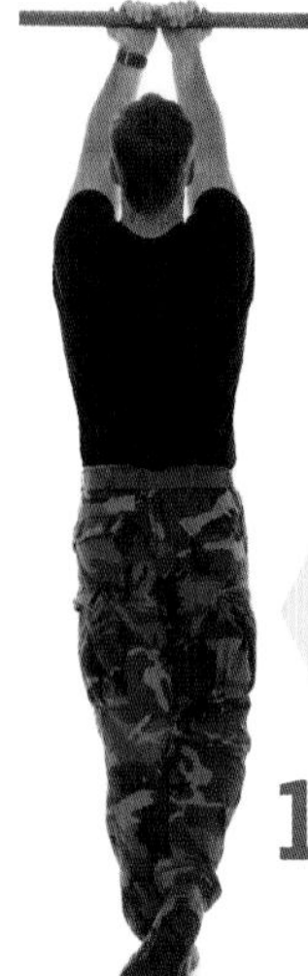

**19** Pull-Up: Reverse Grip pages 80–81

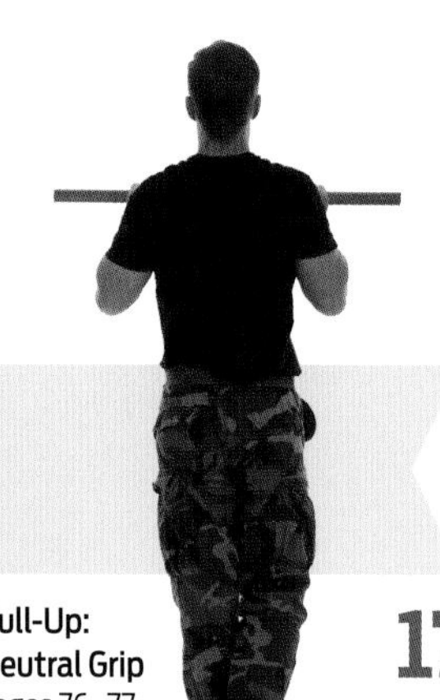

**18** Pull-Up: Neutral Grip pages 76–77

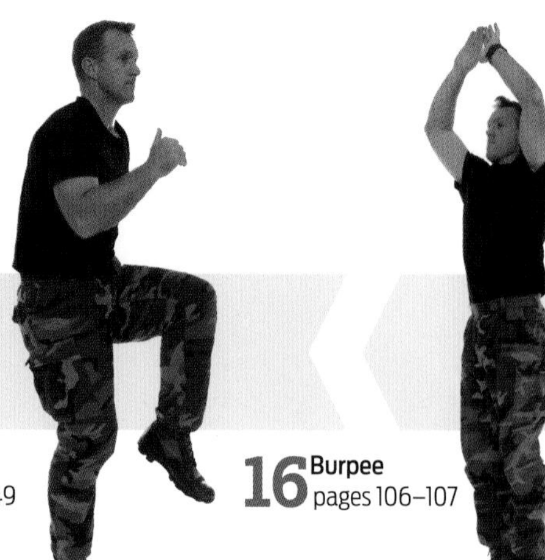

**17** Up-Down pages 148–149

**16** Burpee pages 106–107

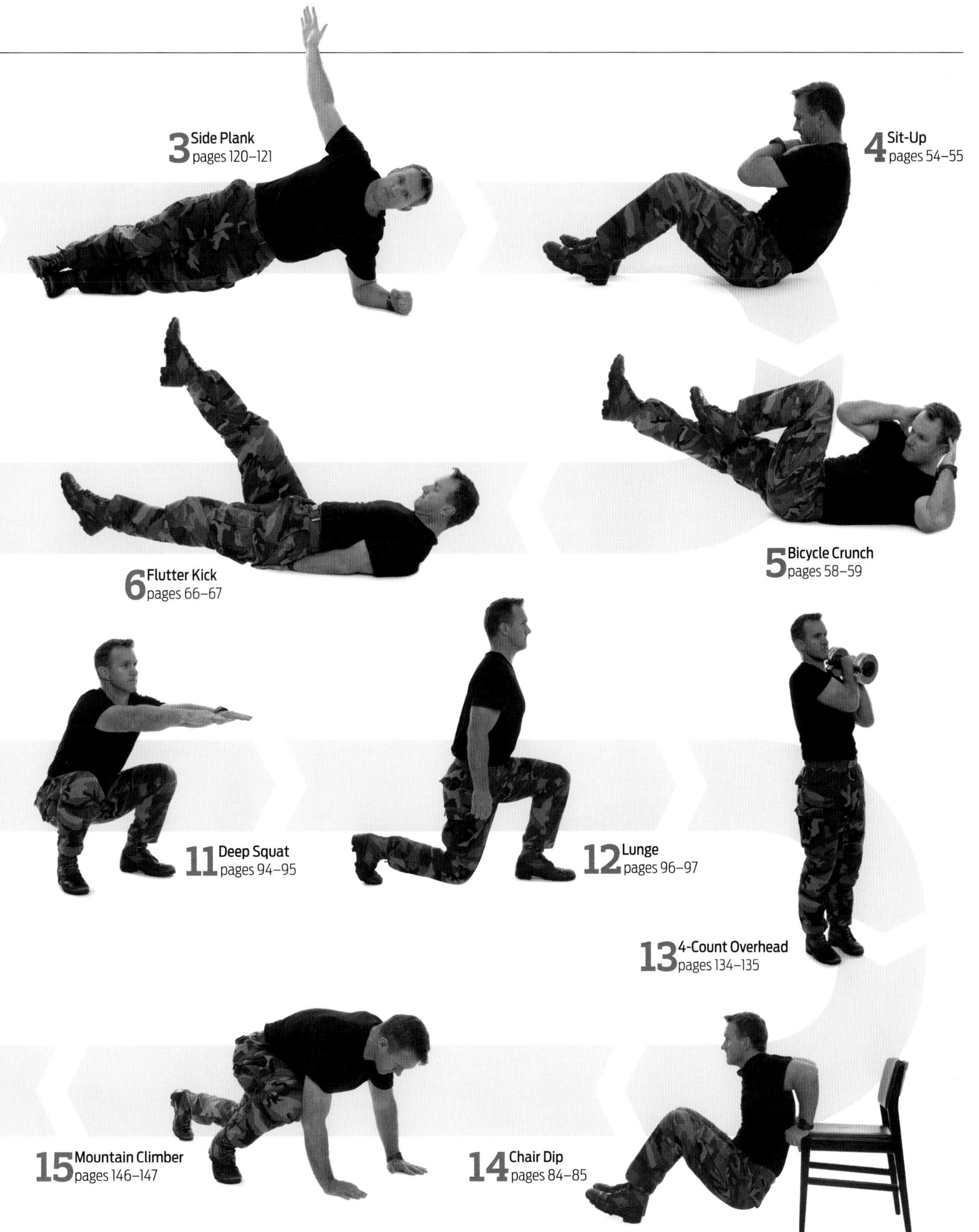
3 Side Plank
pages 120–121
4 Sit-Up
pages 54–55
6 Flutter Kick
pages 66–67
5 Bicycle Crunch
pages 58–59
11 Deep Squat
pages 94–95
12 Lunge
pages 96–97
13 4-Count Overhead
pages 134–135
15 Mountain Climber
pages 146–147
14 Chair Dip
pages 84–85

**CIRCUIT BRAVO**

- One-Arm Dumbbell Row x 15 each side
- One-Arm T-Row x 15 each side
- Triceps Push-Up x 20
- Walking Lunge x 20 each leg
- Alligator Crawl for 30 seconds
- Bicycle Crunch x 20 each side
- DFRB x 5
- V-Up x 20
- Pull-Up: Neutral Grip x 10
- Shoulder Crusher x 5
- Knees to Chest x 20
- Sprawl Push-Up x 20
- Slalom Skier x 20 each leg
- Speed Skater x 20
- Pull-Up: Mountain-Climber Grip x 10
- Deep Squat x 20
- Good Morning, Darling x 20
- Crab Crawl for 15 seconds
- Bear Crawl for 15 seconds
- Turtle Shell for 30 seconds
- Penguin Crunch x 20 each side
- Obliques x 20 each side
- Shoulder Flexing x 20
- Skip Rope to recover

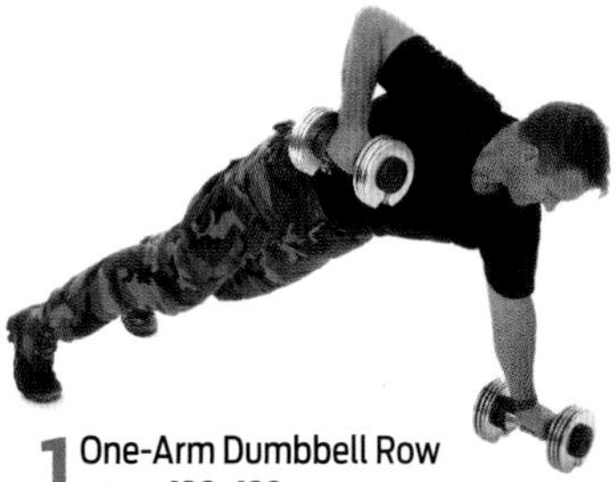

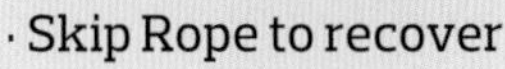

**1** One-Arm Dumbbell Row
pages 138–139

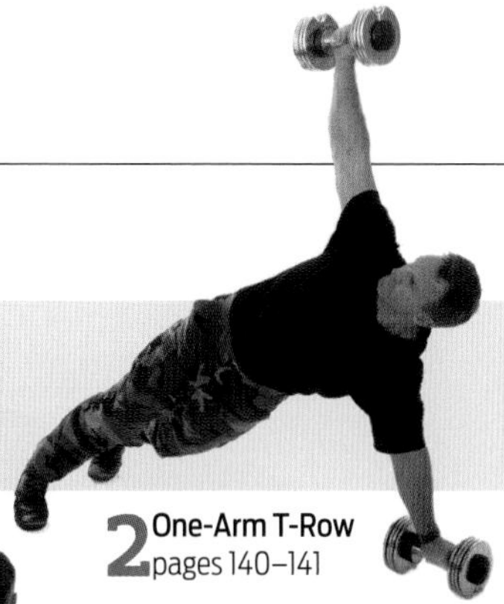

**2** One-Arm T-Row
pages 140–141

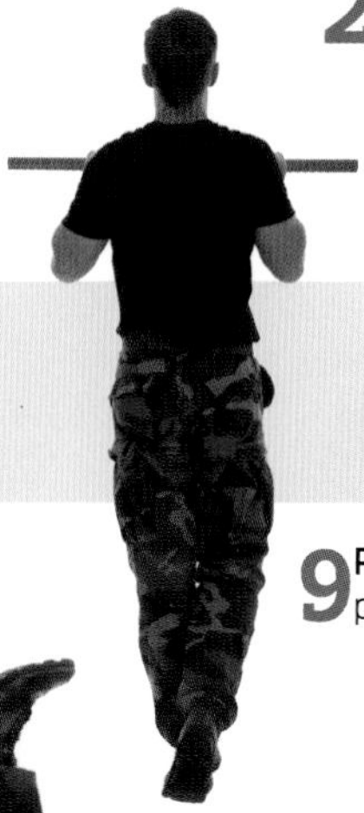

**9** Pull-Up: Neutral Grip
pages 76–77

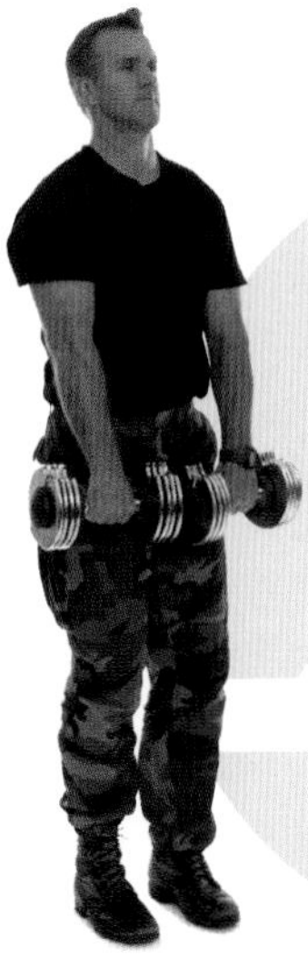

**10** Shoulder Crusher
pages 132–133

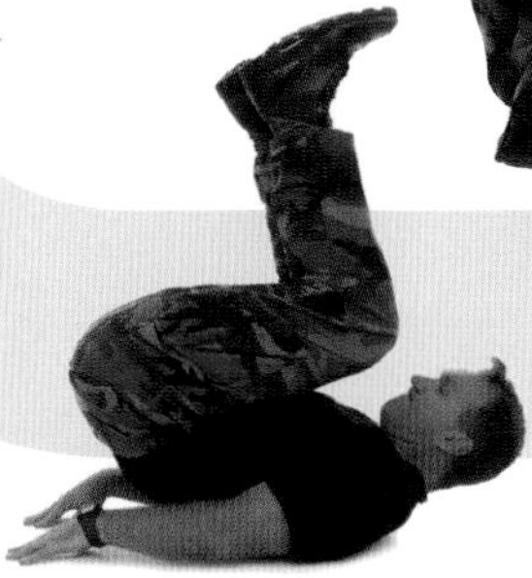

**11** Knees to Chest
pages 68–69

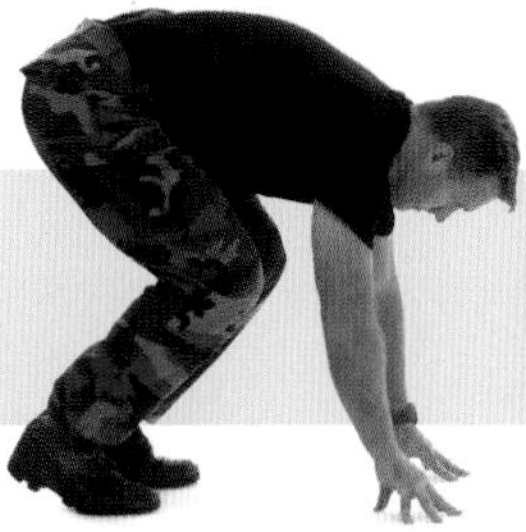

**12** Sprawl Push-Up
pages 50–51

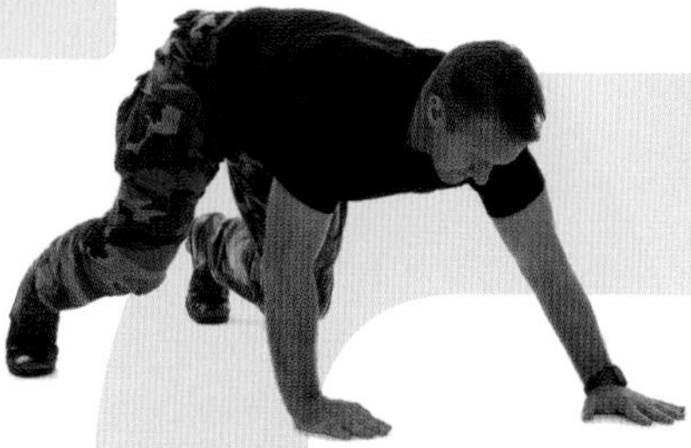

**19** Bear Crawl
pages 124–125

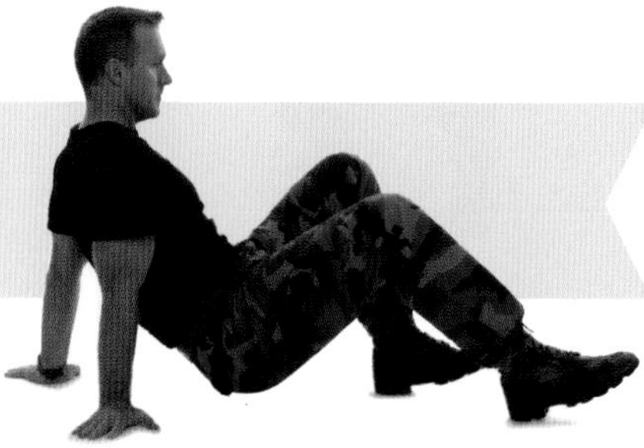

**18** Crab Crawl
pages 126–127

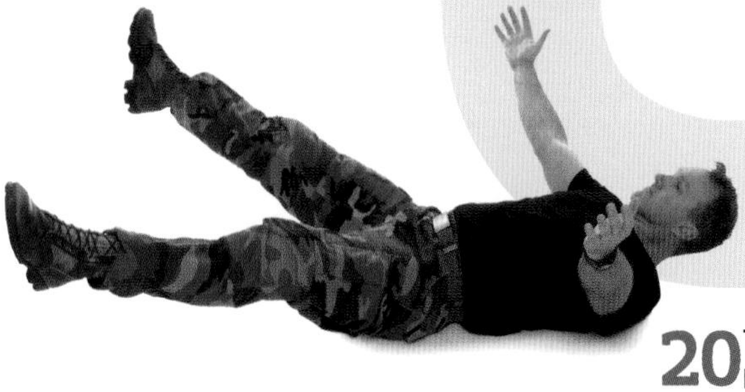

**20** Turtle Shell
pages 62–63

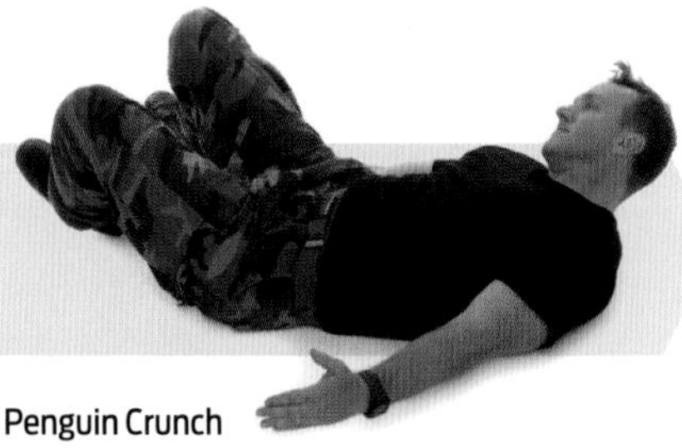

**21** Penguin Crunch
pages 60–61

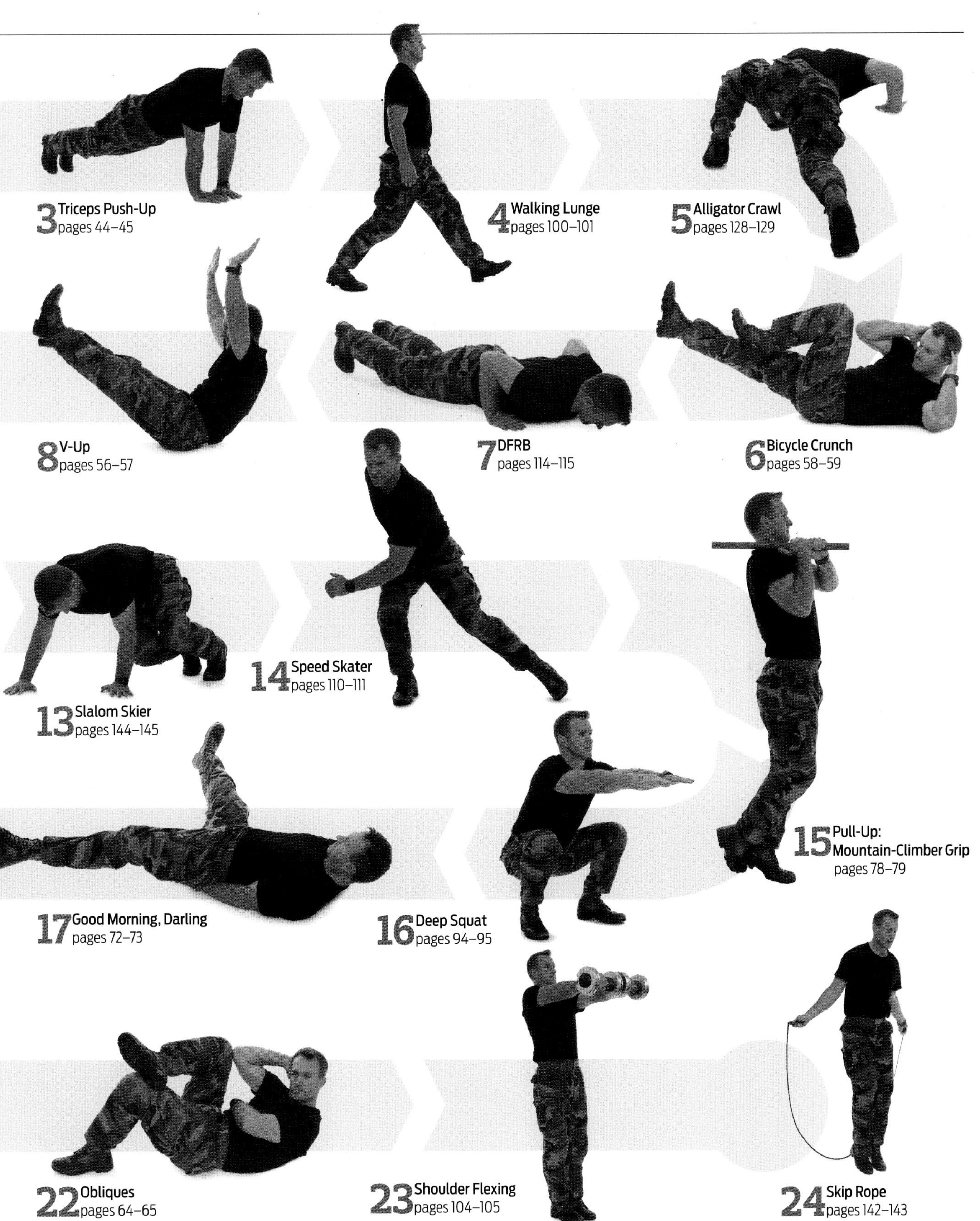
3 Triceps Push-Up
pages 44–45
4 Walking Lunge
pages 100–101
5 Alligator Crawl
pages 128–129
8 V-Up
pages 56–57
7 DFRB
pages 114–115
6 Bicycle Crunch
pages 58–59
13 Slalom Skier
pages 144–145
14 Speed Skater
pages 110–111
15 Pull-Up: Mountain-Climber Grip
pages 78–79
17 Good Morning, Darling
pages 72–73
16 Deep Squat
pages 94–95
22 Obliques
pages 64–65
23 Shoulder Flexing
pages 104–105
24 Skip Rope
pages 142–143

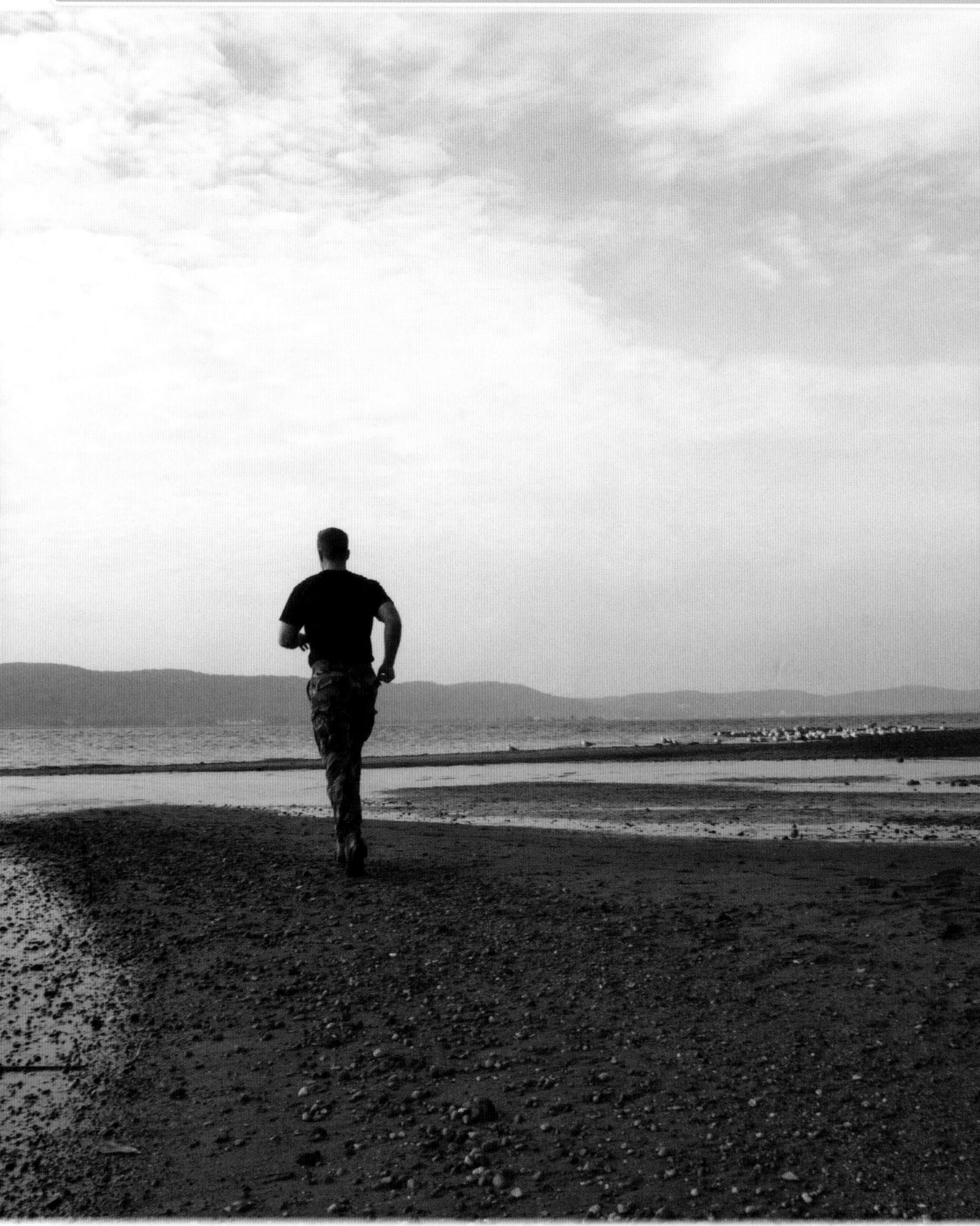

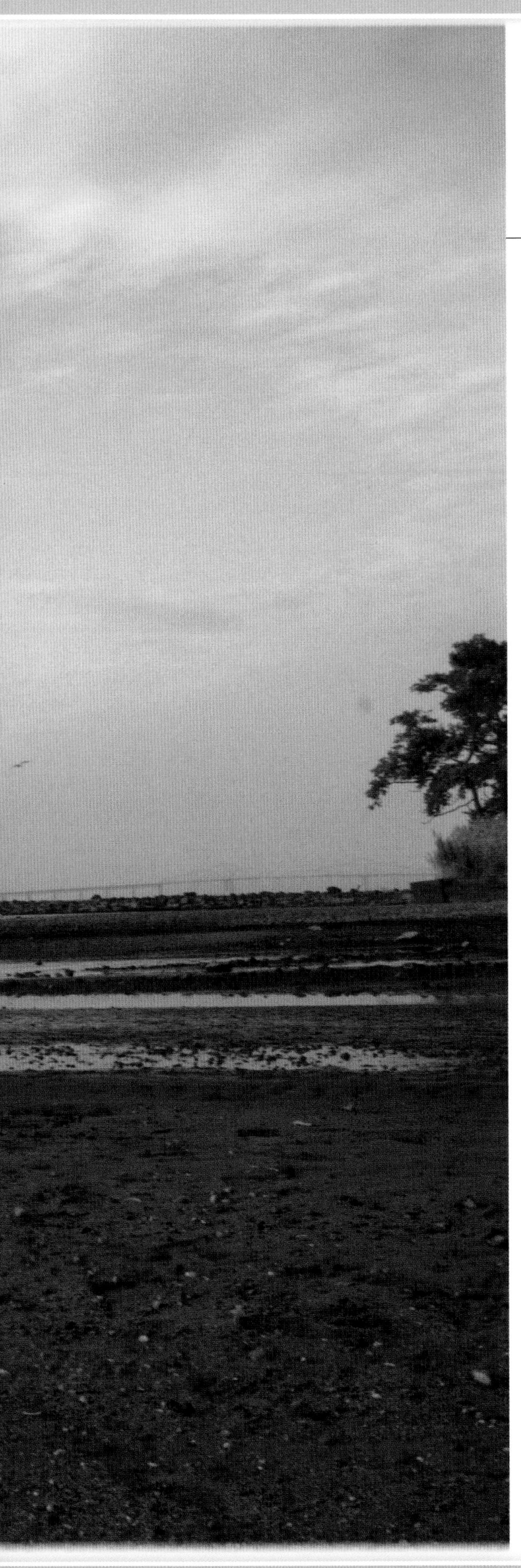

# Conclusion

Welcome to the warrior journey—it will be one that lasts a lifetime as you continually strive to master both your body and mind. We began with how to adopt a warrior mindset, which allows you to control your destiny and become the best you can be, whether your endeavor is getting fit or just getting through the day. Being a student of both body and mind allows you to perform the exercises for fitness and health while also acquiring the skills necessary for success in all aspects of life.

Understanding the body means you must also understand nutrition. It is more than just the taste of your food—it impacts sport and fitness performance and, especially, your overall health. To truly thrive, you must learn and practice proper nutrition, ignoring the fog of marketing meant to sell products rather than produce health. Gaining the knowledge of nutrition has life-altering implications, and this book serves as the beginning of that learning process.

To stay in top physical condition, special forces teams swim, run, and perform PT daily. The exercises and workouts found in this book are used by conventional and military special operations forces all over the world for their PT. These are some of the toughest movements known. Practice them and perfect your form. Once you begin performing the workouts featured in this book, you will find each one will provide months and months of tough training. This book can be a resource for years of tough physical and mental training that will make your mind and body bulletproof.

Now get to it, and stay the course!

# Glossary

## GENERAL TERMINOLOGY

**abduction:** Movement away from the body.

**adduction:** Movement toward the body.

**aerobic:** Exercise that requires a sustained elevated heart rate.

**anaerobic:** Exercise that does not require long periods of sustaining an elevated heart rate.

**anterior:** Located in the front.

**autosuggestion:** Influencing of one's own attitudes, behavior, or physical condition by mental processes other than conscious thought.

**ballistic exercise.** See *dynamic exercise.*

**BUD/S:** The U.S. Navy SEAL Basic Underwater Demolition School, a 24-week training challenge that develops the SEAL candidates' mental and physical stamina and leadership skills.

**cardiovascular exercise:** Any exercise that increases the heart rate, making oxygen and nutrient-rich blood available to working muscles.

**cool-down:** An exercise performed at the end of the workout session that works to cool and relax the body after more vigorous exertion.

**core stabilizer:** An exercise that calls for resisting motion at the lumbar spine though activation of the abdominal muscles and deep stabilizers; improves core strength and endurance.

**core strengthener:** An exercise that allows for motion in the lumbar spine, while working the abdominal muscles and deep stabilizers; improves movement such as running or walking.

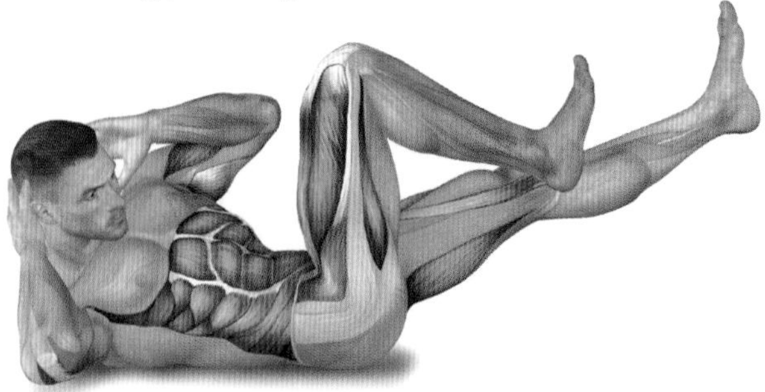

**core:** Refers to the deep muscle layers that lie close to the spine and provide structural support for the entire body. The core is divisible into two groups: major core and minor core muscles. Major muscles reside on the trunk and include the belly area and the mid and lower back. This area encompasses the pelvic floor muscles (levator ani, pubococcygeus, iliococcygeus, pubo-rectalis, and coccygeus), the abdominals (rectus abdominis, transversus abdominis, obliquus externus, and obliquus internus), the spinal extensors (multifidus spinae, erector spinae, splenius, longissimus thoracis, and semispinalis), and the diaphragm. The minor core includes the latissimus dorsi, gluteus maximus, and trapezius (upper, middle, and lower). Minor core muscles assist the major muscles when the body engages in activities or movements that require added stability.

**crunch:** A common abdominal exercise that calls for curling the shoulders toward the pelvis while lying supine with hands behind head and knees bent.

**dead hang:** Lowering your body until your arms are perfectly straight during a Pull-Up.

**dumbbell:** A basic piece of resistance equipment that consists of a short bar on which plates are secured. A person can use a dumbbell in one hand or both hands.

**dynamic exercise:** Dynamic exercise involves continuous movement of both joints and muscles. *Also known as* "ballistic."

**extension:** The act of straightening.

**extensor muscle:** A muscle serving to extend a body part away from the center of the body.

**external rotation:** The act of moving a body part away from the center of the body.

**flexion:** The bending of a joint.

**flexor muscle:** A muscle that decreases the angle between two bones, as bending the arm at the elbow or raising the thigh toward the stomach.

**hand weights:** Small weights that can be incorporated into exercises to add resistance to an exercise.

**hyperextension:** An excessive joint movement in which the angle formed by the bones of that joint is opened, or straightened, beyond its normal range of motion. This movement may make the joint unstable and increase the risk for dislocation or other potential injuries.

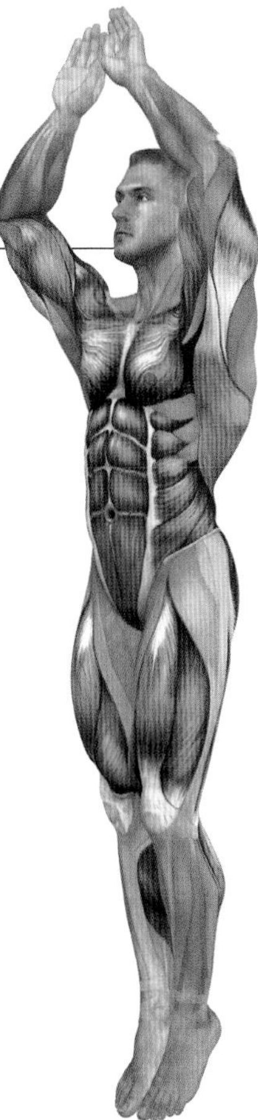

**iliotibial band (ITB):** A thick band of fibrous tissue that runs down the outside of the leg, beginning at the hip and extending to the outer side of the tibia just below the knee joint. The band functions in concert with several of the thigh muscles to provide stability to the outside of the knee joint.

**isometric exercise:** See *static exercise.*

**kipping:** Swinging your body during a Pull-Up.

**lateral:** Located on, or extending toward, the outside.

**lumbar spine:** The lower part of the spine.

**medial:** Located on, or extending toward, the middle.

**mindset:** A fixed mental attitude or disposition that predetermines a person's responses to and interpretations of situations.

**muscle fiber:** One of the structural cells of a muscle. Three main types are involved in exercise: Type 1 is aerobic. These fibers are red because they use a lot of red, oxygenated blood. Type 2a is anaerobic. They are white due to a lack of blood supply. Type 2b is a combination. They are pink. They have less blood and use less oxygen than type 1 fibers and more blood and more oxygen than type 2a fibers.

**neutral:** Describes the position of the legs, pelvis, hips, or other part of the body that is neither arched nor curved forward.

**posterior:** Located behind.

**pronate:** In running, the flattening of the foot as it hits the ground.

**qi:** The basic life-force energy present in all beings as well as the universe.

**range of motion:** The distance and direction a joint can move between the flexed position and the extended position.

**rotator muscle:** One of a group of muscles that assists the rotation of a joint, such as the hip or the shoulder.

**self-actualization:** To fully realize one's potential.

**special forces:** Military units units highly trained to perform unconventional, often high-risk missions.

**special operations:** Military operations that are considered unconventional, usually carried out by dedicated special forces units.

**squat:** An exercise movement that calls for moving the hips back and bending the knees and hips to lower the torso and an accompanying weight, and then returning to the upright position. A squat primarily targets the muscles of the thighs, hips, buttocks, and hamstrings.

**static exercise:** A form of exercise that exerts muscles at high intensities, without movement of your joints. *Also known as* "isometric."

**stress inoculation:** A method of military training that prepares recruits to cope with the aftermath of exposure to stressful events, such as those faced in combat, and to "inoculate" them to the effects of future and ongoing stressors.

**supinate:** In running, the rolling inward of the foot as it hits the ground.

**thoracic spine:** The middle part of the spine.

**visualization:** The ability to envision the act of surmounting a problem or achieving a goal.

**warm-up:** Any form of light exercise of short duration that prepares the body for more intense exercise.

**yin and yang:** A concept originating that explains the harmony and interdependence of opposites.

## LATIN TERMINOLOGY

*The following glossary list explains the Latin terminology used to describe the body's musculature. In some instances, certain words are derived from Greek, which is therein indicated.*

### Chest

**coracobrachialis:** Greek *korakoeidés*, "ravenlike," and *brachium*, "arm"

**pectoralis (major and minor):** *pectus*, "breast"

### Abdomen

**obliquus externus:** *obliquus*, "slanting," and *externus*, "outward"

**obliquus internus:** *obliquus*, "slanting," and *internus*, "within"

**rectus abdominis:** *rego*, "straight, upright," and *abdomen*, "belly"

**serratus anterior:** *serra*, "saw," and *ante*, "before"

**transversus abdominis:** *transversus*, "athwart," and *abdomen*, "belly"

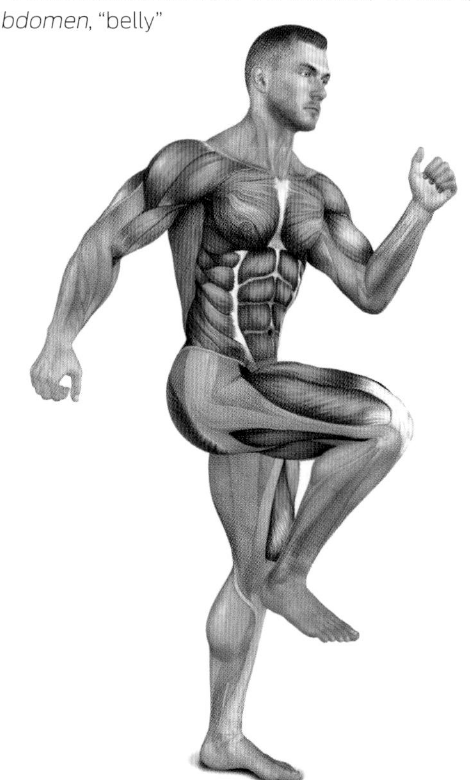

### Neck

**scalenus:** Greek *skalénós*, "unequal"

**semispinalis:** *semi*, "half," and *spinae*, "spine"

**splenius:** Greek *splénion*, "plaster, patch"

**sternocleidomastoideus:** Greek *stérnon*, "chest," Greek *kleís*, "key," and Greek *mastoeidés*, "breastlike"

### Back

**erector spinae:** *erectus*, "straight," and *spina*, "thorn"

**latissimus dorsi:** *latus*, "wide," and *dorsum*, "back"

**multifidus spinae:** *multifid*, "to cut into divisions," and *spinae*, "spine"

**quadratus lumborum:** *quadratus*, "square, rectangular," and *lumbus*, "loin"

**rhomboideus:** Greek *rhembesthai*, "to spin"

**trapezius:** Greek *trapezion*, "small table"

### Shoulders

**deltoideus (anterior, medial, and posterior):** Greek *deltoeidés*, "delta-shaped"

**infraspinatus:** *infra*, "under," and *spina*, "thorn"

**levator scapulae:** *levare*, "to raise," and *scapulae*, "shoulder [blades]"

**subscapularis:** *sub*, "below," and *scapulae*, "shoulder [blades]"

**supraspinatus:** *supra*, "above," and *spina*, "thorn"

**teres (major and minor):** *teres*, "rounded"

### Upper arm

**biceps brachii:** *biceps*, "two-headed," and *brachium*, "arm"

**brachialis:** *brachium*, "arm"

**triceps brachii:** *triceps*, "three-headed," and *brachium*, "arm"

### Lower arm

**anconeus:** Greek *anconad*, "elbow"

**brachioradialis:** *brachium*, "arm," and *radius*, "spoke"

**extensor carpi radialis:** *extendere*, "to extend," Greek *karpós*, "wrist," and *radius*, "spoke"

**extensor digitorum:** *extendere*, "to extend," and *digitus*, "finger, toe"

**flexor carpi pollicis longus:** *flectere*, "to bend," Greek *karpós*, "wrist," *pollicis*, "thumb," and *longus*, "long"

**flexor carpi radialis:** *flectere*, "to bend," Greek *karpós*, "wrist," and *radius*, "spoke"

**flexor carpi ulnaris:** *flectere*, "to bend," Greek *karpós*, "wrist," and *ulnaris*, "forearm"

**flexor digitorum:** *flectere*, "to bend," and *digitus*, "finger, toe"

**palmaris longus:** *palmaris*, "palm," and *longus*, "long"

**pronator teres:** *pronate*, "to rotate," and *teres*, "rounded"

## Hips

**gemellus (inferior and superior):** *geminus*, "twin"

**gluteus maximus:** Greek *gloutós*, "rump," and *maximus*, "largest"

**gluteus medius:** Greek *gloutós*, "rump," and *medialis*, "middle"

**gluteus minimus:** Greek *gloutós*, "rump," and *minimus*, "smallest"

**iliopsoas:** *ilium*, "groin," and Greek *psoa*, "groin muscle"

**obturator externus**: *obturare*, "to block," and *externus*, "outward"

**obturator internus:** *obturare*, "to block," and *internus*, "within"

**pectineus:** *pectin*, "comb"

**piriformis:** *pirum*, "pear," and *forma*, "shape"

**quadratus femoris:** *quadratus*, "square, rectangular," and *femur*, "thigh"

## Upper leg

**adductor longus:** *adducere*, "to contract," and *longus*, "long"

**adductor magnus:** *adducere*, "to contract," and *magnus*, "major"

**biceps femoris:** *biceps*, "two-headed," and *femur*, "thigh"

**gracilis:** *gracilis*, "slim, slender"

**rectus femoris:** *rego*, "straight, upright," and *femur*, "thigh"

**sartorius:** *sarcio*, "to patch" or "to repair"

**semimembranosus:** *semi*, "half," and *membrum*, "limb"

**semitendinosus:** *semi*, "half," and *tendo*, "tendon"

**tensor fasciae latae:** *tenere*, "to stretch," *fasciae*, "band," and *latae*, "laid down"

**vastus intermedius:** *vastus*, "immense, huge," and *intermedius*, "between"

**vastus lateralis:** *vastus*, "immense, huge," and *lateralis*, "side"

**vastus medialis:** *vastus*, "immense, huge," and *medialis*, "middle"

## Lower leg

**adductor digiti minimi:** *adducere*, "to contract," *digitus*, "finger, toe," and *minimum* "smallest"

**adductor hallucis:** *adducere*, "to contract," and *hallex*, "big toe"

**extensor digitorum:** *extendere*, "to extend," and *digitus*, "finger, toe"

**extensor hallucis:** *extendere*, "to extend," and *hallex*, "big toe"

**flexor digitorum:** *flectere*, "to bend," and *digitus*, "finger, toe"

**flexor hallucis:** *flectere*, "to bend," and *hallex*, "big toe"

**gastrocnemius:** Greek *gastroknémía*, "calf [of the leg]"

**peroneus:** *peronei*, "of the fibula"

**plantaris:** *planta*, "the sole"

**soleus:** *solea*, "sandal"

**tibialis anterior:** *tibia*, "reed pipe," and *ante*, "before"

**tibialis posterior:** *tibia*, "reed pipe," and *posterus*, "coming after"

# Icon Index

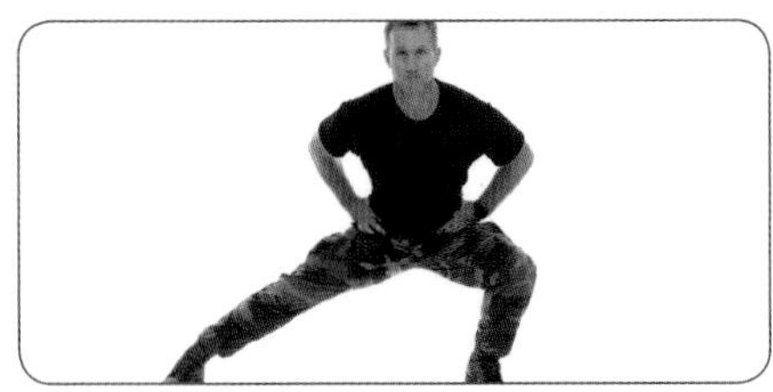
Lateral Lunge with Squat


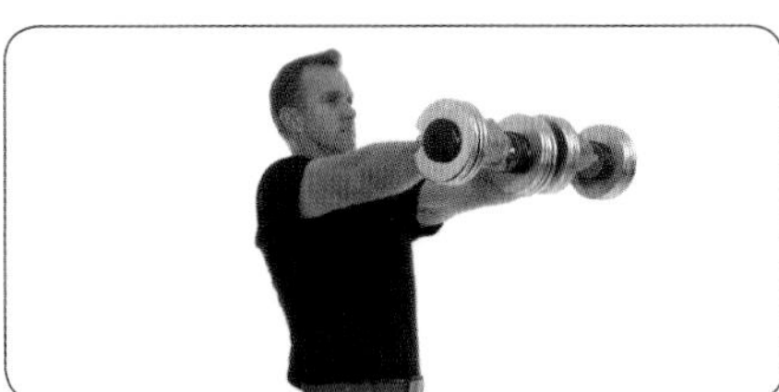
Shoulder Flexing


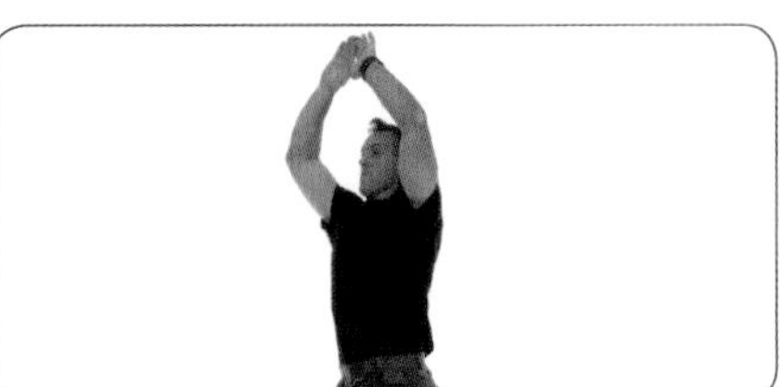
Burpee


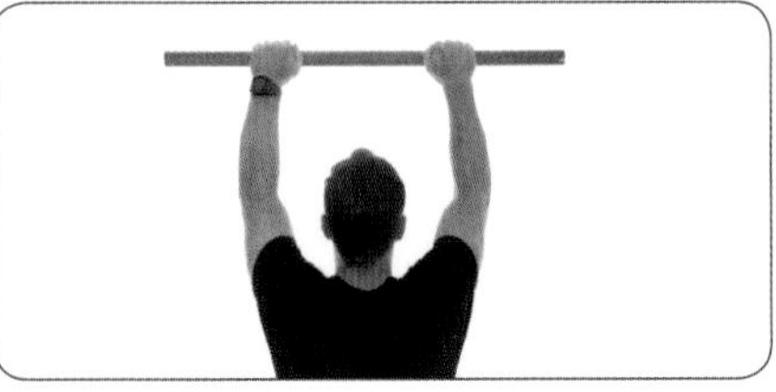
Burpee with Pull-Up


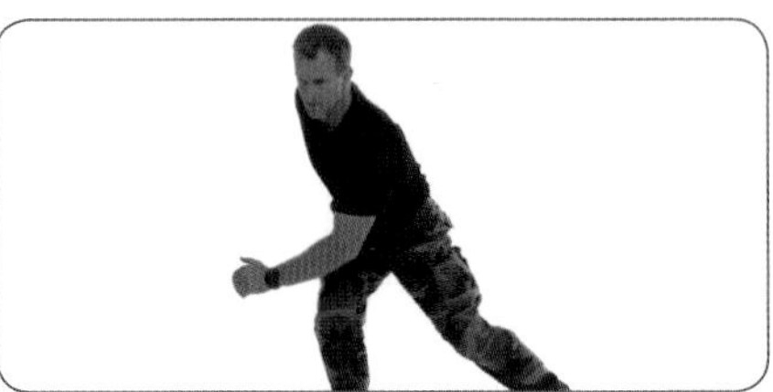
Speed Skater


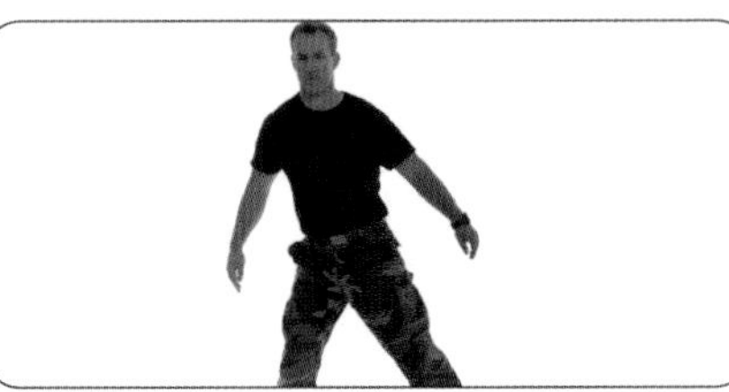
Straight-Leg Skater


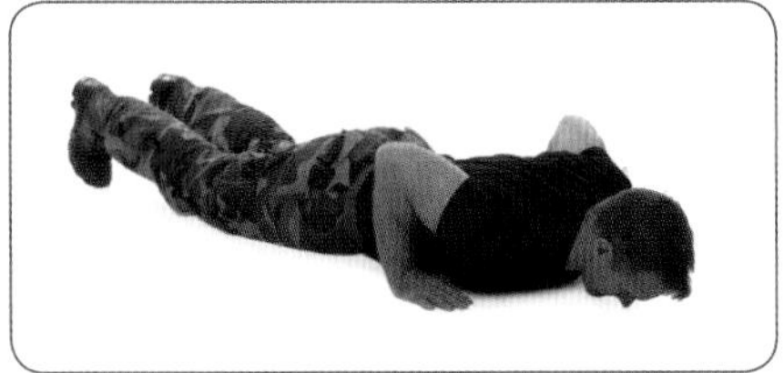
DFRB


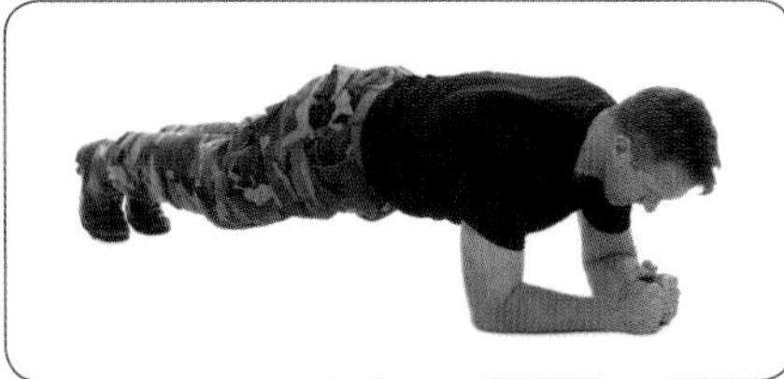
Plank


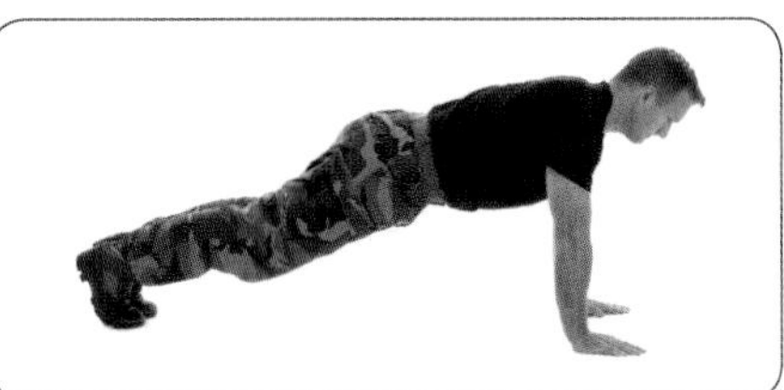
High Plank


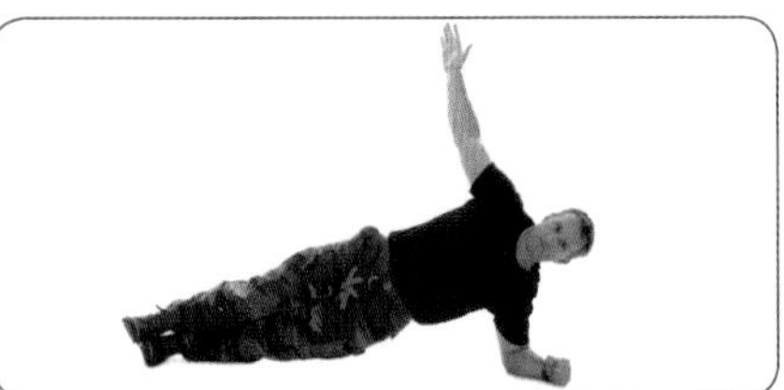
Side Plank


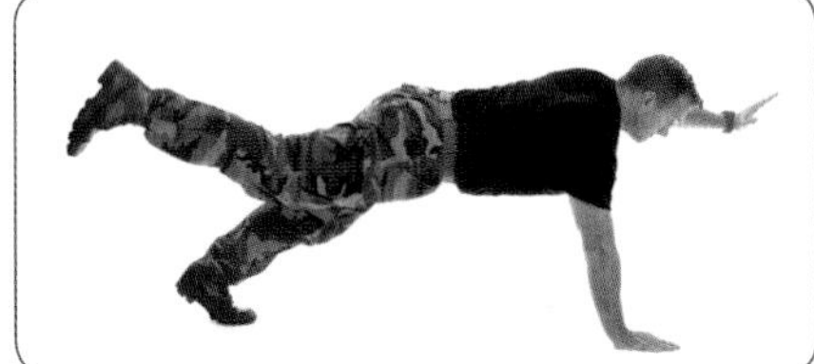
Bird Dog


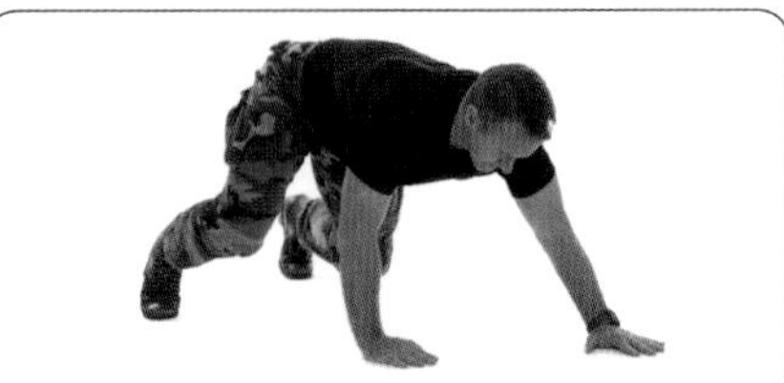
Bear Crawl


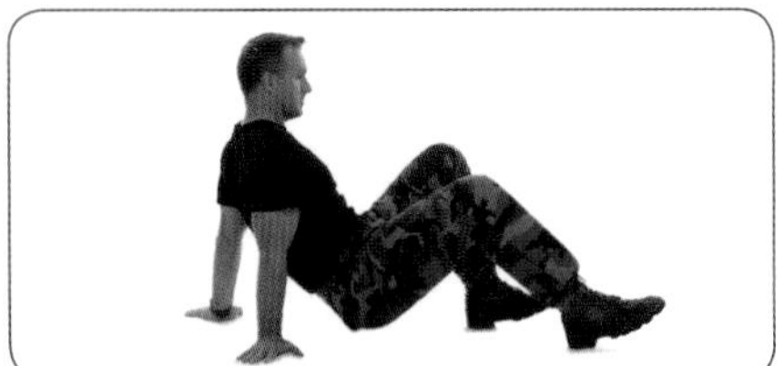
Crab Crawl


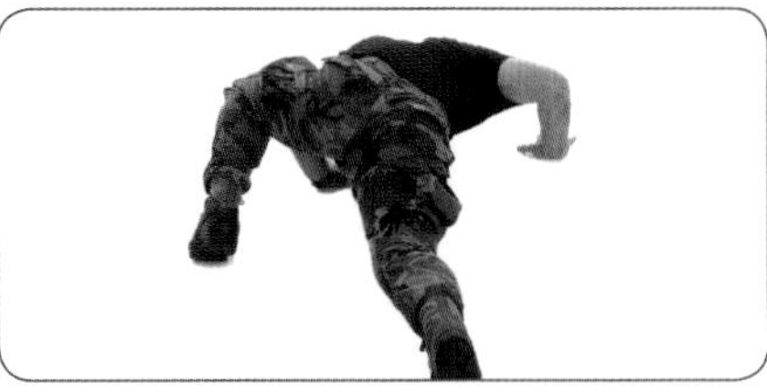
Alligator Crawl


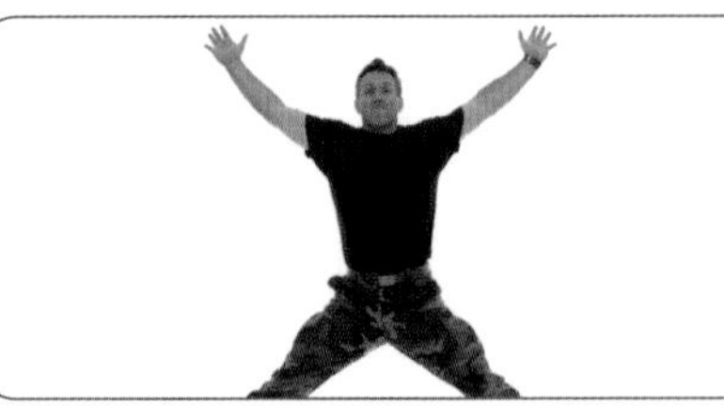
Star Jump

# About the Author

Stephen M. Erle, DC, CSCS, USAW, spent eight years serving in the United States Navy Reserve while also working as the training director for a civilian SEAL training program. There he trained hundreds of recruits for Basic Underwater Demolition/SEAL Training.

Dr. Erle has worked in private practice as a physiotherapist and chiropractor and is also a Certified Strength and Conditioning Coach, Olympic Lifting Sport Performance Coach and Certified Personal Trainer. He has also taught Tactical Combat Casualty Care. In his over 25 years of training and coaching, he has trained and treated Professional football players, collegiate athletes, SEAL Team and Army SF personnel.

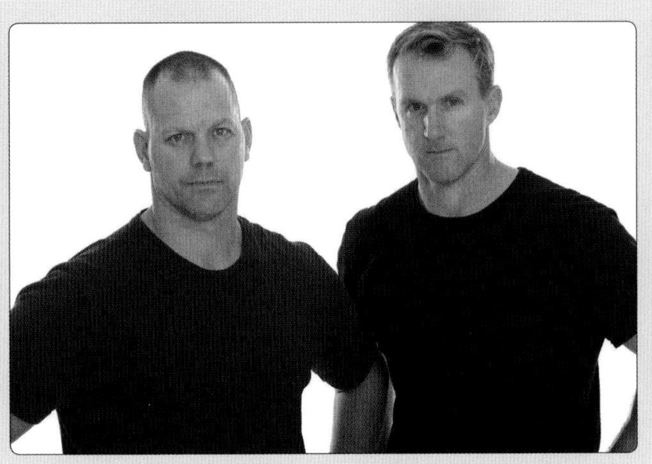

## Credits

*All photographs by Jonathan Conklin Photography, Inc., except:*

Page 8 (box) Photographer's Mate 1st Class (AW) Shane T. McCoy/U.S. Navy; 9 Photographer's Mate 2nd Class Eric S. Logsdon/U.S. Navy; 10 (top) U.S. Navy; 10 (box) Mass Communication Specialist 2nd Class Shauntae Hinkle-Lymas/U.S. Navy; 11 Photographer's Mate 1st Class (AW) Shane T. McCoy/U.S. Navy; 12 Netfalls - Remy Musser/Shutterstock; 13 U.S. Army; 14 djem/Shutterstock; 15 Chris Curtis/Shutterstock; 16 (top) OPOLJA/Shutterstock; 16 (bottom) sacura/Shutterstock; 17 graja/Shutterstock; 19 Oleg Zabielin/Shutterstock; 20 (box) Masa Oz/Shutterstock; 21 (box) SOMKKU/Shutterstock; 22 Senior Airman Matthew Bruch/U.S. Air Force; 23 Mayoca Design; 24 Staff Sergeant J. L. Wright Jr./U.S. Marine Corps; 25 Karen Prince; 26 (top left) Olga Miltsova/Shutterstock; 26 (middle left) margouillat photo/Shutterstock; 26 (bottom left) Dionisvera/Shutterstock; 26 (top right) Denis Kuvaev/Shutterstock; 26 (bottom right) Marcin Balcerzak/Shutterstock; 27 Maxisport/Shutterstock; 28 Frances L Fruit/Shutterstock; 29 (box top left) Valentina Razumova/Shutterstock; 29 (box middle left) Andrey Starostin/Shutterstock; 29 (box bottom left) Anna Kucherova/Shutterstock; 29 (box top center) Karramba Production/Shutterstock; 29 (box middle center) viviamo/Shutterstock; 29 (box bottom center) Alexey V Smirnov/Shutterstock; 29 (box top right) Norman Chan/Shutterstock; 29 (box middle right) Viktar Malyshchyts/Shutterstock; 29 (box bottom right) SOMMAI/Shutterstock; 152–153 Karen Prince; 154 (box) Pal Teravagimov/Shutterstock; 155 (left) miqu77/Shutterstock; 155 (box) EpicStockMedia/Shutterstock; 156 (left) jeep2499/Shutterstock; 156 (right) Mitch Gunn/Shutterstock; 157 (top left, bottom left, top right) Stew Smith; 157 (box) Chief Mass Communication Specialist Dave Kaylor/U.S. Navy; 158 (box) Phiseksit/Shutterstock; 159 (bottom left) Karen Prince; 159 (box) Maridav/Shutterstock; 160 (box) Mass Communication Specialist 2nd Class Kyle D. Gahlau/U.S. Navy; 161 (box) Karen Prince; 182–183 Karen Prince.

*All anatomical illustrations by Hector Aiza/3 D Labz Animation India, except:*

Small insets and full-body anatomy (pages 38–39) by Linda Bucklin/Shutterstock; pages 13, 158 (top right; middle right), 159 (top left) Sebastian Kaulitzki/Shutterstock.

# About the model

Stewart "Stew" Smith is a graduate of the U.S. Naval Academy, a former Navy SEAL, and has trained thousands of students for Navy SEAL, Special Forces, SWAT, FBI, ERT, and many other military, law enforcement, and fire fighter professions. This has included working for eight years as a Special Ops Team Coach at the U.S. Naval Academy that assists in the preparation of future candidates for SEAL, EOD, and MARSOC training. Stew also runs a non-profit called Heroes of Tomorrow where he provides free training for people seeking tactical professions.


## Acknowledgments

I would like to thank my SEAL team friends whom have allowed me to work with them for so many years. Don Mann, Don Shipley, Brett Hess, Stew Smith, Fred Kolberg, Kory Knowles, and Army Ranger Jeff Soule, as well as civilian Lou Font and Police Chief Jan Wright. It has been my honor and to work alongside such amazing professionals.

Thank you to my wife, Amber, who allows me to leave her and our girls to go play and train with my friends. You are my best friend.

~ Steve Erle